Macquarie Monographs in Cognitive Science

A Special Issue of
Aphasiology

Progressive language impairments: Intervention and management

Edited by

Lyndsey Nickels
Macquarie University, Sydney, Australia

and

Karen Croot
University of Sydney, Sydney, Australia

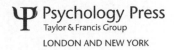
Psychology Press
Taylor & Francis Group
LONDON AND NEW YORK

First published 2009 by Psychology Press
27 Church Road, Hove, East Sussex, BN3 2FA

Simultaneously published in the USA and Canada
by Psychology Press
711 Third Avenue, New York, NY 10017

Psychology Press is an imprint of the Taylor & Francis Group, an informa business

British Library Cataloguing in Publication Data

A catalogue record for this book is available from the British Library

ISBN 13: 978-1-84872-701-4
ISSN 0268-7038

Cover design by Hybert Design
Typeset in China by Charlesworth

PROGRESSIVE LANGUAGE IMPAIRMENTS: INTERVENTION AND MANAGEMENT

Macquarie Monographs in Cognitive Science

Series Editor: MAX COLTHEART

The Macquarie Monographs in Cognitive Science series will publish original monographs dealing with any aspect of cognitive science.

Each volume in the series will cover a circumscribed topic and will provide readers with a summary of the current state-of-the-art in that field.

A primary aim of the volumes is also to advance research and knowledge in the field through discussion of new theoretical and experimental advances.

APHASIOLOGY

Volume 23   Number 2   February 2009

CONTENTS

APHASIOLOGY

SUBSCRIPTION INFORMATION

Subscription rates to Volume 23, 2009 (12 issues) are as follows:
To institutions (full subscription): £1,339.00 (UK);   €1,768.00 (Europe); $2,221.00 (Rest of the world).
To institutions (online only):   £1,272.00 (UK);   €1,680.00 (Europe); $2,110.00 (Rest of the world).
An Institutional subscription to the print edition also includes free access to the online edition for any number of concurrent users across a local area network.
Subscriptions purchased at the personal (print only) rate are strictly for personal, non-commercial use only. The reselling of personal subscriptions is strictly prohibited. Personal subcriptions must be purchased with a personal cheque or credit card. Proof of personal status may be requested. For full information please visit the Journal's homepage.
To individuals: £563.00 (UK);   €744.00 (Europe); $935.00 (Rest of the world).
A subscription to the print edition includes free access for any number of concurrent users across a local area network to the online edition, ISSN 1464-5041.
Print subscriptions are also available to individual members of the British Aphasiology Society (BAS), on application to the Society.
Aphasiology now offers an iOpenAccess option for authors. For more information, see: www.tandf.co.uk/journals/iopenaccess.asp

For a complete and up-to-date guide to Taylor & Francis's journals and books publishing programmes, visit the Taylor and Francis website: http://www.tandf.co.uk/

Aphasiology (USPS 001413) is published monthly by Psychology Press, 27 Church Road, Hove, BN3 2FA, UK. The 2009 US Institutional subscription price is $2,221.00. Periodicals Postage Paid at Jamaica, NY 11431, by US Mailing Agent Air Business Ltd, c/o Worldnet Shipping USA Inc., 149-35 177th Street, Jamaica, New York, NY 11434, USA. US **Postmaster**: Send address changes to *Aphasiology* (PAPH), Air Business Ltd, C/O Worldnet Shipping USA Inc., 149-35 177th Street, Jamaica, New York, NY 11434, USA.
All subscriptions are payable in advance and all rates include postage. Journals are sent by air to the USA, Canada, Mexico, India, Japan and Australasia. Subscriptions are entered on an annual basis, i.e., from January to December. Payment may be made by sterling cheque, dollar cheque, international money order, National Giro, or credit card (AMEX, VISA, Mastercard).

Orders originating in the following territories should be sent direct to the local distributor.
India: Universal Subscription Agency Pvt. Ltd, 101–102 Community Centre, Malviya Nagar Extn, Post Bag No. 8, Saket, New Delhi 110017.
Japan: Kinokuniya Company Ltd, Journal Department, PO Box 55, Chitose, Tokyo 156.
USA, Canada and Mexico: Psychology Press, a member of Taylor & Francis, 325 Chestnut St, Philadelphia, PA 19106, USA
UK and other territories: Psychology Press, c/o T&F Customer Services, Informa UK Ltd, Sheepen Place, Colchester, Essex, CO3 3LP, Tel: +44 (0)20 7017 5544; Fax: +44 (0)20 7017 5198; UK. E-mail: tf.enquiries@tfinforma.com

Typeset by H. Charlesworth & Co. Ltd., Wakefield, UK, and printed by Hobbs the Printers Ltd., Totton, Hants, UK. The online edition can be reached via the journal's website: http://www.psypress.com/aphasiology

Back issues: Taylor & Francis retains a three-year back issue stock of journals. Older volumes are held by our official stockists: Periodicals Service Company, 11 Main Street, Germantown, NY 12526, USA, to whom all orders and enquiries should be addressed. Tel: +1 518 537 4700; Fax: +1 518 537 5899;
E-mail: psc@periodicals.com; URL: http://www.periodicals.com/tandf.html

APHASIOLOGY, 2009, 23 (2), 123–124

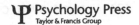

Editorial

Progressive language impairments: Intervention and management

A special issue of *Aphasiology*

Lyndsey Nickels
Macquarie University, Sydney, NSW, Australia

Karen Croot
University of Sydney, NSW, Australia

What are progressive language impairments? They comprise a broad range of symptoms involving impaired language processing, ranging from impaired knowledge of the concepts underlying language to impaired ability to articulate speech, and encompassing a wide range of difficulties in comprehending, formulating, or producing language in spoken or written form. By definition, these symptoms worsen over time as a result of neurodegenerative disease, although the rate of decline varies radically and may sometimes include relatively long periods during which change is minimal. We use the term "progressive language impairments" in order to focus on the *symptoms* occurring in a range of disorders and diseases described under a number of syndrome labels including primary progressive aphasia (fluent and nonfluent), semantic dementia, and progressive anomia. We choose to do this as these syndrome labels may carry different connotations for different researchers and clinicians—in particular, for some researchers and clinicians they have implications for the underlying pathological mechanisms. The progressive language impairments described in this special issue of *Aphasiology* can occur as a result of a variety of pathologies including frontotemporal lobar degeneration or Alzheimer's disease. The people with progressive language impairments reported here typically experienced language impairments as the most prominent initial symptom, however progressive language impairments can also occur in the context of more generalised dementia. See Croot (2009, this issue) for further discussion.

What then of intervention for progressive language impairments, the focus of this volume? Language impairments have a profound effect on those affected: that intervention is appropriate for language impairments is not questioned for children with developmental language impairments or adults with language impairments

Address correspondence to: Lyndsey Nickels, Macquarie Centre for Cognitive Science, Macquarie University, Sydney, NSW, Australia. E-mail: nickels@maccs.mq.edu.au

© 2009 Psychology Press, an imprint of the Taylor & Francis Group, an Informa business
http://www.psypress.com/aphasiology   DOI: 10.1080/02687030801943021

acquired as a result of trauma, stroke, infection, tumour, or surgery. If treatment is denied or not available for the language impairments of these populations, it is a matter of grave concern. Yet our experience has taught us that the same values are not applied to those individuals whose language impairments progressively worsen over time. We know of one man who showed severe progressive word retrieval impairments but otherwise intact cognitive processing, yet who was turned away from an outpatient speech pathology service. He was told, "There is nothing we can do". We have observed the difference in the quality of life of two gentlemen with similar progressive language impairments—one man had a family who actively sought ways for him to continue in his role as a father and grandfather. They explained his communicative problems to his grandchildren, encouraged communication strategies, fostered nonverbal hobbies, and ensured that as far as possible he remained engaged and included. The other man's family misunderstood the nature of his impairments, believing he suffered from a severe dementia. His lifestyle became restricted, opportunities for communication were limited, and his quality of life suffered as a function of social isolation. We were appalled by the injustice of these examples—as the confused family of the man who was refused intervention asked us, "If speech pathologists can't help us, who can?"

The aim of this volume is to demonstrate that there *is* something we *can* and *should* do. In fact there are many things at many levels: impairment-directed interventions, activity/participation-directed interventions, and education and support programmes to train and resource clients and carers. By implementing such interventions, we can do our best to ensure that families and healthcare services, in cooperation with people with progressive language impairments, understand the nature of the problems, facilitate communication skills, maximise communication opportunities, and optimise quality of life. We hope that this special issue will facilitate understanding of the potential for intervention and overcome any remaining prejudice that intervention is not appropriate for these individuals.

REFERENCE

Croot, K. (2009). Progressive language impairments: Definitions, diagnoses, and prognoses. *Aphasiology*, 22, 302–326.

APHASIOLOGY, 2009, 23 (2), 125–160

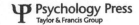

Impairment- and activity/participation-directed interventions in progressive language impairment: Clinical and theoretical issues

Karen Croot
University of Sydney, Sydney, NSW, Australia

Lyndsey Nickels
Macquarie University, Sydney, NSW, Australia

Felicity Laurence
Flinders University, Adelaide, SA, Australia

Margaret Manning
St Margaret's Rehabilitation Hospital, Adelaide, SA, Australia

Background: There is a broad constellation of clinical syndromes in which the most prominent initial and ongoing symptom is deterioration in spoken or receptive language processing, reading, writing, or semantic knowledge. Despite the core language impairments, people with these disorders are likely to be under-referred for speech pathology services (Taylor, Kingma, Croot, & Nickels, 2009 this issue), and there is limited published research on speech pathology interventions in these disorders.
Aims: This paper reviews the published impairment- and activity/participation-directed interventions in semantic dementia and progressive aphasia to determine the current evidence base for clinical decisions about client suitability and selection of treatment goals, methods, and measures. We also identify questions that need to be addressed in future therapy research.
Methods & Procedures: We reviewed 15 reports of impairment-directed behavioural, pharmacological, and repeated transcranial magnetic stimulation treatments that implemented some level of experimental control. We reviewed a further 10 reports of interventions generally carried out without experimental control, targeting impairments, activity/participation limitations, education, carer training, or a mixture of these approaches.
Outcomes & Results: In the impairment-directed studies almost all participants showed improvement on treated items immediately post-treatment. Improvement was specific to treated items in most word retrieval studies, but there is a possibility that greater generalisation to other items or other language tasks/contexts may have occurred in treatments not targeting naming, and/or for clients with articulatory impairments. Without ongoing practice of therapy activities, treatment gains declined for all

Address correspondence to: Karen Croot, School of Psychology A18, University of Sydney, NSW, Australia 2006. E-mail: karenc@psych.usyd.edu.au

Thanks to Elizabeth Armstrong and Regina Jokel for helpful comments on an earlier draft of the paper. Lyndsey Nickels was funded by a National Health and Medical Research Council Senior Research Fellowship during the preparation of this paper.

http://www.psypress.com/aphasiology   DOI: 10.1080/02687030801943179

participants over a period varying from 2 months to between 6 months and 1 year. There was only one experimentally controlled activity/participation-directed intervention reported for people with progressive language impairments, although other reports of activity/participation-directed interventions described increased communicativeness and communication effectiveness for participants following intervention. Consistent with the aims of activity/participation-interventions, these interventions appear to have a greater impact on everyday communication outside the clinic than impairment-directed interventions, but these impacts need to be investigated and documented. *Conclusions*: These studies highlight the need for rigorous research design to identify treatment, generalisation, and maintenance effects (Rapp & Glucroft, 2009 this issue), and to identify outcomes that go beyond improvement in the clinic on targeted words, language structures, and behaviours. It is important to tailor interventions closely to individual client needs, involve the spouse/carer in intervention, and ensure that clients have appropriate expectations about therapy. The patterns of therapy gain, limited generalisation, and decline following cessation of therapy activities in impairment-directed studies raise questions about the learning mechanism(s) involved. They also have implications for client suitability, and for choice of therapy items, and therapy delivery and duration.

Keywords: Primary progressive aphasia; Frontotemporal dementia; Semantic dementia; Treatment; therapy.

The past decade has seen a rapid growth in understanding the speech, language, and communication changes associated with various types of dementia (Bayles & Tomoeda, 1997; Bourgeois, 1991; Clare, 2001; Lubinski, 1995; Ripich & Horner, 2004; Royal College of Speech and Language Therapists, 2005). Of particular interest to speech pathology practice is the fact that a number of neurodegenerative diseases may result in clinical syndromes in which the most prominent initial and ongoing symptom is deterioration in language processing. The best known of these syndromes are *primary progressive aphasia* as defined by Mesulam and colleagues (Mesulam, 2001, 2003; Mesulam, Grossman, Hillis, Kertesz, & Weintraub, 2003), *semantic dementia*, characterised by severe anomia, comprehension deficits, and impaired object recognition due to loss of semantic memory (Snowden, Goulding, & Neary, 1989), and *nonfluent progressive aphasia* (Gorno-Tempini et al., 2004), in which nonfluent spontaneous speech, anomia, and speech sound production errors are the typical presenting symptoms. A wide range of other syndrome labels have also been used for progressive language impairments, including pure progressive anomia, primary progressive conduction aphasia, primary progressive apraxia of speech, language- or temporal-variant frontotemporal dementia, etc. (see Croot, 2009 this issue, for more details about syndromes involving progressive language impairment).

Despite the central nature of the language symptoms, in the past some speech pathologists have not perceived that they have a role in the management of people with progressive language impairments. Even now, speech pathologists may remain uncertain about the best management pathway for these individuals (Taylor et al., 2009 this issue). However, as McNeil and Duffy (2001, p. 475) note, the "presenting *speech and language complaints can be strikingly similar to those of people with stroke-induced aphasia*" (their emphasis). They therefore argue that decisions about treatment in progressive language impairments can be based on the same philosophical, clinical, theoretical, and practical considerations that apply in stroke-related aphasia. Although the nature of the disease process requires that clinicians modify treatment goals and approaches over time in response to (or even in anticipation of) disease progression (Rogers, King, & Alarcon, 2000), this is hardly a new skill: modifying therapy in response to changing client ability or circumstances is standard practice and is required for any speech pathology client group (McNeil & Duffy, 2001). Individuals with progressive language impairment often present with additional cognitive, behavioural, or motor disorders, or develop these with disease progression (see Croot, 2009 this issue, for an overview). Therefore, as in stroke-related aphasia, the speech pathologist needs to be alert for co-occurring disorders, taking them into account in therapy planning and referring the individual for other healthcare services as needed.

The challenge for the speech pathology profession in working with clients with progressive language impairment is to apply, and as necessary adapt, the knowledge-base derived mainly from stroke-related aphasia to this emerging area of practice. Moreover, people with progressive language impairments are almost certainly under-referred for speech pathology services (Taylor et al., 2009 this issue). Therefore speech pathologists also have a role in promoting the suitability and availability of services for these clients to referring medical practitioners.

The need to provide speech pathology services for clients with progressive language impairments has been a clinical reality for some years (e.g., Craenhals, Raison-Van-Ruymbeke, Rectem, Seron, & Laterre, 1990; Holland, McBurney, Moossy, & Reinmuth, 1985; McNeil, Small, Masterson, & Tepanta, 1995; Northen, Hopcutt, & Griffiths, 1990; Schneider, Thompson, & Luhring, 1996). Nevertheless, there are few published studies of speech pathology interventions in this population, although the rate at which new studies are being reported is accelerating (see Appendix Tables 1 to 3). Pressing clinical questions about client suitability for the various therapy options, and about therapy efficacy, timing, and dose, await evidence-based answers. In the absence of published evidence-based practice guidelines, individual clinicians must evaluate the evidence, together with the theoretical and philosophical rationales for the various alternatives, in order to make a reasonable choice about the intervention(s) they will offer (Alarcon, Duffy, McNeil, & Rogers, 2000).

There are three main sources of information available to inform treatment planning for clients with progressive language impairments. First, *descriptions of previous interventions* currently constitute the best empirical information on which to base clinical decisions about client suitability, and treatment goals, methods, materials, and measures. In addition, *psycholinguistic and learning theories* can inform about how a particular treatment may work and for whom it is/is not suitable. Finally, *expert opinion papers* are a rich resource that offer suggestions about best practice based on extensive clinical and research experience with these and allied disorders (McNeil & Duffy, 2001; Robinson, 2001; Rogers et al., 2000; Snowden & Griffiths, 2000; Thompson & Johnson, 2006).

The aim of this paper is to assist clinicians to make choices about speech pathology service provision. We do this by summarising published intervention studies and identifying the theoretical issues that influence therapy planning. Along the way we highlight some questions that need to be addressed in future therapy research. We have organised the review according to whether the reported interventions were primarily directed towards remediating the client's "impairment", or improving their activity/participation levels. The terms impairment and "activity/participation" are taken from the World Health Organisation health classification system (as described in the practice guidelines of the American Speech-Language-Hearing Association, 2001). Impairment-directed interventions are designed to rehabilitate psychological or physical functioning of body structures (e.g., retrieval of lexical items, processing of syntactic structures within the language system, motor

control of speech articulators, neuronal function in language areas, etc.). Activity/
participation-directed interventions aim to improve an individual's ability to
perform a particular task or action or participate in a desired life situation (e.g.,
express basic needs, participate in a conversation or a game of cards).

IMPAIRMENT-DIRECTED STUDIES

We include in this review of impairment-directed studies only published treatment
studies that implemented a level of experimental control. Some studies were carried
out in the context of clinical speech pathology therapy provision, others as
experimental studies in laboratory settings outside the clinical arena. Studies using
behavioural therapies are summarised in Appendix Tables 1 and 2. One of these
(McNeil et al., 1995) compared the effect of a behavioural treatment alone with
behavioural plus pharmacological treatment in a single case. There is another study
reporting a pharmacological treatment only with a group of seven participants
(Reed, Johnson, Thompson, Weintraub, & Mesulam, 2004). Finally, one pioneering
study targeted a person's impaired verb production using repetitive transcranial
magnetic stimulation (rTMS, Finocchiaro et al., 2006). Most of the impairment-
based studies used single-case designs (Bier et al., 2009 this issue; Finocchiaro et al.,
2006; Frattali, 2004; Funnell, 1995; Graham, Patterson, Pratt, & Hodges, 1999;
Heredia, Sage, Ralph, & Berthier, 2009 this issue; Jokel, Rochon, & Leonard, 2002;
McNeil et al., 1995; Rapp & Glucroft, 2009 this issue; Schneider et al., 1996), with
two studies replicating the same therapy across more than one participant (Jokel,
Cupit, Rochon, & Leonard, 2009 this issue; Louis et al., 2001).

IMPAIRMENT-DIRECTED BEHAVIOURAL INTERVENTIONS

The pattern of treatment-specific effects across impairment-directed behavioural
interventions is unmistakeable. Despite the range of participants, interventions used,
and therapy designs, all participants (except one man, discussed somewhat briefly by
Graham et al., 1999; Graham, Patterson, Pratt, & Hodges, 2001) improved on
treated items compared to baseline and/or untreated items immediately post-
treatment. However, generalisation to untreated items or situations was more
restricted. We will now examine the studies in more detail.

Therapy design

All the impairment-directed studies reported took at least some steps to ensure that
change subsequent to intervention could be attributed to the intervention, rather
than to some uncontrolled factor. The simplest form of experimental control was to
include two sets of items (treatment and control sets) matched on factors thought to
influence treatment, in an ABA design. Performance was initially measured on both
sets, then one set was treated over some period, with performance measured again on
both sets at the end of treatment (e.g., Funnell, 1995; Heredia et al., 2009 this issue).

The most common experimental control involved a cross-over or multiple
baselines across behaviours or sets design (Frattali, 2004; Graham et al., 1999; Jokel
et al., 2009 this issue; Jokel et al., 2002; Jokel, Rochon, & Leonard, 2006; Laurence,
Manning, & Croot, 2002; McNeil et al., 1995; Schneider et al., 1996), in which
treatment commenced at different times on different behaviours (e.g., use of gestures

to indicate future versus past tense in Schneider et al.) or on different sets of items (e.g., nouns versus verbs in Frattali, 2004). This design typically also involves several measures of the treatment targets prior to intervention, which are then used to identify the trajectory of change prior to intervention.

Rigorous intervention design is essential because ultimately the quality of evidence that the therapy was effective depends on the quality of the experimental control. Highly informative single-case and single-case series designs can be implemented in a clinical setting with careful planning (Wilson, 1987, 1997), and there are excellent options for statistical analysis of clinically based single-case studies (Gorman & Allison, 1996). Rapp and Glucroft (2009 this issue) provide an excellent discussion of issues regarding the design of treatment studies for people with neurodegenerative disease. Following treatment there may be improvement above baseline levels of accuracy. If this occurs it is considered to be evidence for the effectiveness of treatment, just as it is in the non-progressive population. However, in those individuals with progressive language impairments stable baseline performance may not be observed, instead there may be a decline in performance before treatment. Given the likelihood of slow decline without treatment, an outcome of no change, or a slowing of deterioration can also indicate that the therapy has had an effect. If treated and untreated items have similar pre-treatment accuracy (and hence difficulty), and following therapy treated items are more accurate than untreated items, then the treatment has had an effect. This is the case even if the treated items are less accurate than they were at baseline. If treated and untreated items are equally accurate following treatment (but below baseline levels) the results are more difficult to interpret. There could be no effects of treatment, or the treatment may have had a benefit that has generalised completely (treated and untreated items all benefit). While an analysis comparing the rate of decline before and during treatment may help clarify the situation, the evidence in this situation remains equivocal.

As therapy may result in slowing of deterioration, rather than a noticeable improvement, it is vital that the person with progressive language impairments and their communication partners understand this possibility. Similarly, it is important to ensure that clients and communication partners understand that treatment will not reverse the progression of disease (McNeil & Duffy, 2001).

One limitation of a number of the impairment-directed studies reviewed is that they report effects over a very small number of items (e.g., Bier et al., 2009 this issue, had only 4 words per condition; Funnell, 1995, had 6; and Rapp & Glucroft, 2009 this issue, had 10 per condition). This makes the results vulnerable to item-specific effects, and lacking in statistical power to discriminate "real" change from variability of performance. However, this aspect of therapy design typically reflects a compromise between an ideal study design allowing high statistical power and the clinical realities of limited clinical time and participant-related constraints. For example, the choice to use small numbers of items in the Bier et al. and Rapp and Glucroft studies was determined by the time it took the participant to become fatigued. In such cases, a direct replication of the therapy effects with different items and/or participant(s) would strengthen the conclusions of the study. Studies using larger numbers of items (e.g., approximately 60 items in Jokel et al., 2002, 2006) are more persuasive with regard to positive treatment effects.

The studies we reviewed varied in mode of therapy delivery, duration of individual sessions, duration of the overall intervention, frequency of therapy activities, and whether or not the participant carried out home practice. Studies also varied on the extent to which and how they evaluated treatment effects, general-isation, and maintenance. All these aspects of therapy design await systematic investigation across numbers of participants with progressive language impairments.

What were the characteristics of the participants?

As shown in Appendix Table 1, the participants in the studies surveyed included both men and women (although more women), of a range of ages (49–77 years), at differing times since the onset of symptoms. All showed abnormal brain imaging for left temporal regions (structure and/or function), with a range of other speech and language regions affected. Some participants showed relative sparing of memory-related medial temporal structures but others did not.

Participants were reported under three syndrome categories: semantic dementia (eight clients), nonfluent progressive aphasia (five clients), and primary progressive aphasia (five clients). However, within these syndrome categories participants had heterogeneous presentations. For example, those described as having nonfluent progressive aphasia presented with speech and language symptoms including slow speech (P1 in Jokel et al., 2009 this issue), hesitant speech (P2 in Jokel et al., 2009 this issue), and grammatical impairments, pronunciation errors, and auditory phonetic/phonological processing deficits (Louis et al., 2001). As discussed below, the extent of semantic impairment varied for the people with semantic dementia. Similarly, although three of the five participants reported under the label of primary progressive aphasia (participant CD in Laurence et al., 2002; Rapp & Glucroft, 2009 this issue; Schneider et al., 1996) met the Mesulam (2001) criteria for this diagnosis, they had diverse symptoms. These included nonfluent progressive aphasia and slow speech (Schneider et al.), prominent early writing difficulties and accompanying naming, calculation, constructional, and attentional deficits (Rapp & Glucroft, 2009 this issue), and prominent anomia with fluent aphasia, subtle pragmatic changes, and semantic and pronunciation errors (participant CD in Laurence et al., 2002). The remaining two had a history of isolated language impairment and prominent anomia for less than 2 years.

Memory and naming abilities

The studies reported a wide range of neuropsychological and language assessments, but there were no tests in common across all studies that would allow direct comparison of all participants on any area of neuropsychological or language function. Most, however, reported participants' performance on at least one measure of delayed recall, on the three-picture version of the Pyramids and Palm Trees test (a nonverbal test of semantic associations, Howard & Patterson, 1992), and on the Boston Naming Test (Kaplan, Goodglass, & Weintraub, 1983). Where these latter measures are not reported, Appendix Table 1 gives results from other tests assessing similar abilities.

Only five participants were impaired on measures of delayed recall (Bier et al., 2009 this issue; Frattali, 2004; Heredia et al., 2009 this issue, Snowdon & Neary, 2002) and all of these individuals had a diagnosis of semantic dementia. Poor delayed recall of recently presented material may be associated with poorer generalisation performance (see below under *Generalisation*).

Approximately half the participants for whom a semantic memory measure was reported were impaired on this measure (8 out of 14; of whom 7 had a diagnosis of semantic dementia and 1 of primary progressive aphasia). However, all but two of these (Snowden & Neary, 2002) were performing above chance levels. Some of the early treatment studies had suggested that perhaps participants with relatively well-preserved semantic processing were most likely to show improved naming following lexical retrieval therapy (Laurence et al., 2002). For example, in the study of Graham et al. (1999), DM relearned members of many semantic categories, while AM, who carried out somewhat similar learning activities, did not. One of the differences between these two men was their score on the three-picture version of the Pyramids and Palm Trees Test (Howard & Patterson, 1992). DM scored 49/52, just inside the normal range, whereas AM (scoring 39/52) was quite impaired relative to controls. Scores in the normal range were also reported for GP (McNeil et al., 1995), and AC and CD (Laurence et al.), and the woman reported by Schneider et al. (1996). However, subsequent studies reported participants whose semantic memory scores were impaired but who nevertheless showed an immediate treatment effect. It now appears, therefore, that AM's comparatively low semantic memory scores do not explain the absence of treatment effect in his case. This may instead be due to an ineffective rehearsal strategy based on the initial letters of words without semantic elaboration (Graham et al., 1999).

With regard to naming performance, all but one (Schneider et al., 1996) of the 15 for whom data are provided were impaired on the reported naming test, with three at floor level (Frattali, 2004; Snowden & Neary, 2002). The participants reported by McNeil et al. (1995) and Rapp and Glucroft (2009 this issue) had relatively mild spoken naming impairments (scoring 46/60 and 48/60 respectively on the Boston Naming Test)—potentially one of the reasons spoken noun naming was not targeted for intervention in these studies. Thus, just as is the case in the literature with non-progressive language impairments, individuals with a variety of degrees of naming and semantic impairment can benefit from impairment-directed interventions targeting word retrieval. However, participants' knowledge of specific words and concepts does seem to be relevant for selection of therapy targets (for further details, see below under *Maintenance*).

The characteristics of people with progressive language impairments who have participated in published impairment-directed therapies suggest that a wide range of individuals may be suitable, as long as they are able to understand the tasks required of them. Some individuals may require certain practical support (McNeil & Duffy, 2001) in terms of assistance in getting to therapy, or setting up or being motivated to carry out home practice activities. In some cases therapists may be requested to implement an impairment-directed therapy because of consumer preferences (as with participant CD in Laurence et al., 2002), or may suggest modifications to the way a client is already practising words using a self-devised strategy, as happened with DM (Graham et al., 1999). More precise information about participant factors that influence treatment, generalisation, and maintenance effects is yet to be established.

Selection of impairments targeted and therapy activities

In the above studies the impairments targeted were in each case either the most prominent, or one of the most prominent, of participants' impairments. This is true even in the "proof of concept" studies (Rapp & Glucroft, 2009 this issue) that primarily aimed to find out whether therapy had any effect in clients with progressive language impairments. A high proportion of investigations targeted word retrieval: two-thirds of the interventions targeted spoken noun retrieval, with other studies targeting written naming, and adjective and verb retrieval. A smaller number of studies targeted other impairments: knowledge of semantic attributes, use of tense markers (gestural and verbal), and auditory-phonological processing.

The focus on word retrieval is unsurprising. Word retrieval is always one of the earliest symptoms noticed by people with progressive language impairments (Mesulam, 2001), and has a marked impact on communication. In addition, in non-progressive aphasia, interventions for word retrieval impairments have been relatively well investigated compared with other language-impairment therapies (for review, see Laine & Martin, 2006; Nickels, 2002; Nickels & Best, 1996a, 1996b; Raymer & Gonzalez Rothi, 2002). Nevertheless, even given the small number of studies so far, there is a range of interventions directed to a range of progressive language impairments. This supports McNeil and Duffy's (2001) claim that impairment-directed therapies developed for use in non-progressive aphasia can be readily utilised in progressive language impairments.

Decisions about whether to use an impairment-directed intervention depend on collaborative decisions by the speech pathologist, the client, and their communication partners (e.g., Jokel et al., 2006). Decisions are guided by the social and functional usefulness of the particular communicative activities that are affected by that impairment (see also below under *Generalisation* and *Maintenance*). For example, Bier et al. (2009 this issue) chose to target TBo's knowledge of semantic attributes of objects as well as object names, on the basis that she would find it more useful to know core facts about objects rather than their names. They give the example that it might be more useful for someone with semantic dementia to know you can eat an apple than to know that it is called "apple".

Once the decision is made to treat a particular impairment, selection of therapy activities and items is influenced by the clinician's hypotheses about the impairment. These often include hypotheses about the level and type of cognitive impairment within a cognitive theory of language word production (e.g., Kay, Lesser, & Coltheart, 1992; Nickels, 2000). Rapp and Glucroft (2009 this issue) explicitly used a cognitive model of spelling to guide the assessments and therapy tasks selected for the participant in their study. Different levels of impairment are generally hypothesised to require different approaches to treatment (Hillis & Caramazza, 1994). For example, a word retrieval impairment that is underpinned by a semantic impairment may be most effectively treated by a task focusing on semantic distinctions between words (Hillis, 1991; Nickels, 2002). In contrast, poor word retrieval in the context of relatively preserved semantics but impaired retrieval of phonological forms from the lexicon is best treated using tasks that provide both semantic and phonological activation (e.g., word–picture matching; repetition of the word in the presence of the picture; Nickels, 2002). In addition to hypotheses about the level of impairment, a clinician may form hypotheses about the nature of the impairment. Representations may be hypothesised to be lost from long-term memory, or to be degraded, or to remain intact while access to those representations is impaired. In practice, distinguishing between these different types of impairment is extremely difficult (see Howard, 1995, for discussion) as severely impaired access may be virtually indistinguishable from loss of representations (but for further discussion see below under *How do the behavioural therapies work?*).

Finally, the structuring and frequency of therapy activities, as well as selection of words, language structures, or concepts to target in therapy, also depend on the clinician's theory about how the therapies work: about how previous knowledge is reinstated and/or knowledge is learned or relearned. These issues are also discussed below under *How do the behavioural therapies work?*

Effects of treatment

As we noted above, all studies found that treated items improved compared to baseline and/or untreated items immediately post-treatment, except for one individual with semantic dementia (AM), discussed by Graham et al. (1999, 2001). Although these results are extremely positive and suggest that impairment-directed therapy with clients with a wide range of progressive language impairments can yield treatment gains, caution is required. First, it is possible that a publication bias has distorted the true proportion of cases in which improvement is likely to be seen (i.e., perhaps only studies that found a treatment effect have been published). Second, even if there is no publication bias, and treatment effects are positive for the majority of participants and interventions, decisions about whether impairment-directed therapies should be incorporated into speech pathology provision for individual clients must take account of the much-less-impressive effects found for generalisation and maintenance.

Generalisation

While treated items showed significant benefits from treatment, the effect of treatment on untreated items was far less impressive across studies. None of the seven people with semantic dementia who participated in word retrieval therapies, and for whom generalisation was evaluated, showed *any* improvement in naming of untreated items. This is entirely consistent with the literature on non-progressive aphasia, where effects of treatment for word retrieval are generally restricted to treated items (Nickels, 2002). One study, that of McNeil et al. (1995) with a man with a 9-month history of progressive anomia, used a word retrieval treatment (a cueing hierarchy for adjective retrieval) and did find some generalisation to untreated stimuli (adjectives, verbs, and prepositions). This is not without precedent and has generally been attributed to individuals using the cueing hierarchy to self-cue when word retrieval fails (Coelho, McHugh, & Boyle, 2000; Nickels & Best, 1996b). However, despite the generalisation to untreated items, McNeil et al. found no generalisation to connected speech or a range of standardised speech and language tasks.

Within treated items, some studies examined whether there was generalisation from the stimuli used in treatment to other stimuli designed to elicit the same items. One participant, CR, was able to name the treated items when they were presented in a different order or on differently coloured and formatted materials (Snowden & Neary, 2002), which has implications for the nature of the learning that took place. Similarly, CUB could name different exemplars of the items to those presented in training (Heredia et al., 2009 this issue), although in this latter case the more typical the exemplar (and perhaps therefore the more visually similar it was to the treated exemplar, e.g., two different pictures of a whole banana compared with a picture showing sliced banana), the more successful she was. CUB's husband also reported generalisation of therapy items to her spontaneous speech, a factor worth noting because it may account for CUB's atypically high maintenance of learning after 6 months without deliberate practice. Future studies could fruitfully address the extent to which improvements in word retrieval, as measured by single word retrieval, generalise to the use of these stimuli in communication. There is some evidence in the literature on non-progressive aphasia, that this can occur (Herbert, Best, Hickin, Howard, & Osborne, 2003). Given that this is critical for the functional utility of word retrieval interventions, it is vital that this should not be overlooked.

At present, therefore, evidence for generalisation from treatments aimed at word retrieval is extremely limited, for both progressive and non-progressive language impairments. For this reason, the stimuli treated *must* be highly functional items for the client (e.g., names of family and friends, emotions), chosen in collaboration with the client and their family/friends. Similarly, the client should be made aware that generalisation may not be a realistic objective of therapy (Bier et al., 2009 this issue), and that over time only a small number of words may be retained, with eventual loss of these also occurring with disease progression.

Only one study reported improvement across a range of untrained language tasks (Louis et al., 2001), for all three participants, but this was a brief report with few data provided and only the briefest information about how these measures were obtained. Interpretation of the generalisation effect in this study is unfortunately further limited because a measure of experimental control for the treatment effect was only reported for one of the three participants, while the actual treatment effect was reported for all three participants combined. Thus the data in the report do not adequately demonstrate that participants' improvements on untrained tasks were related to improvements on the intervention. However, the limitations of this report aside, two other studies with greater experimental control and stronger data also found some evidence of generalisation; those of McNeil et al. (1995, described above) and Schneider et al. (1996). The woman described by Schneider generalised use of verbal and gestural future tense markers and verbal past tense markers to untrained sentences in the therapy task. Subsequent to therapy, she also produced a higher proportion of sentences with the trained structure in a narrative task than she had produced before therapy.

The studies of Louis et al. (2001) and Schneider et al. (1996) were similar in that both involved teaching techniques that could be directly applicable to language in many contexts. For example, the study of Louis et al. focused on receptive processing of formant information in spoken language comprehension, and the gestures taught by Schneider et al. were appropriate to mark future or past tense for any verbs. In contrast, the studies focusing on word retrieval typically focused on facilitating retrieval of individual lexical items (or relearning the association between the concept and/or picture and the phonological form). Hence, the type of therapy directly relates to the generalisation expected (and found). The word retrieval study that showed generalisation (McNeil et al., 1995) may also have involved a strategy that could be generalised across stimuli (most likely in addition to a specific facilitatory effect for untreated items).

A more speculative observation at this point in time is that four of the five people reported to show generalisation to untreated items (Louis et al., 2001; Schneider et al., 1996) had the type of articulation deficits that Josephs et al. (2006) suggested are likely to be apraxia of speech (although described in different qualitative terms by the different authors). Further, while the fifth participant who showed generalisation

(McNeil et al., 1995) did not have apraxia of speech, he did have an early and rapidly progressing spastic dysarthria, as evidenced by mild hypernasality, strained-strangled speech, and slow diadochokinetic rate. Prominent articulation deficits (e.g., apraxia of speech, voice changes) are likely to arise from abnormal brain function in different regions of the brain from those most affected in semantic dementia. It remains to be seen whether this different distribution of neuropathology, typically associated with episodic memory difficulties in the semantic dementia but not in the former group, also contributes to the different patterns of generalisation seen across the two groups.

Finally, it must be noted that there is a certain ambiguity in evaluating generalisation in neurodegenerative disease. There is always the possibility that items to which there is no apparent generalisation may actually have deteriorated more quickly without treatment (Rapp & Glucroft, 2009 this issue; Schneider et al., 1996).

Maintenance

Across the impairment-directed studies reviewed, treatment gains declined substantially for almost all participants over a period varying from 2 months (Participant CD, Laurence et al., 2002) to somewhere between 6 months and 1 year (Jokel et al., 2009 this issue; Rapp & Glucroft, 2009 this issue) following cessation of treatment activities. This occurred regardless of clinical syndrome or intervention type. The exceptions were CUB (Heredia et al., 2009 this issue) who retained 82% of treated items at 6 months, and CR (Snowden & Neary, 2002) who scored 65% correct on naming approximately 8 months after treatment ceased.

Heredia et al. (2009 this issue) discuss a number of possible reasons for CUB's superior performance, including rapid learning of items she had been unable to name (she reached ceiling on 28/28 items within 3 days of commencing therapy) with consequent errorless rehearsal of these items for almost a month afterwards, discussed further below in relation to learning mechanisms. CUB also generalised use of treated items to spontaneous speech, suggesting at least some ongoing comprehension and rehearsal of them. Participant CR's comparatively good maintenance was attributed to the concurrent learning of item names and definitions that were personally meaningful to her (linked to their location in her environment and her experience with them, e.g., "This is a duck. It's like the one in your conservatory. You see them on the pond when you go to the park"; Snowden & Neary, 2002, p. 1722). A number of other studies also suggest a role for a "meaningfulness" factor in maintenance of therapy gains by people with semantic dementia. AK (Jokel et al., 2006) showed a stronger treatment effect in naming, and better maintenance of items she could still comprehend but not name, than items she could neither comprehend nor name. Bier et al. (2009 this issue) found better initial generation of general attributes than specific attributes by TBo, but better maintenance of specific attributes than general attributes. People with semantic dementia typically lose more specific knowledge about objects first, with more general knowledge preserved longer (Hodges, Graham, & Patterson, 1995), thus the specific attributes TBo was able to generate potentially reflected a greater level of comprehension than did the general attributes, which may explain why they were maintained longer.

Snowden and Griffiths (2000) therefore advocate that therapy for people with semantic dementia should take place in their own surroundings and using their own belongings, not in a clinic using line drawings or photographs of objects. Use of a client's own objects avoids some of the difficulties a person with semantic dementia is likely to face in generalising from one exemplar to another, and the familiar surroundings provide meaningful context which will potentially support maintenance of knowledge. For the same reasons, Snowden and Griffiths suggest that carers should be educated about the value of brand loyalty when shopping (so that the appearance of household products remains constant when they are replaced), of storing objects in the same place at home, and of carrying out routine activities, such as shopping, in well-known places. As well as enabling people with semantic dementia to carry out activities of daily living more easily, there are safety implications in trying to ensure that items and surroundings are maximally understandable. Snowden and Griffiths recount as a warning an episode in which one woman with semantic dementia mistakenly used bleach, rather than bath bubbles, when preparing a bath for herself.

Given the consistent finding of loss of therapy gains following cessation of treatment activities, one obvious clinical decision would be to plan for the client to simply continue rehearsing the treated words and being exposed to them in day-to-day language use, until the disease progresses to a point where they are no longer maintained even with rehearsal. Such a plan would again highlight the need to target highly functional, personally meaningful words, and to probe maintenance of knowledge on an ongoing basis. In practice, the set of words most likely to be functionally useful and the set of words most likely to be maintained tend to overlap, because personal relevance, frequent exposure to items in everyday life (including use in conversation), and level of existing semantic knowledge for target items are all hypothesised to be related (Heredia et al., 2009 this issue; Snowden & Neary, 2002). In clients with progressive language impairments, if continuing rehearsal is the best way for a participant to maintain highly functional items, studies should not aim to evaluate maintenance without rehearsal without extremely strong ethical justification.

Motivation to practice and personality change

The potential need for ongoing rehearsal raises a final important consideration when planning impairment-directed therapy. If therapy relies on the client carrying out homework tasks, the client needs to be sufficiently motivated to complete these tasks. However, DM (Graham et al., 1999), CD (Laurence et al., 2002), and the man reported by Northen et al. (1990) showed noticeable distress at rehearsing treatment words/carrying out impairment-based therapy in the face of ongoing decline in their abilities. Graham et al. (1999, p. 377) describe DM's therapy as a "two-edged sword", writing that "although this perpetual homework had a beneficial effect on DM's anomia, it seems to have had the opposite effect on his psychological well-being". Further, both AK (Jokel et al., 2006) and CUB (Heredia et al., 2009 this issue) were noted to be obsessed about relearning previously known words, although distress per se is not mentioned in these reports. The possibility of psycho-emotional distress must be discussed with clients and carers in advance and monitored during the course of treatment. It is difficult to know in these cases to what extent distress and obsessive practice may be associated with grief and anxiety in the face of neurodegenerative disease, or with personality change caused by pathology in frontal brain regions. Personality changes are often reported in association with progressive language impairments, with estimates of 46–75% of clients becoming depressed, apathetic, or developing behavioural fixations (Chow, Miller, Boone, Mishkin, & Cummings, 2002; Kertesz, McMonagle, Blair, Davidson, & Munoz, 2005). Personality changes, and grief and insight, together with premorbid personality and motivational factors, will all influence a client's response to therapy, so must be taken into account in treatment planning. Psychiatric assessment is a central part of diagnosis in some clinical settings (Hodges, Berrios, & Breen, 2000), and referral for psychiatric and/or counselling services must remain an option for client and carers with ongoing review.

How do these behavioural therapies work?

A number of the impairment-directed studies discuss the mechanisms by which the therapy is hypothesised to work. These discussions take into account not just theories about the structure and processing characteristics of the language system, but theories of memory function and learning.

Before we discuss specific accounts of the mechanisms for improvement, there is an interesting contrast between studies that focus on progressive versus non-progressive language impairments. In both sets of studies there is a substantial focus on word retrieval. However, the terms that are used to describe the effects of the same treatment techniques tend to be rather different. In the non-progressive literature the treatment is generally described as "improving word retrieval" (e.g., Hickin, Best, Herbert, Howard, & Osborne, 2002) or "priming" retrieval (e.g., Martin & Laine, 2000) of names (but see Fillingham, Sage, & Lambon Ralph, 2005, 2006). In contrast, in the progressive literature there is a tendency instead to talk about "learning" or "relearning" of names (Bier et al., 2009 this issue; Graham et al., 1999; Heredia et al., 2009 this issue; Snowden & Neary, 2002). This use of different terminology seems to imply that in non-progressive aphasia word forms remain "intact but unavailable", whereas in progressive language impairments word forms are "lost" and have to be relearned. As discussed above, this is a difficult distinction to determine experimentally, and to date, for the majority of individuals who have been treated, no attempt has been made to determine whether there is loss or inaccessibility of word form representations. Thus, we would urge caution in over-interpreting these terms in the absence of a clear debate regarding whether one mechanism can account for the data better than the other.

Below we outline four of the mechanisms discussed in the studies reviewed here: a temporary memory system supported by medial temporal lobe structures, the role of multiple retrievals, errorless learning mechanisms, and the linking of target items to existing knowledge.

Graham et al. (1999, 2001), and Heredia et al. (2009 this issue) suggest that the ability to retrieve object names after therapy is due to the relearning of these names within a temporary memory system. This system is supported by medial temporal lobe structures that are relatively undamaged by the neurodegenerative disease compared with longer-term stores supported by other cortical regions that may have been almost decimated by disease. Failure to consolidate learning in long-term stores distributed in neocortex explains why treatment gains are not maintained after therapy activities stop. According to Heredia et al., these long-term stores are also hypothesised to support generalisation, explaining why limited generalisation occurs, at least in participants with semantic dementia.

Several studies discuss the hypothesised benefit of multiple retrievals of information in therapy. Bier et al. (2009 this issue) found no difference between spaced retrieval training (in which the interval between retrievals is carefully controlled and expands as the participant responds correctly) and a technique they called "simple repetition", which utilised the same number of retrievals without the expanding retrieval interval. In both techniques, retrieval of information relevant to different items was interleaved, a procedure thought to support learning of multiple associations (McClelland, McNaughton, & O'Rielly, 1995). According to McClelland et al., interleaving the presentation of target items with that of similar items over many presentations allows information about individual items to be learned gradually. By contrast, participants DM and CUB were provided with a fairly rigid rehearsal order that did not involve interleaving (Graham et al., 1999; Heredia et al., 2009 this issue). The effect of number of retrievals (and the interaction between this and interleaving of target items) needs to be systematically investigated to establish whether there is further support for this hypothesis.

Errorless learning (discouraging the participant from guessing and thus making errors) is another factor thought to play a role in the success of spaced retrieval training in dementia of the Alzheimer type and vascular dementia (Brush & Camp, 1998), and in relearning of forgotten associations in dementia of the Alzheimer type (Clare, Wilson, Breen, & Hodges, 1999; Wilson, Baddeley, Evans, & Shiel, 1994). Frattali (2004) and Snowden and Neary (2002) deliberately utilised errorless learning in their intervention design. Graham et al. (1999) noted that the rigidly ordered rehearsal that DM carried out involved errorless learning. In addition, Heredia et al. (2009 this issue) reported that CUB was getting the names of the therapy items correct by day 3, then continued to rehearse them in what was effectively an errorless paradigm for almost a month. In fact, only two of the eight impairment-directed interventions reported for people with semantic dementia did *not* utilise errorless learning, both of which had very small sets of items (Bier et al., 2009 this issue: four items in spaced retrieval, four in simple repetition; Funnell, 1995: six vegetable names), requiring replication to rule out item-specific effects.

Although it initially appeared that people with semantic dementia had well-preserved episodic memory (Hodges, Patterson, Oxbury, & Funnell, 1992), subsequent research demonstrated impaired performance on episodic memory tests (Simons & Graham, 2000), and atrophy to medial temporal structures associated with episodic memory (Mummery et al., 1999). Lambon Ralph and Fillingham (2007), propose that there are two learning systems. One involves the strengthening of associations between frequently paired stimuli and responses (a simple Hebbian learning system), and another modulates this Hebbian learning depending on whether a response proves to be correct or incorrect. If a person's ability to use this second modulatory system is impaired (because they cannot detect or encode errors), they are left only with the simple (unmodulated) Hebbian system that learns erroneous responses just as effectively as correct responses. In this situation, errorless learning is beneficial because it ensures that only associations between correct stimuli and responses are strengthened. The hypothesis that errorless learning supports (re)learning in semantic dementia requires systematic investigation.

Whether there is also a benefit in errorless learning for people with syndromes of non-fluent or primary progressive aphasia awaits investigation, because all the interventions to date with people diagnosed with these syndromes (Appendix

Table 2) have involved errorful learning (in which the client has the opportunity to give a response, even if it is incorrect). Interestingly, however, for non-progressive aphasia, treatment for word retrieval is not found to be more effective when errorless learning is utilised (Fillingham et al., 2005, 2006). This could be because these participants have sufficiently preserved memory and executive skills to support the modulatory learning system proposed by Lambon Ralph and Fillingham (2007).

A final mechanism that potentially contributes to participants' improvement on naming tasks relates to linking target items to existing knowledge. Meaningfulness of items to be learned, degree of item-specific knowledge retained by the participant, and use of therapy activities that activate a wide semantic network including the network supporting semantic features and lexical knowledge, are all factors associated with item-specific improvement in the naming studies surveyed. Once again, perhaps this relates to the distinction between relearning and re-accessing representations. Those items for which there is retained knowledge (e.g., richer semantics) are more likely to be retained themselves, and require facilitation of access, rather than requiring relearning of semantic information and/or relearning of the links between meaning and form. In the non-progressive literature there is a preponderance of explanations for improvement in word retrieval that rely on improving access through "priming" (strengthening links between representations or increasing resting levels of activation of representations themselves, e.g., Biedermann & Nickels, 2008; Howard, 2000). It is therefore plausible that improvement that is dependent on improving access is easier to attain than improvement requiring complete or substantial relearning, although both mechanisms may account for improved word retrieval.

CUB's results are particularly interesting because she showed longer maintenance than the other participants with semantic dementia. Heredia et al. (2009 this issue) consider whether any of the following factors might provide an explanation: amount of therapy, number of items treated, therapy method and items selected, severity of semantic memory impairment, degree of brain atrophy, and differences in occupation or education prior to illness, but they conclude that the most likely factor is generalisation to spontaneous speech (see above). The effects of all of these factors await systematic investigation. Information about CUB's generalisation of treated items to spontaneous speech relied on her husband's report; in fact, none of the studies we reviewed included a measure of language use in an everyday setting: clearly this is important for future research.

The theories discussed above to some extent make different predictions about what manipulations in therapy activities will be most beneficial, thus future clinical research studies need to tease these apart. Until the results are in, the best chance of clinical success will be to combine as many of these factors as possible and practicable, as in the example of the intervention with CUB.

IMPAIRMENT-DIRECTED PHARMACOLOGICAL INTERVENTIONS

To date there are only two papers reporting pharmacological interventions aimed to improve language abilities in primary progressive aphasia, neither of which show strong promise. McNeil et al. (1995), as discussed above, targeted adjective retrieval in a single-case design that alternated a combined pharmacological–behavioural intervention with behavioural intervention only and withdrawal phases. Dextroamphetamine was administered on the basis of research showing greater recovery of function following cerebral lesion with dextroamphetamine plus behavioural treatment than behavioural treatment alone (McNeil et al., 1995). There was no strong evidence for a benefit of the combined treatment above that of the behavioural treatment alone, although the researchers noted a trend for the combined treatment to be associated with increased generalisation.

The second study (Reed et al., 2004) trialled bromocriptine with six people with primary progressive aphasia diagnosed according to the criteria of Mesulam (2001). Bromocriptine, a dopamine agonist used in treating Parkinson's disease, was selected because it has been associated with improved speech production in nonfluent aphasia caused by left hemisphere stroke (Raymer et al., 2001). The study had a double-blind, placebo-controlled, crossover design, and measured language abilities on naming, word fluency, and a narrative task. Most of the measures did not suggest any benefit from the bromocriptine. However, mean length of utterance was found to be greater in the bromocriptine condition compared with placebo, but nonetheless declined for the group over the 5-month course of the study. The researchers concluded that bromocriptine might have slightly slowed the participants' language deterioration but that the effect was limited.

IMPAIRMENT-DIRECTED rTMS INTERVENTION

A small number of recent studies have begun to demonstrate benefits of repetitive transcranial magnetic stimulation (rTMS) on language function in people with acquired language impairments (Cotelli et al., 2006; Naeser et al., 2005). This technique has also shown some benefit for a 60-year-old man diagnosed with primary progressive aphasia according to the Mesulam (2001) criteria (Finocchiaro et al., 2006). Repetitive TMS is hypothesised to inhibit or excite neuronal function, depending on whether the stimulation is low versus high frequency, respectively. In the study of Finocchiaro et al., high-frequency rTMS was applied to a left inferior frontal region hypothesised to be involved in verb processing, in five sessions held over consecutive days. The man with primary progressive aphasia improved on a verb-naming task but not on two memory span tasks, with the benefits lasting approximately 46 days after the first round of TMS, and approximately 31 days after the second round of TMS. A "sham" treatment served as a control, in which, unknown to the participant, the magnet was angled away from the scalp, but all other aspects of treatment delivery were unchanged. Although the man improved substantially relative to baseline after the two rTMS treatments, there was no change after the sham treatment. These technologies are very much in their infancy, and all applications of therapeutic rTMS are at present highly experimental and limited in scope—but we should follow the progress of rTMS as a potential alternative or addition to behavioural approaches for impairment-based intervention.

ACTIVITY/PARTICIPATION-DIRECTED INTERVENTION STUDIES

There are 11 papers that describe activity/participation-directed interventions, education, and carer training in some detail (summarised in Appendix Table 3). A number of other reports (e.g., Béland & Ska, 1992; Hart, Beach, & Taylor, 1997; Thompson, Ballard, Tait, Weintraub, & Mesulam, 1997) mention speech therapy (including use of a communication book, articulatory-kinematic training, and pacing and contrastive stress exercises), but with insufficient detail to be included in

Appendix Table 3. Some of the interventions reviewed combined impairment-directed approaches with activity/participation-directed activities (Holland et al., 1985; L. L. Murray, 1998; Northen et al., 1990). One was a group therapy (four participants) in which the clinicians developed aphasia-friendly formats for viewing and discussing half-hour episodes of a television series dealing with the life events of contemporary Australians (Cartwright & Elliott, 2009 this issue).

The literature suggests that written and pictorial information (communication books, boards and cards, encouraging the person and/or their communication partner to write, or draw pictures or symbols), gesture and sign (pantomime and communicative gesture, Amerind and American Sign Language), and other augmentative and alternative (AAC) technologies (text-to-speech machines, emergency wrist devices) may all have the potential to help maximise the communication potential of a person with progressive language impairments. Most of the studies also mention speech pathology sessions dedicated to carer training or counselling, and/or group sessions in which the person with progressive language impairments has the opportunity to practise communication techniques, interact socially with others with aphasia or dementia, and receive feedback and peer support. Discourse analysis has been used to identify functional communication needs and sources of communication breakdown as the basis for training the person with progressive language impairments and their communication partner, and to measure the success of conversation training techniques (L. L. Murray, 1998; Wong, Anand, Chapman, Rackley, & Zientz, 2009 this issue).

The activity/participation-directed studies that we reviewed highlight the importance of tailoring the intervention to the individual client and context. Cress and King (1999) reported a number of benefits of the AAC approaches introduced with participant CE. Using a receptive communication board, CE was able to comprehend around 70% of the necessary routine messages his family wished to communicate. Significantly, CE still responded to messages communicated via the board 1 year later, when he no longer demonstrated comprehension of verbal material. CE also "tended to express more complex messages and more communicative turns with a wider variety of listeners when using communication boards than without them" (Cress & King, 1999, p. 256), and continued to use his expressive communication board at 1-year follow-up to manage conversation topics. However, a noteworthy feature of the intervention was the speech pathologist's close social relationship with CE, which allowed her to spend intensive time with CE and his family over a month-long period to introduce the AAC techniques. She was also able to facilitate CE's use of these techniques outside the home, at bowling, restaurants, parties and musical events. Similarly, Rogers et al. (2000) describe how FA, who had given up playing poker with close friends, was able to begin playing again with assistance from his wife and friends, using communication cards (e.g., types of poker game, bidding rules) also individually tailored for use with those partners in that situation. Again similarly, Cartwright and Elliot (2009 this issue) prepared in advance a glossary of key words that would be used in each group television-watching session, and a summary of the plot of each episode that the group watched together. In the latter two studies, enjoyment of the activity by all communication participants (person with aphasia, spouse, friends, speech pathologist) was reported as one major outcome of the intervention.

Rogers and colleagues (Rogers & Alarcon, 1998; Rogers et al., 2000) have written most extensively on activity/participation approaches to intervention in progressive language impairments, and give a number of case examples. They stress the importance of three principles: (1) implement goals in anticipation of decline, (2) use dyad-focussed therapy, and (3) use augmentative techniques that rely on preserved abilities to increase participation. Rogers et al. provide suggestions for assessing impairments, activities, and participation in progressive language impairments, and discuss potentially useful content for inclusion in communication books and ways to address acceptance issues. They underscore the suggestion above that transfer of AAC approaches outside the clinic is maximised when the speech pathologist dedicates regular time to facilitating typical interactions between the client and his or her regular communication partners using AAC.

At this point in time the case reports and anecdotes summarised in Appendix Table 3 indicate that activity/participation approaches with people with progressive language impairments show great promise. To date, however, there are almost no published formal evaluations of these interventions that would allow future activity/ participation therapy planning for these clients to be evidence based. Future activity/ participation interventions must be designed to allow clinicians/researchers to show that apparent improvements in a client's activity/participation levels are reliable, and can be unambiguously attributed to the intervention(s) implemented (e.g., using control groups/participants or control sets of items or behaviours). Wilson (1987, 1997) provides an excellent summary of research designs that can be readily used in clinical settings. In this context, the aphasia-friendly television-viewing intervention designed by Cartwright and Elliot (2009 this issue) is innovative and exemplary in describing the intervention methods and measures in detail, and in comparing participants' performance before and after intervention within participant, within group, and to a control group, on several discourse measures.

Future activity/participation-directed interventions in this population must also meet the challenge of assessing whether clients show improvements in activity/ participation levels outside the clinic. This is equally an issue in non-progressive aphasia (Turner & Whitworth, 2006) and quantitative and qualitative measures of functional communicative success developed for people with aphasia (e.g., Armstrong & Mortensen, 2006), dementia (e.g., Lubinski & Orange, 2000), and traumatic brain injury (Togher, McDonald, Code, & Grant, 2004) could all be adapted for use with people with progressive language impairment. Work is just beginning in this area with people with progressive language impairment. Rogers et al. (2000) discuss potential assessments for use with this population, and the discourse intervention with Bobby V (Wong et al., 2009 this issue) makes an important contribution by specifying clearly a framework within which communicative effectiveness can be evaluated.

Finally, many of the reports summarised in Appendix Table 3 also refer to additional benefits of communication intervention for the person with progressive language impairments and their communication partners. These include improved quality of life, a decreased sense of isolation (Thompson & Johnson, 2006), increased feeling of personal control (McNeil & Duffy, 2001; Robinson, 2001; Thompson & Johnson, 2006), enhanced sense of purpose and goal in life (McNeil & Duffy, 2001), participant and speech pathologist enjoyment (Cartwright & Elliott, 2009 this issue), and neuroprotective benefits of cognitive stimulation provided by therapy (Cartwright & Elliott, 2009 this issue). All of these potential positive outcomes of therapy await formal evaluation (e.g., use of standardised scales, questionnaires, and tailor-made outcome measures) and documentation in peer-reviewed articles.

ISSUES RELEVANT TO ALL INTERVENTIONS

Involvement of spouse/carer

A spouse/carer may have a number of roles in maximising health, social, and communication opportunities and speech therapy outcomes of the person with progressive language impairments, perhaps even taking on a case manager-type role (Robinson, 2001). Given the potential burden of caring for someone with progressive disease (J. Murray, Schneider, Banerjee, & Mann, 1999), education programmes for people with dementia typically include components that focus on caring for the carer (Northen et al., 1990; Ripich, 1994). The Primary Progressive Aphasia Program at the Cognitive Neurology and Alzheimer's Disease Center at North Western University, Chicago, offers educational lectures and small group discussion with input from medical staff, psychologists, and social workers, followed up by monthly carer support meetings (Cognitive Neurology & Alzheimer's Disease Center, 2006). As one of the healthcare team, the speech pathologist has a role in monitoring a carer's coping abilities and referring to extra services (general practitioner, social work, occupational therapy, psychology, respite services, support groups etc.) as required.

A spouse/carer in good health is an invaluable informant about the functional relevance of potential therapy activities, and about key items to treat in impairment-directed interventions or include in a communication book. If changes in insight and personality occur with disease progression, the spouse/carer is likely to be the most sensitive observer of these, and one of the people most affected by them. A number of anecdotes reporting successful activity/participation-directed interventions (Appendix Table 3) highlight the role of the spouse/carer in transferring communication strategies from the clinical setting to everyday life. As mentioned above, Rogers et al. (2000) suggest that speech pathologists dedicate at least 5–10 minutes per client per week in the clinic to observing and facilitating communication between clients and their communication partners using augmentative and alternative communication tools, to assist transfer of these skills outside the clinic. However, primary carers (spouse, adult children) may see the speech pathology appointment time as an opportunity for respite (Cathleen Taylor & Rachel Miles Kingma, personal communication, 19 June 2007), so it may be important to discuss with them the potential benefits of their participation in speech pathology sessions.

Participants may be less likely to carry out home practice activities if they live alone or do not otherwise have a spouse or carer who is committed and able to help them with home therapy activities. In two contrasting examples, Rapp and Glucroft (2009 this issue) noted that CB, who was living alone, did not consistently complete her homework tasks, whereas CUB (Heredia et al., 2009 this issue) asked her husband for names and information about therapy items, and this may have assisted transfer of these items to her spontaneous speech. Older clients and their carers may also need assistance, instruction, and reassurance in learning to use computer-delivered therapy activities or other technologies such as those reported by Heredia et al. (2009 this issue), Jokel et al. (2009 this issue), and Cartwright and Elliot (2009 this issue). For example, to address these sorts of difficulties in their aphasia-friendly television viewing intervention, Cartwright and Elliot provided a glossary, and spoken and pantomimed explanations of terminology associated with using a DVD player.

Participant characteristics and co-occurring deficits

Future reports also need to document clients' non-language characteristics in detail to establish which client factors are associated with particular therapy outcomes. The suitability of particular interventions (impairment-directed as well as activity/participation-directed) for particular clients will depend on the client's and partners' cognitive abilities, on personality and motivational factors, and on attitudes and access to particular communication modes and opportunities (Turner & Whitworth, 2006).

Individuals with co-occurring behaviour, motor, and/or mood disturbances will also require referral to neurology, psychiatry, psychology, physiotherapy, and occupational therapy services (Robinson, 2001). Additional behavioural and pharmacological interventions may be required, as well as interventions directed at enhancing the participants' mobility and safety in their environment, including assessment of swallowing (Gregory & Lough, 2001; Rahman, Sahakian, Hodges, Rogers, & Robbins, 1999; Robinson, 2001; Royal College of Speech & Language Therapists, 2005)

Replication

Finally, replication for all the therapies reported is extremely important. First, a successful replication reduces the possibility that an effect reported in a single-case study (almost all the studies reviewed here) is peculiar to that study (clinician and/or participant effects). A limitation of the single-case design used in most of the studies that we reviewed is the impossibility of knowing to what extent the observed results can be generalised to other clients, whereas a series of replications would begin to indicate the client group(s) for whom a positive outcome from therapy might be expected. The currently limited replication of impairment-directed interventions with people with progressive language impairments therefore urges caution in assuming results for one participant will be observed in another. For example, in the Jokel et al. study in this issue, both participants received the same intervention, but P2 took far longer than P1 to reach criterion and the treatment effect and maintenance were not as strong. In the study of McNeil et al. (1995), a cueing hierarchy for adjective retrieval in an antonym task did not yield the same results as a similarly designed synonym task.

CONCLUDING COMMENTS

Taylor et al. (2009 this issue) highlight the need for a speech pathology management pathway for people with progressive language impairments. As part of a multidisciplinary dementia health and social care service, such a pathway will need to be eclectic, considering the relative merits of impairment-directed, activity/participation-directed, and combined approaches on an individual basis for each client. There is a pressing need for client and carer education, peer support, and for counselling about communication, disruptive behaviour, personality change, carer burden, and grief and end-of-life issues. Therapy options already in use in the context of stroke-related aphasia are appropriate for use with people with progressive language impairments. These should be selected on the basis of comprehensive initial assessment and ongoing review, and proactively implemented in anticipation of decline, rather than solely matched to the client's current needs (Rogers & Alarcon, 1998; Rogers et al., 2000).

In sum, it is clear that treatment for progressive language impairments can be of great benefit. However, intervention needs to encompass the individual's communicative needs in everyday contexts, and to anticipate future needs. We hope that clinicians embrace this challenge and that services for this population become more widespread. Similarly, we hope that the clinical research base will increase, enabling future clinical decisions about therapy design to be both theoretically and empirically motivated.

REFERENCES

Alarcon, N. B., Duffy, J. R., McNeil, M. R., & Rogers, M. (2000, 16–19 November). *Aphasia grand rounds: Primary progressive aphasia.* Paper presented at the American Speech Hearing Association Annual Conference, Washington DC.

American Speech-Language-Hearing Association (2001). *Scope of practice in Speech-Language pathology [Scope of practice].* Available from www.asha.org/policy.

Armstrong, E., & Mortensen, L. (2006). Everyday talk: Its role in assessment and treatment for individuals with aphasia. *Brain Impairment, 7*(3), 175–189.

Bayles, K. A., & Tomoeda, C. K. (1997). *Improving function in dementia and other cognitive-linguistic disorders: Guide and resource book.* Tucson, AZ: Canyonlands.

Béland, R., & Ska, B. (1992). Interaction between verbal and gestural language in progressive aphasia: A longitudinal case study. *Brain and Language, 43,* 355–385.

Biedermann, B., & Nickels, L. (2008). The representation of homophones: More evidence from the remediation of anomia. *Cortex, 44,* 276–293.

Bier, N., Macoir, J., Gagnon, L., Van der Linden, M., Louveaux, S., & Desrosiers, J. (2009). Known, lost, and recovered: Efficacy of formal-semantic therapy and spaced retrieval method in a case of semantic dementia. *Aphasiology, 22,* 210–235.

Bourgeois, M. S. (1991). Communication treatment for adults with dementia. *Journal of Speech and Hearing Research, 34,* 831–844.

Brush, J. A., & Camp, C. A. (1998). Using spaced retrieval as an intervention during speech language therapy. *Clinical Gerontologist, 19*(1), 51–64.

Cartwright, J., & Elliott, K. A. E. (2009). Promoting strategic television viewing in the context of progressive language impairment. *Aphasiology, 22,* 266–285.

Chow, T. W., Miller, B. L., Boone, K., Mishkin, F., & Cummings, J. L. (2002). Frontotemporal dementia classification and neuropsychiatry. *The Neurologist, 8,* 263–269.

Clare, L. (Ed.). (2001). *Cognitive rehabilitation in dementia.* Hove, UK: Psychology Press.

Clare, L., Wilson, B. A., Breen, K., & Hodges, J. R. (1999). Errorless learning of face–name associations in early Alzheimer's disease. *Neurocase, 5,* 37–46.

Coelho, C. A., McHugh, R. E., & Boyle, M. (2000). Semantic feature analysis as a treatment for aphasic dysnomia: A replication. *Aphasiology, 14*(2), 133–142.

Cognitive Neurology & Alzheimer's Disease Center (CNADC). (2006). *Primary progressive aphasia (PPA) program [electronic version].* Retrieved 31 January 2007 from Northwestern University, Cognitive Neurology and Alzheimer's Disease Center website: www.brain.northwestern.edu/ppa/ppa.html.

Coltheart, M., Kay, J., & Lesser, R. (1995). *Evaluación del Procesamiento Lingüístico en la Afasia.* Hove UK: Psychology Press.

Cotelli, M., Vanenti, R., Cappa, S. F., Geroldi, C., Zanetti, O., & Rossini, P. M. et al. (2006). Transcranial magnetic stimulation improves action naming in Alzheimer's patients. *Archives of Neurology, 63,* 1602–1604.

Craenhals, A., Raison-Van-Ruymbeke, A. M., Rectem, D., Seron, X., & Laterre, E. C. (1990). Is slowly progressive aphasia actually a new clinical entity? *Aphasiology, 4*(5), 485–509.

Cress, C. J., & King, J. M. (1999). AAC Strategies for people with primary progressive aphasia without dementia: Two case studies. *AAC Augmentative and Alternative Communication, 15,* 248–259.

Croot, K. (2009). Progressive aphasia: Definitions, diagnoses, and prognoses. *Aphasiology, 22,* 302–326.

Dunn, L. M., Dunn, L. M., & Whetton, C. (1982). *British Picture Vocabulary Scale: Long form.* Windsor, UK: NFER-Nelson.

Fillingham, J. K., Sage, K., & Lambon Ralph, M. (2005). Further explorations and an overview of errorless and errorful therapy for aphasic word-finding difficulties: The number of naming attempts during therapy affects outcome. *Aphasiology, 19,* 567–614.

Fillingham, J. K., Sage, K., & Lambon Ralph, M. (2006). The treatment of anomia using errorless learning. *Neuropsychological Rehabilitation, 16,* 129–154.

Finocchiaro, C., Maimone, M., Brighina, F., Piccoli, T., Giglia, G., & Fierro, B. (2006). A case study of primary progressive aphasia: Improvement on verbs after rTMS treatment. *Neurocase, 12,* 317–321.

Frattali, C. (2004). An errorless learning approach to treating dysnomia in frontotemporal dementia. *Journal of Medical Speech-Language Pathology, 12*(3), xi–xxiv.

Funnell, E. (1995). A case of forgotten knowledge. In R. Campbell & M. A. Conway (Eds.), *Broken memories: Case studies in memory impairment* (pp. 225–236). Oxford, UK: Blackwell.

Goodglass, H., & Kaplan, E. (1983). *The assessment of aphasia and related disorders* (2nd ed.). Philadelphia: Lea & Febiger.

Gorman, B. S., & Allison, D. B. (1996). Statistical alternatives for single-case designs. In R. D. Franklin, D. B. Allison, & B. S. Gorman (Eds.), *Design and analysis of single-case research* (pp. 159–214). Mahwah NJ: Lawrence Erlbaum Associates Inc.

Gorno-Tempini, M. L., Dronkers, N. F., Rankin, K. P., Ogar, J. M., Phrengrasamy, L., & Rosen, H. J. et al. (2004). Cognition and anatomy in three variants of primary progressive aphasia. *Annals of Neurology, 55,* 335–346.

Graham, K. S., Patterson, K., Pratt, K. H., & Hodges, J. R. (1999). Relearning and subsequent forgetting of semantic category exemplars in a case of semantic dementia. *Neuropsychology, 13*(3), 359–380.

Graham, K. S., Patterson, K., Pratt, K. H., & Hodges, J. R. (2001). Can repeated exposure to "forgotten" vocabulary help alleviate word-finding difficulties in semantic dementia? An illustrative case study. *Neuropsychological Rehabilitation, 11*(3/4), 429–454.

Gregory, C., & Lough, S. (2001). Practical issues in the management of early onset dementia. In J. R. Hodges (Ed.), *Early-onset dementia: A multidisciplinary approach* (pp. 449–469). Oxford, UK: Oxford University Press.

Hart, R. P., Beach, W. A., & Taylor, J. R. (1997). A case of progressive apraxia of speech and non-fluent aphasia. *Aphasiology, 11*(1), 73–82.

Helm-Estabrooks, N. (2001). *Cognitive Linguistic Quick Test.* San Antonio, TX: Harcourt Assessment.

Herbert, R., Best, W., Hickin, J., Howard, D., & Osborne, F. (2003). Combining lexical and interactional approaches to the treatment of word-finding deficits in aphasia. *Aphasiology, 17,* 1163–1186.

Heredia, C. G., Sage, K., Ralph, M., & Berthier, M. (2009). Relearning and retention of verbal labels in a case of semantic dementia. *Aphasiology, 22,* 192–209.

Hickin, J., Best, W., Herbert, R., Howard, D., & Osborne, F. (2002). Phonological therapy for word-finding difficulties: A re-evaluation. *Aphasiology, 16,* 981–999.

Hillis, A. E. (1991). Effects of separate treatments for distinct impairments within the naming process. *Clinical Aphasiology, 19,* 255–265.

Hillis, A. E., & Caramazza, A. (1994). Theories of lexical processing and rehabilitation of lexical deficits. In M. J. Riddoch & G. W. Humphreys (Eds.), *Cognitive neuropsychology and cognitive rehabilitation* (pp. 449–482). Hove, UK: Lawrence Erlbaum Associates Ltd.

Hodges, J. R., Berrios, G., & Breen, K. (2000). The multidisciplinary memory clinic approach. In G. E. Berrios & J. R. Hodges (Eds.), *Memory disorders in psychiatric practice* (pp. 101–121). Cambridge, UK: Cambridge University Press.

Hodges, J. R., Graham, N., & Patterson, K. (1995). Charting the progression in semantic dementia: Implications for the organisation of semantic memory. *Memory, 3,* 463–495.

Hodges, J. R., & Patterson, K. (1995). Is semantic memory consistently impaired early in the course of Alzheimer's disease? Neuroanatomical and diagnostic implications. *Neuropsychologia, 33,* 441–459.

Hodges, J. R., Patterson, K., Oxbury, S., & Funnell, E. (1992). Semantic dementia: Progressive fluent aphasia with temporal lobe atrophy. *Brain, 115,* 1783–1806.

Holland, A. L., McBurney, D. H., Moossy, J., & Reinmuth, O. M. (1985). The dissolution of language in Pick's disease with neurofibrillary tangles: A case study. *Brain and Language, 24,* 36–58.

Howard, D. (1995). Lexical anomia (or the case of the missing lexical entries). *Quarterly Journal of Experimental Psychology, 48*A, 999–1023.

Howard, D. (2000). Cognitive neuropsychology and aphasia therapy: The case of word retrieval. In I. Papathanasiou (Ed.), *Acquired neurogenic communication disorders: A clinical perspective.* London: Whurr.

Howard, D., & Patterson, K. (1992). *Pyramids and Palm Trees: A test of semantic access from pictures and words.* Bury St Edmunds, UK: Thames Valley Test Company.

Jokel, R., Cupit, J., Rochon, E., & Leonard, C. (2009). Re-learning lost vocabulary in non-fluent progressive aphasia with Mosstalk Words®. *Aphasiology, 22,* 175–191.

Jokel, R., Rochon, E., & Leonard, C. (2002). Therapy for anomia in semantic dementia. *Brain and Cognition, 49*(2), 241–244.

Jokel, R., Rochon, E., & Leonard, C. (2006). Treating anomia in semantic dementia: Improvement, maintenance, or both? *Neuropsychological Rehabilitation, 16*(3), 241–256.

Josephs, K. A., Duffy, J. R., Strand, E. A., Whitwell, J. L., Layton, K. F., & Parisi, J. E. et al. (2006). Clinicopathological and imaging correlates of progressive aphasia and apraxia of speech. *Brain, 129,* 1385–1398.

Kaplan, E., Goodglass, H., & Weintraub, S. (1983). *Boston Naming Test.* Philadelphia: Lea & Febiger.

Kay, J., Lesser, R., & Coltheart, M. (1992). *Psycholinguistic Assessments of Language Processing in Aphasia.* Hove, UK: Lawrence Erlbaum Associates Ltd.

Kertesz, A. (1979). *Aphasia and associated disorders: Taxonomy, localization, and recovery.* New York: Grune & Stratton.

Kertesz, A., McMonagle, P., Blair, M., Davidson, W., & Munoz, D. (2005). The evolution and pathology of frontotemporal dementia. *Brain, 128,* 1996–2005.

Laine, M., & Martin, N. (2006). *Anomia: Clinical and theoretical aspects.* Hove, UK: Psychology Press.

Lambon-Ralph, M. A., & Fillingham, J. K. (2007). The importance of memory and executive function in aphasia: Evidence from the treatment of anomia using errorless and errorful learning. In A. Meyer, L. Wheeldon, & A. Krott (Eds.), *Automaticity and control in language porocessing* (pp. 193–216). Hove, UK: Psychology Press.

Laurence, F., Manning, M., & Croot, K. (2002, July). *Impairment-based interventions in primary progressive aphasia: Theoretical and clinical issues.* Paper presented at The 10th International Aphasia Rehabilitation Conference: Past, Present and Future, Brisbane, Australia.

Louis, M., Espesser, R., Rey, V., Daffaure, V., Di Cristo, A., & Habib, M. (2001). Intensive training of phonological skills in progressive aphasia: A model of brain plasticity in neurodegenerative disease. *Brain & Cognition, 46*(1–2), 197–201.

Lubinski, R. (Ed.). (1995). *Dementia and communication.* San Diego, CA: Singular.

Lubinski, R., & Orange, J. B. (2000). A framework for the assessment and treatment of functional communication in dementia. In L. E. Worrall & C. M. Frattali (Eds.), *Neurogenic communication disorders: A functional approach* (pp. 220–246). New York: Thieme.

Martin, N., & Laine, M. (2000). Effects of contextual priming on impaired word retrieval. *Aphasiology, 14*(1), 53–70.

Mazaux, J., & Orgogozo, J. (1972). *Echelle d'évaluation de l'aphasie (BDAE).* Issy-Les-Moulineaux: Editions EAP.

McClelland, J., McNaughton, B. L., & O'Rielly, R. C. (1995). Why there are complementary learning systems in the hippocampus and neocortex: Insights from the successes and failures of connectionist models of learning and memory. *Psychological Review, 102*(3), 419–457.

McNeil, M. R., & Duffy, J. R. (2001). Primary progressive aphasia. In R. Chapey (Ed.), *Language intervention strategies in adult aphasia* (4th ed., pp. 472–486). Baltimore: Lippincott, Williams & Wilkins.

McNeil, M. R., Small, S. L., Masterson, R. J., & Tepanta, R. D. (1995). Behavioural and pharmacological treatment of lexical-semantic deficits in a single patient with primary progressive aphasia. *American Journal of Speech-Language Pathology, 4,* 76–93.

Mesulam, M-M. (2001). Primary progressive aphasia. *Annals of Neurology, 49,* 425–432.

Mesulam, M-M. (2003). Primary progressive aphasia – A language-based dementia. *New England Journal of Medicine, 349*(16), 1535–1542.

Mesulam, M-M., Grossman, M., Hillis, A. E., Kertesz, A., & Weintraub, S. (2003). The core and halo of primary progressive aphasia and semantic dementia. *Annals of Neurology, 54*(Suppl. 5), S11–S14.

Mummery, C. J., Patterson, K., Wise, R. J. S., Vandenbergh, R., Price, C. J., & Hodges, J. R. (1999). Disrupted temporal lobe connections in semantic dementia. *Brain, 122,* 61–73.

Murray, J., Schneider, J., Banerjee, S., & Mann, A. (1999). Eurocare: A cross-national study of co-resident spouse carers for people with Alzheimer's disease: II – A qualitative analysis of the experience of caregiving. *International Journal of Geriatric Psychiatry, 14,* 662–667.

Murray, L. L. (1998). Longitudinal treatment of primary progressive aphasia: A case study. *Aphasiology, 12*(7/8), 651–672.

Naeser, M., Martin, P., Nicholas, M., Baker, E. H., Seekins, H., & Helm-Estabrooks, N. et al. (2005). Improved naming after TMS treatments in a chronic, global aphasia patient – case report. *Neurocase, 11*, 182–193.

Nickels, L. (2000). *A sketch of the cognitive processes involved in the comprehension and production of single words*. Retrieved 2 March 2007 from http://www.maccs.mq.edu.au/~lnickels/model.doc.

Nickels, L. (2002). Therapy for naming disorders: Revisiting, revising and reviewing. *Aphasiology, 16*, 935–980.

Nickels, L., & Best, W. (1996a). Therapy for naming disorders (Part 1): Principles, puzzles, and progress. *Aphasiology, 10*(1), 21–47.

Nickels, L., & Best, W. (1996b). Therapy for naming disorders (Part II): Specifics, surprises, and suggestions. *Aphasiology, 10*(2), 109–136.

Northen, B., Hopcutt, B., & Griffiths, H. (1990). Progressive aphasia without generalised dementia. *Aphasiology, 4*(1), 55–65.

Rahman, S., Sahakian, B. J., Hodges, J. R., Rogers, R. D., & Robbins, T. W. (1999). Specific cognitive deficits in mild frontal variant frontotemporal dementia. *Brain, 122*, 1469–1493.

Rapp, B., & Glucroft, B. (2009). The benefits and protective effects of behavioural treatment for dysgraphia in a case of primary progressive aphasia. *Aphasiology, 22*, 236–265.

Raymer, A. M., Bandy, D., Adair, J. C., Schwartz, R. L., Williamson, D. J., & Gonzalez Rothi, L. J. et al. (2001). Effects of bromocriptine in a patient with crossed nonfluent aphasia: A case report. *Archives of Physical Medicine and Rehabilitation, 82*(1), 139–144.

Raymer, A. M., & Gonzalez Rothi L., J. (2002). Clinical diagnosis and treatment of naming disorders. In A. E. Hillis (Ed.), *The handbook of adult language disorders*. Hove, UK: Psychology Press.

Reed, D. A., Johnson, N. A., Thompson, C., Weintraub, S., & Mesulam, M-M. (2004). A clinical trial of bromocriptine for treatment of primary progressive aphasia. *Annals of Neurology, 56*(5), 750.

Rey, A. (1964). *L'examen clinique en psychologie*. Paris: Presses Universitaires de France.

Ripich, D. N. (1994). Functional communication with AD patients: A caregiver training programme. *Alzheimer Disease and Related Disorders, 8*(Suppl. 3), 95–109.

Ripich, D. N., & Horner, J. (2004). The neurodegenerative dementias: Diagnosis and interventions. *The ASHA Leader, 9*(8), 4–5, 14.

Robinson, K. M. (2001). Rehabilitation applications in caring for patients with Pick's disease and frontotemporal dementias. *Neurology, 56*, S56–S58.

Rogers, M. A., & Alarcon, N. B. (1998). Dissolution of spoken language in primary progressive aphasia. *Aphasiology, 12*(7/8), 635–650.

Rogers, M. A., King, J. M., & Alarcon, N. B. (2000). Proactive management of primary progressive aphasia. In D. R. Beukelman, K. M. Yorkston, & J. Reichle (Eds.), *Augmentative and alternative communication for adults with acquired neurologic disorders* (pp. 305–337). Baltimore: Brookes.

Royal College of Speech & Language Therapists (2005). *Speech and language therapy provision for people with dementia*. Retrieved 25 January 2007 from www.rcslt.org/resources/publications/dementia_paper.pdf.

Scheull, H., & Sefer, J. W. (1973). *Differential diagnosis of aphasia with the Minnesota Test*. Minneapolis, MN: University of Minnesota Press.

Schneider, S. L., Thompson, C. K., & Luhring, B. (1996). Effects of verbal plus gestural matrix training on sentence production in a patient with primary progressive aphasia. *Aphasiology, 10*, 297–317.

Simons, J. S., & Graham, K. S. (2000). New learning in semantic dementia: Implications for cognitive and neuroanatomical models of long-term memory. *Revue de Neuropsychologie, 10*(1), 199–215.

Snowden, J. S., Goulding, P. J., & Neary, D. (1989). Semantic dementia: A form of circumscribed cerebral atrophy. *Behavioural Neurology, 2*, 167–182.

Snowden, J. S., & Griffiths, H. (2000). Semantic dementia: Assessment and management. In W. Best, K. Bryan, & J. Maxim (Eds.), *Semantic processing: Theory and practice* (pp. 180–203). London: Whurr.

Snowden, J. S., & Neary, D. (2002). Relearning of verbal labels in semantic dementia. *Neuropsychologia, 40*, 1715–1728.

Taylor, C., Miles Kingma, R., Croot, K., & Nickels, L. (2009). Speech pathology services for primary progressive aphasia: Exploring an emerging area of practice. *Aphasiology, 22*, 161–174.

Thompson, C. K., Ballard, K. J., Tait, M. E., Weintraub, S., & Mesulam, M-M. (1997). Patterns of language decline in non-fluent primary progressive aphasia. *Aphasiology, 11*(4/5), 297–321.

Thompson, C. K., & Johnson, N. (2006). Language interventions in dementia. In D. K. Attix & K. A. Welsh-Bohmer (Eds.), *Geriatric neuropsychology: Assessment and intervention* (pp. 315–332). New York: Guildford Press.

Togher, L., McDonald, S., Code, C., & Grant, S. (2004). Training communication partners of people with traumatic brain injury: A randomised controlled trial. *Aphasiology, 18*(4), 313–335.

Turner, S., & Whitworth, A. (2006). Conversational partner training programmes in aphasia: A review of key themes and participants' roles. *Aphasiology, 20*(6), 483–510.

Warrington, E. K. (1984). *Recognition Memory Test*. Windsor, UK: NFER Nelson.

Wechsler, D. (1981). *Wechsler Adult Intelligence Scale – Revised. Test manual*. New York: Psychological Corporation.

Wechsler, D. (1987). *Wechsler Memory Scale – Revised manual*. San Antonio, TX: Psychological Corporation.

Wilson, B. (1987). Single-case experimental designs in neuropsychological rehabilitation. *Journal of Clinical and Experimental Neuropsychology, 9*, 527–544.

Wilson, B. (1997). Research and evaluation in rehabilitation. In B. Wilson & D. L. McLellan (Eds.), *Rehabilitation studies handbook* (pp. 161–187). Cambridge, UK: Cambridge University Press.

Wilson, B., Baddeley, A., Evans, J., & Shiel, A. (1994). Errorless learning in the rehabilitation of memory impaired people. *Neuropsychological Rehabilitation, 4*, 307–326.

Wong, S. B. C., Anand, R., Chapman, S. B., Rackley, A., & Zientz, J. (2009). When nouns and verbs degrade: Facilitating communication in semantic dementia. *Aphasiology, 22*, 286–301.

APPENDIX TABLE 1

Summary of demographic characteristics and clinical presentations of participants in the reviewed impairment-directed studies

Studies grouped by clinical syndrome	Participant	Age, Sex	Prominent symptoms	Time post-onset	Brain imaging	Neuropsychology		
						Delayed recall	Semantic processing	Naming
Semantic dementia								
Funnell, 1995	Mrs P	63, F	semantic dementia[1]	3 yrs	CT: L temporal, SPECT: frontotemporal	Rey figure recall ✓, RMT faces: 42/50 ✗	BPVT: at 5yrs;6 mo level ✗	Semantic Battery:[2] 14/48 ✗
Graham et al., 1999, 2001	DM	61, M	anomia, impaired comprehension; progressed to semantic dementia[1]	4 yrs	MRI: L temporal	complex figure ✓	P&PT: 49/52 pics ✓	Semantic Battery:[2] 34/48 ✗
Jokel et al., 2002, 2006	AK	63, F	semantic dementia[1]	7 yrs	SPECT: L temporal, MRI: bitemporal L > R, L ventral frontal	nonverbal cognition ✓	PALPA synonym judgement: 56/60[6] 3, P&PT 37/52 pics[7] ✗	BNT: 8/60 [6] ✗, 5/60 [7] ✗
Snowden & Neary 2002	KB	64, F	semantic dementia[1] especially visual knowledge	3 yrs	SPECT, MRI: bitemporal, R > L, including medial temporal structures	RMT 30/50 words ✗, 25/50 faces ✗	P&PT: 35/52 words ✗, 25/52 pics ✗	BNT: 0/60 ✗
	CR	57, F	semantic dementia[1]	3 yrs	SPECT, MRI: bitemporal, L > R, relative preservation of hippocampus	RMT: 29/50 words ✗, 29/50 faces ✗	P&PT: 29/52 words ✗, 29/52 pics ✗	BNT: 4/60 ✗
Frattali, 2004		66, M	anomia, word-by-word reading, impaired auditory comprehension & word recognition & auditory memory, behaviour change	n/a	PET: L frontotemporal & ant. insula, MRI: inf medial L temporal, mostly spared hippocampus	verbal memory on DRS and WMS ✓	auditory word recognition: 3/6 colours ✗, 4/6 body parts ✗	BNT: 1/60 ✗

APPENDIX TABLE 1
(Continued.)

Studies grouped by clinical syndrome	Participant	Age, Sex	Prominent symptoms	Time post-onset	Brain imaging	Neuropsychology		
						Delayed recall	Semantic processing	Naming
Bier et al., 2009 this issue	TBo	70, F	semantic dementia[1]	5 yrs	SPECT, MRI: L sylvian fissure, L frontal	all tests ✓, except hard form of Doors Test[4] ✗	P&PT: 36/52 words ✗, 37/52 pics ✗	76/127 [5] ✗
Heredia et al., 2009 this issue	CUB	53, F	semantic dementia[1]	2 yrs	MRI: bitemporal, focal on L, mild on R	visual memory ✗	P&PT: 31/52 words ✗, 33/52 pics ✗	EPLA: 13/60 ✗
Nonfluent progressive aphasia								
Louis et al., 2001	64, F		all 3: nonfluent aphasia (agrammatic, pronunciation errors[8], anomia), impaired auditory processing and auditory working memory	n/a	n/a	n/a	n/a	n/a
	71, F			n/a	n/a	n/a	n/a	n/a
	77, F			n/a	n/a	n/a	n/a	n/a
Jokel et al., 2009 this issue	P1	58, F	nonfluent aphasia, slow and anomic speech	3-4 yrs	SPECT: L temporal	story recall ✓	P&PT: 51/52 pics ✓	BNT: 26/60 ✗
	P2	75, F	nonfluent aphasia, hesitant and anomic speech	n/a	SPECT: bitemporal	story recall ✓	P&PT: 50/52 pics ✓	BNT: 29/60 ✗
Primary progressive aphasia								
McNeil et al., 1995	GP	61, M	anomia, mild spastic dysarthria, mild aphasia	9 mo	SPECT: L temporo-parietal, MRI: L temporal	short passage story recall ✓, complex figure story recall ✓	P&PT: 49/52 pics ✓	BNT: 46/60 ✗
Schneider et al., 1996		62, F	nonfluent aphasia (agrammatic, pronunciation errors[8], anomia), slow reading & spelling	2.5 yrs	SPECT, MRI: L perisylvian	WMS ✓	category naming:[3] ✓	BNT: 59/60 ✓

APPENDIX TABLE 1
(Continued.)

Studies grouped by clinical syndrome	Participant	Age, Sex	Prominent symptoms	Time post-onset	Brain imaging	Neuropsychology		
						Delayed recall	Semantic processing	Naming
Laurence et al., 2002	CD	49, F	fluent aphasia, anomia, reading and writing difficulties, semantic & pronunciation errors	30 mo	SPECT, MRI: L temporal	words & complex figure ✓	P&PT: 49/52 words ✓, 35/52 pics ✗	BNT: 33/60 ✗
	AC	63, F	mild anomia, fluent aphasia, semantic errors, pragmatic changes	1 yr	MRI: L temporal	n/a	P&PT: 50/52 pics ✓	35/60 BNT ✗
Rapp & Glucroft, 2009 this issue	CB	60, F	dysgraphia, anomia, dyscalculia, attention deficits, mild constructional deficits	8 yrs	MRI: temporo-parietal, L > R	RAVLT and Rey copy ✓	PPVT: 68%ile ✗	BNT: 48/60 ✗

Abbreviations for tests: BNT = Boston Naming Test (Kaplan & Goodglass, 1983); BPVS = British Picture Vocabulary Scale (Dunn, Dunn & Whetton, 1982); EPLA = Evaluación del Procesamiento Lingüístico en la Afasia (Coltheart, Kay & Lesser, 1995); PALPA = Psycholinguistic Assessment of Language Processing in Aphasia (Kay, Lesser & Coltheart); P&PT = Pyramids and Palm Trees test (Howard & Patterson, 1992); RAVLT = Rey Auditory Verbal Learning Test (Rey, 1964); RMT = Recognition Memory Test (Warrington, 1984); WMS = Wechsler Memory Scale (Wechsler, 1987)

Other abbreviations: ant. = anterior; CT = computerised tomography; F = female; inf. = inferior; L = left; M = male; mo = months; MRI = magnetic resonance imaging; n/a = not available; PET = positron emission tomography; pics = pictures; R = right; SPECT = single photon emission computed tomography; vol. = volume; yrs = years; %ile = percentile ✓ = within normal limits/judged to be unimpaired for this participant; ✗ = judged to be impaired for this participant

Notes: [1] As defined by the Lund criteria (Neary, 1998); [2] Semantic Battery (Hodges & Patterson, 1995); [3] Test of Adolescent Word Finding (German, 1990 in Schneider et al., 1996); [4] Baddeley (1994); [5] Locally developed naming test using pictures from Snodgrass & Vanderwart (1980); [6] Seven months before study; [7] Five months after study; [8] Deficits potentially described by other researchers as apraxia of speech

APPENDIX TABLE 2

Summary of interventions and results in the reviewed impairment-directed studies

Studies grouped by clinical syndrome	Participant	Impairment treated	Description of intervention	Treatment effect	Generalisation	Maintenance
Semantic dementia						
Funnell, 1995	Mrs P	Vegetable naming	1 session pairing vegetable and name 10 times each. Home practice: self-test with vegetable, written name and description; EF	YES: 6/5 correct	NO, not to other less familiar vegetables	1 week: 6/6; 1-2 months: 5/6; 8 months: 3/6. Practice over this period not described but vegetables not in season
Graham et al., 1999, 2001	DM	Noun retrieval	Rehearsing members of semantic categories (name+picture) in home practice, 30 mins/ day × 2 weeks; EL	YES	NO	40% at 10 weeks
Jokel et al., 2002, 2006	AK	Naming	Picture+reading name aloud+read personally relevant description. Home practice 30 mins/ day × 6 days; EL	YES: –N–C 18/30 (60%); –N–C 11/30 (37%)	NO	4 weeks: –N+C43%*, –N–C 23%; 6 months: –N+C 30%, –N–C 13%. *statistically reliable effect
Snowden & Neary 2002	KB	Naming	errorless pairing of picture with spoken and written name, 3 times per set on 2 occasions; EL	YES for items with partial knowledge. YES (marginal) for items about which KB had no preserved knowledge	Not reported. KB continued to learn name of new people and medicines in everyday life	2 weeks: YES; 4 months: NO
	CR	Naming & recall of definitions	studied picture, written name and information relevant to personal experience in 2 treatment sessions. Home practice 20 mins/day × 3 weeks; EL	YES, on Day 20	Day 20: YES, to reverse presentation order. Day 60: YES, 20/20 to reverse presentation order, 15/20 to materials altered in colour, format. Day 250: YES, 8/20 on altered materials	Day 60: 20/20 naming, 13/20 definitions (with 2 days' study before). Day 250: 13/20 naming, 10/20 definitions.

APPENDIX TABLE 2
(Continued.)

Studies grouped by clinical syndrome	Parti-cipant	Impairment treated	Description of intervention	Treatment effect	Generalisation	Maintenance
Frattali, 2004		Noun and verb retrieval	Conversation about semantic features and associates of photo graphed items. 12 × 2 hour sessions over 3 months; EL	YES on 20 treated nouns and 20 treated verbs	NO, not to untreated nouns and verbs, nor to performance on neuropsychological tests	3 months: NO
Bier et al., 2009 this issue	TBo	Naming & learning semantic attributes	8 items, formal-semantic therapy using cueing hierarchy and semantic feedback. 3 sessions spaced retrieval compared with 3 sessions simple repetition; EF	YES: picture names YES: specific attributes NO: general attributes Spaced retrieval equal to simple repetition.	NO, not on naming to within-category items or another naming test or letter fluency task	Naming: NO, loss of treatment gains over 5-week period. Better maintenance of specific attributes
Heredia et al., 2009 this issue	CUB	Naming	computer-based presentation of picture alone then picture+read aloud written name, home practice daily for 1 month; EL	YES: 28/28 treated items	YES: 92% correct on other exemplars of treated items. YES: to spontaneous speech (anecdotal report)	1 month: YES 27/28; 6 months: YES 23/28 with no deliberate practice
Nonfluent progressive aphasia						
Louis et al., 2001	3 Ps	auditory-phonological processing	Tapping syllables, phoneme discrimination and segmentation of tokens slowed by 166%. 15-20 mins/day × 42 days; EF	YES in data pooled across 3 Ps	YES: Improved performance for at least 1 of the 3 Ps on several French BDEA subtests. 1 reduced phoneme errors, 1 improved on reading and repetition.	One P was given a phase of treatment with tokens at normal speed: performance declined

APPENDIX TABLE 2
(Continued.)

Studies grouped by clinical syndrome	Parti-cipant	Impairment treated	Description of intervention	Treatment effect	Generalisation	Maintenance
Jokel et al., 2009 this issue	P1	Naming	MossTalk Words® Cued Naming of 3 lists of 14 words, 1 hour 3 ×/week for 4 weeks per list; EF	YES: all 3 lists	NO, not to Philadelphia Naming Test	1 month: YES; 6 months: NO; all 3 lists
	P2	Naming	MossTalk Words® Cued Naming, 3 lists of 14-15 words, 1 hour 2x/week for 12 weeks per list; EF	YES: all 3 lists	NO, not to Philadelphia Naming Test	1 month: YES 2 lists, NO 1 list; 6 months: NO 2 lists, MARGINAL 1 list
Primary progressive aphasia						
McNeil et al., 1995	GP	Adjective retrieval	Cueing hierarchy + pharmacological treatment (dextroamphetamine); 31 × 2-hour sessions over 5 months; EF	YES, but pharmaco-logical treatment + cueing hierarchy no clear advantage over cueing hierarchy alone	YES, some to untrained adjectives, and to untrained verbs and prepositions. NO, not to connected speech	declined at approximately 3 months without rehearsal
Schneider et al., 1996		Use of gestural and verbal forms for nouns, verbs and tense markers	Verbal + gesture training of target structures in sentences × 18 sessions. Home practice with pictures of gestures; EF	YES	YES, to untrained verbs & untrained sentences. NO, not to untrained tenses. Increased use of trained sentence form in story retell.	3 months: gesture maintained but verbal forms not maintained
Laurence et al., 2002	CD	Naming	Spoken word-picture matching, Home practice 30 items once per day × 2 weeks; EF	YES	NO, not to untrained items in another naming test	return to baseline level in 5-9 weeks without practice

APPENDIX TABLE 2
(Continued.)

Studies grouped by clinical syndrome	Parti-cipant	Impairment treated	Description of intervention	Treatment effect	Generalisation	Maintenance
Laurence et al., 2002 (Cont.)	AC	Naming	Written word-picture matching with semantic distractors. 40 high frequency items × 6 weeks, low frequency items × 4 weeks. Daily home practice; EF	YES, on written and spoken naming for high and low frequency words	NO, not to picture description task	11 weeks: High frequency spoken naming still 100%; 12 weeks: low frequency spoken naming at baseline levels; 14 weeks: high frequency written naming at 42%
Rapp & Glucroft, 2009 this issue	CB	Dysgraphia	4 sets: Trained (spell-study-spell) biweekly 3 hour sessions over 15 weeks, Repeated: spelled in each session; Homework (copy and self-test) sporadic; Control (Not Trained); EF	YES: 10% gain in Trained, Repeated and Homework stable, decline on Control	NO	6 months: YES, Trained, Repeated & Homework better than Control; 12 months: NO

EF = errorful learning; EL = errorless learning; mins = minutes; −N−C not named and not comprehended; −N+C not named but partially comprehended
P(s) = participant(s); BDEA = Boston Diagnostic Aphasia Examination (French adaptation; Mazaux & Orgogozo, 1971)

APPENDIX TABLE 3

Summary of activity/participation-directed interventions in the reviewed studies

Studies grouped by clinical syndrome	Participant	Age, Sex	Clinical presentation	Time post-onset	Duration of therapy	Brain imaging	Neuropsychology	Therapy components
Primary progressive aphasia								
Cress & King (1999)	CE	60, M	BDAE impaired on commands, complex ideation, repetition, sentence comprehension, naming, verbal fluency; used gesture and vocalisations to supplement/substitute for speech	7 years	1 mo AAC development, 1 year follow-up	MRI: focal L temporal	Visual processing and learning, arithmetic, sensorimotor skills, complex attention, orientation WNL	In context of close social relationship therapist developed communication boards, and spent 1 hour with CE 3-4 times/week; 3-6 hours with CE and family & 1-3 occasions/week outside the home e.g. bowling
Cress & King (1999)	MC	59, F	Mod-severe non-fluent aphasia on WAB, high level of fillers, repetitions & restarts, used self-generated communicative strategies e.g. oral spelling, written information in purse, questions to repair breakdown	6 years	Approx 3 sessions	MRI: L temporal	Reading comprehension better than auditory comprehension; delayed verbal memory WNL	(i) Words written when she couldn't understand, (ii) communication book with maps, family tree, house layout, pets, relationships (iii) names and pictures of food items on file cards filed in categories, taken out for shopping list and matched to items in supermarket
Murray (1998)	DD	65, F	Stuttering, slurred, agrammatic speech, word-finding difficulties, auditory & reading comprehension impairment	4 years	2.5 years	PET: L fronto-parietal	Complex figure delayed copy WNL; Auditory word recognition 57/60; BNT 19/20	(i) Activities involving listening to, reading, speaking and writing sentences and paragraphs; (ii) "back to the drawing board" communicative use of pictures; (iii) functional communication including spouse training, support group and Dyna Vox AAC device

APPENDIX TABLE 3
(Continued.)

Studies grouped by clinical syndrome	Parti-cipant	Age, Sex	Clinical presentation	Time post-onset	Duration of therapy	Brain imaging	Neuropsychology	Therapy components
Pattee, Von Berg & Ghezzi (2006)		57, F	PPA with AOS: <20% of speech intelligible, preserved receptive language	n/a	9 weeks	PET: L temporal	Preserved non-language cognition implied	Elicited agent-action-object sentences and Wh-questions using TTS and ASL. Utterances in both modes were similarly informative, but P preferred ASL because it felt more "normal". Accepted AAC electronic wrist device for emergencies.
Rogers, Alarcon & King (2000)	FA	M	Fluent aphasia	4 years	n/a	n/a	n/a	AAC (communication notebook, gestures, strategies for specific situations e.g. poker including wife's assistance)
Thompson & Johnson (2006)	RP	M, 58	Difficulty understanding words and expressing his thoughts, independent ADLs, social withdrawal outside family, WAB: anomic aphasia, word-finding diffiulties, semantic paraphasias	4 years	n/a	PET: bilateral temporal (L > R), frontal and parietal	non-verbal congition WNL	Communicative gesture, self-cueing strategies and ways of compensating for word-finding difficulties, emergency communication card, education in communication strategies for family
Nonfluent primary progressive aphasia								
Rogers & Alarcon (1998)	OD	71, M	Anomia, AOS, telegraphic speech, short phrases	2 years	4 years	MRI: widening L sylvian fissure	BNT≈19; WAIS perf IQ, immediate & delayed Rey Figure copy, Trail-Making test, Halstead-Reitan Category Test & WMT WNL	Proactive intervention: (i) anticipate future decline by targeting more severe impairment than currently experienced, (ii) dyad-oriented, (iii) activity-participation focus led to increasing use of AAC including gesture, writing, drawing, partner training, communication book, AAC device

APPENDIX TABLE 3
(Continued.)

Studies grouped by clinical syndrome	Parti-cipant	Age, Sex	Clinical presentation	Time post-onset	Duration of therapy	Brain imaging	Neuropsychology	Therapy components
Rogers, Alarcon & King (2000)	NA	M	Nonvocal communicator, required AAC for comprehension of even simple utterances	10 years	n/a	n/a	n/a	AAC (communication notebook, introduction card, Dyna Vox, drawing, written symbols, gesture & facial expression); language group
Pick's disease								
Holland, McBurney, Moossy, & Reinmuth (1985)	Mr E	68, M	Slow, deliberate speech, long pauses, anomia, phonological paraphasias	0 years	6 weeks (4 yrs post); brief Amerind trial (10 yrs post)	EEG: atypical L temporal & frontal	MTDDA: normal reading & writing, impaired auditory comprehension & auditory memory	4 years post onset: education, auditory comprehension/attention, articulation 10 years post onset: Amerind sign training, learned 50 signs but did not use them communicatively at home
Semantic dementia								
Wong, Anand, Chapman, Rackley & Zientz (2009 this issue)	Bobby V	61, M	Anomia, fluent empty speech, semantic paraphasias. Phonology, syntax, repetition unimpaired	n/a	4 years	SPECT: L temporal	P&PT, RAVLT, drawing: WNL	Discourse intervention guided by Halliday's (1977) 6 functions of communication. Individual and group sessions with client; education and training with spouse
Slowly progressive aphasia without generalised dementia								
Northen, Hopcutt & Griffiths (1990); Goulding et al. (1990)	—	M, 64	Effortful speech with fluent islands, effortful syllable repetition, right-sided tremor and rigidity	18 mo	4.5 years	SPECT: L frontal, temporal, parietal & sub-cortical	Non-verbal cognition WNL	Discontinued impairment-based treatment because of participant distress, introduction of AAC and focus on training spouse and care staff at home/care premises and counselling spouse

APPENDIX TABLE 3
(Continued.)

Studies grouped by clinical syndrome	Parti-cipant	Age, Sex	Clinical presentation	Time post-onset	Duration of therapy	Brain imaging	Neuropsychology	Therapy components
Progressive language impairment								
Cartwright & Elliot (2009 this issue)	P1 P2 P3 P4	F, 65; F, 59; F, 66; M, 62	Heterogeneous language presentations: 3 with nonfluent speech, one semantic dementia	10 weeks	n/a	n/a	CLQT language severity score: 2 severe, 1 moderate, 1 mild	Group programme with aphasia-friendly TV viewing, supported discussion of episode content and themes relevant to participants

Abbreviations for tests: BDAE Boston Diagnostic Aphasia Examination (Goodglass & Kaplan, 1983); CLQT Cognitive Linguistic Quick Test (Helm-Estabrooks, 2001); MTDDA Minnesota Test for Differential Diagnosis of Aphasia (Scheull & Sefer, 1973); WAB Western Aphasia Battery (Kertesz, 1979); WAIS Wechsler Adult Intelligence Scale (Wechsler, 1981); WMT Wechsler Memory Scale (Wechsler, 1987)

Other abbreviations: AAC = augmentative and alternative communication; ASL = Americal Sign Language; EEG: electroencephalogram; F = female;L = left; M = male; mo = months; MRI = magnetic resonance imaging; n/a = not available; P = participant; PPA = primary progressive aphasia; perf = performance; PET = positron emission tomography; pics = pictures; R = right; SPECT = single photon emission computed tomography; TTS = Text to Speech; WNL = within normal limits; yr(s) = year(s); %ile = percentile

APHASIOLOGY, 2009, 23 (2), 161–174

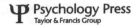

Speech pathology services for primary progressive aphasia: Exploring an emerging area of practice

Cathleen Taylor and Rachel Miles Kingma

War Memorial Hospital, Waverley, NSW, Australia

Karen Croot

University of Sydney, Sydney, NSW, Australia

Lyndsey Nickels

Macquarie University, Sydney, NSW, Australia

Background: Primary progressive aphasia (PPA) is a clinical dementia syndrome characterised by the gradual dissolution of language without impairment of other cognitive domains for at least the first 2 years of illness (Mesulam, 2001). In recent years the authors had observed an increase in the number of referrals of individuals with a queried diagnosis of PPA to their speech pathology service. However, they perceived a lack of information on the best management path for these individuals.

Aims: The aim of this study was to collate information about current service provision for clients with PPA living in the Australian state of New South Wales (NSW) and their caregivers. This information would identify current referral rates and speech pathology management of this population. This information, when combined with a review of the literature and an examination of overseas service provision, would be used to develop a framework for future speech pathology service provision for progressive aphasia.

Method & Procedures: Data relating to individuals with queried or confirmed PPA was collected from speech pathologists via a survey. Speech pathology services with an adult neurological caseload were surveyed in rural and metropolitan regions across NSW. Questions asked for information relating to referral patterns, demographics, and interventions provided.

Outcomes & Results: Responses from the survey indicated that only a small number of clients with PPA are referred to speech pathologists state-wide. At facilities where individuals were referred with queried PPA, all respondent speech pathologists provided some form of intervention. All clients were assessed and various intervention types were delivered including individual therapy, group therapy, intermittent review, and client and carer education. Overwhelmingly respondents talked of an emerging field of practice, and the need for more accessible information for clinicians and people with PPA and their carers.

Conclusion: PPA appears to be an area of under-referral for speech pathologists in NSW. We would like to see increased referrals to speech pathology services and promotion of the role of the speech pathologist on dementia care teams. There is

Address correspondence to: Cathleen Taylor, Speech Pathology, War Memorial Hospital, 125 Birrell St., Waverley, NSW, 2024, Australia. E-mail: taylorca@sesiahs.health.nsw.gov.au

Many thanks to Sandra Weintraub and Darcy Morhardt for generously sharing details of the CNADC PPA program. Lyndsey Nickels was funded by an NHMRC Senior Research Fellowship during the preparation of this manuscript.

http://www.psypress.com/aphasiology   DOI: 10.1080/02687030801943039

evidence that speech pathology intervention with this population can be effective. It is recommended that intervention targets both impairment and activity-participation levels but also we stress the importance of education and support that is specifically tailored to those with progressive language disorders.

Keywords: Primary progressive aphasia; Speech pathology; Language; Intervention.

The term primary progressive aphasia (PPA) was first used by Mesulam (1982). In an overview of progress in understanding PPA, Mesulam (2001, p. 425) defined this gradually worsening aphasia as a "focal dementia characterised by an isolated and gradual dissolution of language function." Duffy (1987, modified in Chapey, 2001, p. 472) similarly defined PPA as:

... aphasia of insidious onset, gradual progression, and prolonged course, without evidence of non-language computational impairments that are shared by a common aetiology to the aphasia, and due to a degenerative condition that presumably and predominantly involves the left (language dominant) peri-sylvian region of the brain.

There is no published diagnostic test of PPA; rather, diagnosis generally follows criteria proposed by Mesulam and colleagues (Mesulam, 1982, 2001; Mesulam & Weintraub, 1992; Weintraub, Rubin & Mesulam, 1990). These criteria are (1) a minimum 2-year history of progressive language disturbance of insidious onset, (2) preservation of other mental functions (although acalculia or limb apraxia may be present), (3) independence in activities of daily living except those dependent on the person's impaired language abilities, and (4) full neurological investigations excluding other causes of aphasia. A broad range of related disorders (including semantic dementia and primary progressive apraxia of speech) also show progressive language deterioration. There may be accompanying speech, motor, behavioural, personality, or other cognitive changes, sometimes emerging within 2 years of the initial language symptoms. Relationships between PPA and related disorders are discussed in Croot (2009, this issue).

PPA as defined by Mesulam and colleagues (see above) describes a clinical syndrome and not a disease process per se. Fluent and non-fluent varieties of PPA are observed, with the clinical picture varying depending on the distribution of the disease in brain tissue. However, despite different clinical presentations of aphasia, all individuals with PPA will have a distinct period of time, which may vary between 2 and 20 years, when they are living with an isolated aphasia and its concomitant effects on activity, participation, and well being (Duffy & Petersen, 1992; Rogers & Alarcon, 1999; Westbury & Bub, 1997). People with PPA "come to medical attention because of the onset of word finding difficulties, abnormal speech patterns and prominent spelling errors" (Mesulam, 2003, p. 1535)—a similar presentation to that of many people with acute onset aphasia who are referred for speech pathology services. There is substantial clinical similarity between individuals with acute onset aphasia and progressive aphasia, with the most important difference being the progressive nature of the latter. Further, because the criteria for a diagnosis of PPA call for relative preservation of non-language cognitive functions, learning might be well maintained by these clients. For these reasons, people with PPA would appear to be entirely appropriate candidates for intervention provided by Speech Pathologists (McNeil & Duffy, 2001).

The impetus for this research was a recent change in the referral pattern to speech pathology services in an aged care assessment and rehabilitation facility in Sydney, New South Wales, Australia. Over the previous 4 years, we had observed an increase in the number of referrals to our service of individuals with a queried diagnosis of PPA (from less than one case per year in the first 3 of these 4 years to six cases (4.5% of caseload) in the fourth year). Although total referral numbers to the clinic were relatively small, the increase was significant—$\chi^2 1$ sample (3 df) = 14.14, $p = .003$— and prompted several questions, including:

- Was this experience of a sharp increase in referral numbers typical?
- What was the current practice of speech pathologists with this client group?

In order to address these questions, we investigated current services to individuals with PPA by surveying speech pathologists across a range of adult healthcare settings throughout the Australian state of New South Wales. Healthcare services in Australia are administered primarily on a state-wide basis through a number of Area Health Services. New South Wales is Australia's most populous state, with approximately 6.7 million people living in an area of around 800,000 km^2. The population is distributed across four geographical regions: major cities (71.4%), inner regional areas (20.6%), outer regional areas (7.3%), and remote or very remote areas (0.7%) (Australian Bureau of Statistics, 2005). A total of 13.5% of the state's population are aged 65 years and over. We had two main reasons to expect that referrals for speech pathology services for people with PPA would be increasing in New South Wales. First, awareness of PPA as a disorder has been growing since Mesulam's (1982) seminal report. In the 10 years before Mesulam's 1982 paper, 2 cases were reported that fitted the criteria for PPA (Schwartz, Marin & Saffran, 1979; Warrington, 1975), whereas in the 10 years following, 57 new cases were reported (Mesulam & Weintraub, 1992). By 2001, Mesulam (2001) was able to propose that PPA may account for 20% of all dementia cases. Second, age is the most important risk factor for dementia (di Carlo, Baldereschi, Inzitari, & Amaducci, 1999), and the population of NSW is ageing as in the rest of the developed world. Henderson and Jorm (1998) reported that Australia-wide there were approximately 130,000 people with dementia in 1998, a number projected to rise to 183,000 in 2006 and 210,000 in 2011.

Our survey aimed to collect information about referral rates and current speech pathology service provision for clients with PPA and their carers living in New South Wales. Given that patients with diagnosed or queried PPA are suitable candidates for speech pathology intervention, we wanted to know whether speech pathology centres throughout New South Wales were being referred such cases, and if so, what services were being provided? We saw this as the first step towards providing improved services for these clients and their carers in the context of our state's health services.

We will first provide details regarding the survey and its results. We will then discuss the implications for service delivery. We conclude the paper with discussion of the broader implications for clinical management of PPA.

METHOD AND PROCEDURES

We collected data regarding speech pathology and PPA using a postal survey. For the purpose of this research we used the definition of PPA first given by Mesulam (1982), and provided this in the preamble to the survey. Questions asked for information about referral patterns, demographics, and interventions provided to patients referred with PPA or queried PPA across the specified 12-month period. All responses were anonymous. The survey questions are provided in the Appendix.

We attempted to ensure that all speech pathologists in New South Wales who were responsible for clinical management of adults with neurological disorders received a survey, by reference to lists of Speech Pathology Area Advisers/ Representatives and Managers of Greater Metropolitan Sydney Speech Pathology Services in New South Wales Health. This effectively covered all Area Health Services of New South Wales. In Metropolitan areas, this generally resulted in surveys being sent direct to the relevant service provider. In rural and remote areas, managers of that area were responsible for forwarding the survey to the relevant individual speech pathologist(s). Surveys were sent to a total of 34 speech pathology sites in rural and metropolitan regions across a variety of settings including; private and public services, acute and subacute hospitals, as well as outpatient and community services.

RESULTS

The survey reply rate was 76.5%. Of the 26 surveys returned, 13 respondents were unable to provide any information as they had not been referred any patients with the disorder within the time period stated.

Client demographics

The 13 affirmative responses described 20 individual cases of PPA: 13 females and 7 males. Responses were received from metropolitan and rural areas, from acute hospital, inpatient rehabilitation, outpatient rehabilitation, domiciliary and private services.

Referral and diagnosis

Consultant neurologists were the largest referral agents to speech pathology, responsible for 50% of referrals. 35% of individuals were referred by geriatricians, 10% by their local medical officer, and one individual (5%) had self-referred.

Respondents reported that in 63% of cases their clinical reports were used by the referring specialist to confirm or discard a diagnosis of PPA. Half (50%) of clients and/or carers had been advised of their diagnosis of PPA before seeing the speech pathologist while the other 50% were unaware of their diagnosis of PPA.

Management and intervention

Figure 1 summarises the types of service delivery provided by respondents to referred PPA clients. All clients with PPA or possible PPA were provided with assessment by the speech pathologists to whom they were referred. In addition, the majority (17/20; 85%) were also provided with individual treatment. Of these, six (35%) were given more than five sessions of treatment. One person received both individual and group treatment.

The treatments described could be broadly categorised as remediation techniques focusing on the language impairment, and activities that aimed to facilitate participation. The impairment-focused remediation techniques included semantic therapy, naming therapy, word-finding strategies, fluency treatment, and nonverbal

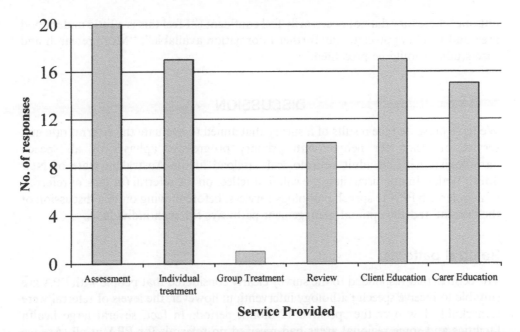

Figure 1. Types of service delivery provided by survey respondents to referred PPA clients.

language-based treatments. The participation-focused activities included the teaching of total communication techniques and/or development of augmentative and alternative communication (AAC) including life books, personal portfolios, and/or communication books. Other interventions included drawing and facilitated conversation. Following individual treatment, 53% (9/17) received regular review of their language.

In addition to assessment, the majority (85%) of clients and carers were provided with education regarding the nature of PPA and language disorders. All three individuals who did not receive treatment received education. One of these individuals was referred on to another speech pathology service, and one was provided with regular review.

Current service provision: Support groups

Overwhelmingly respondents noted a lack of appropriate sources of support and information for people with PPA and their carers, and commented that no support groups were available. In particular, many remarked that current services were not adequate for this client group. One Speech Pathologist wrote, "Clients do not fit into existing support groups – either stroke support or dementia care." Another commented, "I think support groups would be very important and wish this service was more readily available in my area."

Current service provision: Speech pathology intervention

The feedback from the surveys gave a clear picture that speech pathologists viewed PPA as an emerging field of practice, and an area in which they felt intervention was appropriate ("We can be a great resource to this client population and their carers") but one where they did not necessarily feel confident ("I feel this is a little understood area and would appreciate any further information available"; "More research and case studies should be presented.").

DISCUSSION

We have presented the results of a survey that aimed to evaluate the referral rate and service provision for people with primary progressive aphasia by all speech pathologists with an adult neurological caseload in the Australian state of New South Wales. In our discussion, we will first reflect on the referral (or lack of referral) of people with PPA to speech pathology services, before moving on to a discussion of the current and the optimal management pathways for such individuals.

Referral patterns

The centres that responded to the survey clearly considered that people with PPA are suitable to receive speech pathology intervention; however, the levels of referral were remarkably low over the specified 12-month period. In fact, several large health facilities and some regional areas had received no referrals for PPA at all. Are we able to assume that significant numbers of people in the regions surveyed are in fact living with PPA but not receiving speech Pathology services?

It is difficult to determine the precise incidence of PPA, as to date we know of no studies of incidence or prevalence of PPA specifically. Mesulam (2001) estimates PPA to account for roughly 20% of all dementias. This is within the bounds of McNeil and Duffy's (2001) observation that one quarter of all dementias are atypical and that some proportion of these will be PPA. It is also consistent with Harvey, Roques, Fox, and Rossor's (1996) epidemiological review suggesting that one in seven cases of early-onset dementia (onset before age 65) is likely to be associated with frontotemporal lobar degeneration, the neuropathology most commonly (but not exclusively) associated with PPA. The current incidence of dementia of all types in the Australian population is 1 per 100 (Access Economics, 2005). For the state of NSW an estimate of 1 per 100 with dementia (Access Economics, 2005) would suggest that 67,000 people in NSW have dementia and, if Mesulam's (2001) estimate is anywhere near correct, this would suggest that perhaps 13,000 people have PPA or a kindred disorder. Yet our survey identified only 20 cases referred to the speech pathologist respondents over the 12-month survey period, in addition to the 6 cases referred to the first two authors' speech pathology service in the same period. Even given the possibility of major sampling error in our survey, and grossly inaccurate estimates of dementia incidence and PPA incidence, these figures can only suggest that people with PPA are substantially under-referred for speech pathology services.

There is currently a growing recognition of—and evidence for—the role of the speech pathologist in the treatment of individuals with communication disorders associated with dementias—e.g., Royal College of Speech and Language Therapists (RCSLT), 2005a, 2005b. Nevertheless, it is still the case that in service delivery models where a speech pathologist is not typically a member of the dementia care team, service provision can become somewhat of a "chance" event. The results of this survey indicate there is a need to promote the role of the speech pathologist in working with people with PPA to the relevant referring agencies. Appropriate specialists need to refer every person diagnosed with PPA for speech pathology services.

The question remains as to why our particular speech pathology service experienced a relative surge in referral numbers for PPA, which appears contrary to the experience of similar centres across the state. We can only speculate as to the reasons. One factor may have been that the local area from which referrals originate has a high number of residents from a high socio-economic, tertiary-educated background (Randwick City Council, 2007), a demographic associated with high rates of proactive health consumers (Deloitte Research, 1999) who may have sought speech pathology services even in situations where a referral for speech pathology was not routinely offered. Healthcare providers are advised to expect health consumers to be increasingly proactive as generational change occurs (Brodaty, 2006), so we should be prepared for increasing levels of interest about services for PPA from people with PPA and their carers. A second factor is that over the years the clinic has developed as a centre with some expertise in speech pathology services for communication in aged care, and referrals were made by physicians who had regularly referred to this clinic for speech pathology services.

Management pathways for PPA

The survey revealed that when clients were referred for SLP services, all centres provided assessment services, and most clients were provided with education and treatment (impairment or activity-participation based). Nevertheless, no clear single management pathway emerged and speech pathologists consistently requested further guidance on service provision for this population. It seems unlikely that this need is restricted to the clinicians of New South Wales or Australia. To the best of our knowledge there are no guidelines worldwide for the clinical management of communication in individuals with progressive aphasia. While in the United Kingdom the RCSLT's Clinical Guidelines publication (2005a) covers a huge range of communication disorders and medical conditions that lead to such disorders, it does not specifically mention primary progressive aphasia. In the section devoted to dementia, the guidelines note that "Dementia is not necessarily a global decline in all functions. In the early stages, some areas of cognition may be relatively spared" (p. 89). The fact that language may be the only area of impairment for some years in some "atypical" dementias is not highlighted, nor are specific clinical guidelines recommended for this group.

There is, however, an RCSLT Position Paper on speech and language therapy provision for people with dementia (RCSLT, 2005b, p. 12) that notes the "crucial role" speech pathologists have in assessing language in frontotemporal dementia, progressive aphasia, language presentations of Alzheimer's Disease, and corticobasal degeneration, especially to assist with differential diagnosis. It argues for the need to assess articulation disturbance in various neurodegenerative diseases, to monitor progression and response to pharmacological treatments, and for the potential efficacy of specific communication interventions in semantic dementia. Although this paper does not provide detailed guidelines about interventions for progressive language impairment, the important points it raises about speech pathology services for dementia in general are highly relevant for these clients.

What information is available about specific programmes for these individuals? In the United States, one group is at the forefront of the development of coherent and systematic management pathways for individuals with PPA. Weintraub and colleagues at the Cognitive Neurology and Alzheimer's Disease Centre, Northwestern University, Chicago, have set up a Primary Progressive Aphasia Program (CNADC PPA Program, Cognitive Neurology and Alzheimer's Disease Centre, 2002b). This programme is a 3–4-day multidisciplinary approach to evaluation, diagnosis, and treatment of PPA. It comprises neurological, neuropsychological, language, and social work evaluation. An integral part of this programme is feedback and recommendations from the speech pathologist regarding tools for improving communication and compensating for difficulties (and referral to local therapists when appropriate). The individuals with PPA and their families also receive educational materials regarding PPA in the form of a handbook (Cognitive Neurology and Alzheimer's Disease Centre, 2002a).

The CNADC PPA Program also provides clear recommendations for treatment (Cognitive Neurology and Alzheimer's Disease Centre, 2002c). In particular, they suggest that direct treatment of the language impairment (particularly word retrieval disorders) should be used. Indeed, there is increasing evidence that direct impairment based treatment can benefit people with progressive language disorders (e.g., McNeil, Small, Masterson & Fossett, 1995; Schneider, Thompson & Luring, 1996, and all papers in this special issue of *Aphasiology*). For example, there is evidence that previously "lost" words can be relearned or re-accessed and that treatment can slow the rate of decline for treated items. In addition, the CNADC PPA program (Cognitive Neurology and Alzheimer's Disease Centre, 2002c) advises that treatment focusing on the use of augmentative and alternative communication strategies (such as the use of gesture, drawing, and communication books) should be provided even in early stages. Both impairment- and participation-focused treatments are suggested to be important and appropriate, but a key point is that the relative focus of the treatment provided will change as language declines (for a lengthy discussion see Rogers, King, & Alarcon, 2000). The change in a person's communicative ability over time emphasises the need for regular review and reassessment of the person with PPA in order to ensure that the treatment and advice is appropriate to their needs at all stages of disease progression. From the survey results, in 53% of PPA cases the speech pathologist included regular review as part of the management plan. We would suggest that, for a progressive disorder that not only impacts communication, but also may include dysphagia as a later stage symptom, regular review is a necessary component of the optimal speech pathology management plan for all PPA clients.

Support and education

The structured individual approach used by the CNADC PPA programme seems a good model for best practice. However, like the respondents in our survey, those involved in the CNADC PPA Program also perceived a need for group education and support (personal communication, Darcy Morhardt, 7 December 2005). They therefore developed a three-part education/support series. Each session was half a day in length and began with an hour of educational lectures covering topics of relevance to PPA, such as "Coping with Common Communication and Behavioral Issues", and "Caring for the Caregiver". Following the lectures, the attendees were divided into small support groups facilitated by social workers, psychiatrists, clinical neuropsychologists, and graduate students. These support groups were designed to offer participants an opportunity to discuss the challenges of providing care for an individual with PPA with other families living in similar situations. At the attendees' request, the programme has been followed by monthly support groups. A similar approach to group education and support has been adopted at other tertiary referral hospitals with large clientele with progressive aphasia. For example, the Pick's disease support group based at the National Hospital, London (Harvey et al., 1996; Pick's Disease Support Group, 2007) and the Cambridge Memory Clinic at Addenbrooke's Hospital, Cambridge, UK (Nestor & Hodges, 2001) also provide support groups and newsletter support for people with progressive aphasia and their carers, and there are education and support programmes linked to major hospitals throughout North America under the umbrella of the Association for Frontotemporal Dementias (2007).

The clinical experience of two of us (Taylor and Kingma) strongly suggests that programmes developed for the carer also need to become an important component of interventions for PPA in Australia. It is clear from the literature on communication in various types of dementia that training the carers of individuals with dementia has positive benefits. For example, Ripich, Ziol, Fritsch, and Durand (1999) looked at training the partners of individuals with Alzheimer's disease to be better communicators. Their results suggest that communication partners of persons with Alzheimer's disease can be trained to structure questions that result in more successful communication. Benefits of partner training, both in more successful communication and reduction of anxiety and depression are further supported by qualitative studies (Greene & Monahan, 1989; Shulman & Mandel, 1988). Within the aphasia treatment literature there is also a body of evidence that supports the positive benefits of partner training (Boles & Lewis, 2003; Booth & Swabey, 1999; Hopper, Holland & Rewega, 2002; Kagan, 1998; Kagan, Black, Duchan, Simmons-Mackie, & Square, 2001; Lock et al., 2001).

As the survey had identified a particular need for support and information services for people with PPA and their carers in an Australian context, two of the authors (Taylor and Kingma) developed an education and support training programme. This programme combined elements inspired by the CNADC PPA Program and the literature on the role of training both communicative partners (described above). The initial pilot programme was conducted over three sessions, with involvement by a neurologist and social worker. There was a heavy emphasis on conversation training, as well as information on nature of the disorder, progression, treatment, support, and life-planning issues. The feedback from the attendees was extremely positive, for example the husband of a woman with PPA said, "I feel now I have a better understanding of what I can do to help my wife communicate. There's a lot more I can do." The service aims to run the programme regularly, continuing to refine the education and carer-training components in light of ongoing research on PPA, and on social approaches to aphasia intervention (Byng, Pound, & Parr, 2000).

A further important issue that emerged from the survey was highlighted by respondents' reports that 50% of patients referred were unaware of their diagnosis of PPA at the time of seeing the speech pathologist at initial assessment. There are obvious difficulties in proceeding with education and management when the patient and/or carer are unaware of the diagnosis. This issue has been discussed by McNeil and Duffy (2001, p. 474) who have reported that "the hiatus in the diagnosis can delay aphasia management and general life planning". Although it is not within the scope of this article to discuss this issue in detail, speech pathologists need to consider the impact of delay in formal diagnosis. As with all of the progressive communication or cognitive disorders, life-planning issues will factor strongly. We need to consider when intervention to address these issues should begin.

Conclusions

The survey we report here was modest to say the least. It surveyed centres in one state of Australia, receiving 26 responses describing services for 20 clients with PPA. These limitations notwithstanding, the PPA incidence estimates (see above) would suggest that there are people living in the community with PPA who are not being referred to speech pathology services, even though there is an increasing literature that describes the benefits of intervention for this group (e.g., Croot, Nickels Laurence, & Manning, 2009 this issue). Our survey indicates that steps need to be taken to improve this situation. We would like to see increased referrals to speech pathology services and to promote the role of the speech pathologist on dementia care teams. Increasing awareness of progressive aphasia and related disorders among consultant neurologists and geriatricians, combined with an ageing population and increasingly proactive consumers will contribute to an increased referral rate over time. The preliminary goal of the survey was to stimulate dialogue among speech pathologists in New South Wales regarding service provision for people with PPA. Our aim in reporting the survey in this paper is to propagate that discussion internationally within the speech pathology profession. We hope many speech pathologists will take up the opportunity to explore optimal management and support pathways for individuals with PPA and their carers.

We end with a comment made by one speech pathologist in response to the survey, which encapsulates the issues for the speech pathology profession in its emerging role with people with primary progressive aphasia: "We need more services, more awareness and more information."

REFERENCES

Access Economics. (2005). *Dementia estimates and projections: Australian states and territories.* Access Economics Pty Ltd. for Alzheimer's Australia.

Association for Frontotemporal Dementias. (2007). *The Association for Frontotemporal Dementias: Home.* Retrieved 31 January 2007 from http://www.ftd-picks.org/.

Australian Bureau of Statistics. (2005). *National Regional Profile: New South Wales.* Retrieved on 7 June 2006 from http://www.abs.gov.au/AUSSTATS/abs@.nsf/9fdb8b444ff1e8e2ca25709c0081a8f9/c673c19381c275afca2571cb000ac6eb!OpenDocument.

Boles, L., & Lewis, M. (2003). Working with couples: Solution focused aphasia therapy. *Asia Pacific Journal of Speech, Language and Hearing, 8*(3), 153–159.

Booth, S., & Swabey, D. (1999). Group training in communication skills for carers of adults with aphasia. *International Journal of Language & Communication Disorders, 34*(3), 291–309.

Brodaty, H. (2006). *Dementia in Australia now.* Plenary session address at The Hammond Care Group's 6th Biennial International Dementia Conference, 29/30 June 2006, Sydney, Australia.

Byng, S., Pound, C., & Parr, S. (2000). Living with aphasia: A framework for interventions. In I. Papathanasiou (Ed.), *Acquired neurogenic communication disorders* (pp. 49–75). London: Whurr.

Chapey, R. (Ed.). (2001). *Language intervention strategies in aphasia and related neurogenic communication disorders* (4th ed.). Baltimore, MD: Lippincott Williams & Wilkins.

Cognitive Neurology and Alzheimer's Disease Centre. (2002b). *Primary Progressive Aphasia (PPA) Program.* Retrieved 31 January 2007 from Northwestern University, Cognitive Neurology and Alzheimer's Disease Centre website: www.brain.northwestern.edu/ppa/ppa.html.

Cognitive Neurology and Alzheimer's Disease Centre. (2002a). *PPA handbook: What is primary progressive aphasia?.* Retrieved 31 January 2007 from Northwestern University, Cognitive Neurology and Alzheimer's Disease Centre website: www.brain.northwestern.edu/ppa/handbook.html.

Cognitive Neurology and Alzheimer's Disease Centre. (2002c). *Treatment: Treatment of communication impairments in primary progressive aphasia.* Retrieved 31 January 2007 from Northwestern University, Cognitive Neurology and Alzheimer's Disease Centre website: http://www.brain.northwestern.edu/ppa/treatment.html.

Croot, K. (2009). Progressive language impairments: Definitions, diagnoses, and prognoses. *Aphasiology, 22,* 302–326.

Croot, K., Nickels, L., Laurence, F., & Manning, M. (2009). Impairment- and activity/participation-directed interventions in progressive language impairment: Clinical and theoretical issues. *Aphasiology, 22,* 125–160.

Deloitte Research. (1999). *The emergence of the E-health consumer.* Retrieved 30 January 2007 from http://lc.etfbl.net/learningcubes/news/documents/Emergence_of_eHealth_Consumer.pdf.

di Carlo, A., Baldereschi, M., Inzitari, D., & Amaducci, L. (1999). Dementias, the dimension of the problem: Epidemiology notes. In S. Govoni, C. L. Bolis, & M. Trabucchi (Eds.), *Dementias: Biological bases and clinical approach to treatment* (pp. 1–18). Milano: Springer-Verlag Italia.

Duffy, J. R. (1987). Slowly progressive aphasia. *Clinical Aphasiology, 16,* 349–356.

Duffy, J. R., & Petersen, R. C. (1992). Primary progressive aphasia. *Aphasiology, 6*(1), 1–15.

Greene, V. L., & Monahan, D. J. (1989). The effect of a support and education program on stress and burden among family caregivers to frail elderly persons. *The Gerontologist, 29,* 472–480.

Harvey, R. J., Roques, P., Fox, N. C., & Rossor, M. N. (1996). Non-Alzheimer dementias in young patients. *British Journal of Psychiatry, 168*(3), 384–385.

Henderson, A. S., & Jorm, A. F. (1998). *Dementia in Australia (Aged and Community Care Service Development and Evaluation Report no 35).* Canberra: Australian Government Publishing Service.

Hopper, T., Holland, A., & Rewega, M. (2002). Conversational coaching: Treatment outcomes and future directions. *Aphasiology, 16,* 745–762.

Kagan, A. (1998). Supported conversation for adults with aphasia: Methods and resources for training conversation partners. *Aphasiology, 12*(9), 816–830.

Kagan, A., Black, S. E., Duchan, J. F., Simmons-Mackie, N., & Square, P. (2001). Training volunteers as conversation partners using "Supported Conversation for Adults with Aphasia" (SCA): A controlled trial. *Journal of Speech, Language, and Hearing Research, 44*(3), 624 638.

Lock, S., Wilkinson, R., Bryan, K., Maxim, J., Edmundson, A., & Bruce, C. et al. (2001). Supporting Partners of People with Aphasia in Relationships and Conversation (SPPARC). *International Journal of Language & Communication Disorders, 36*(Suppl), 25–30.

McNeil, M. R., & Duffy, J. R. (2001). Primary progressive aphasia. In R. Chapey (Ed.), *Language intervention strategies in aphasia and related neurogenic communication disorders* (4th ed., pp. 472–486). Baltimore, MD: Lippincott Williams & Wilkins.

McNeil, M. R., Small, S. L., Masterson, R. J., & Fossett, T. R. D. (1995). Behavioral and pharmacological treatment of lexical-semantic deficits in a single patient with primary progressive aphasia. *American Journal of Speech-Language Pathology, 4,* 76–87.

Mesulam, M. M. (1982). Slowly progressive aphasia without dementia. *Annals of Neurology, 11,* 592–598.

Mesulam, M. M. (2001). Primary progressive aphasia. *Annals of Neurology, 49,* 425–432.

Mesulam, M. M. (2003). Current concepts: Primary progressive aphasia – a language-based dementia. *The New England Journal of Medicine, 349*(16), 1535–1542.

Mesulam, M-M., & Weintraub, S. (1992). Spectrum of primary progressive aphasia. *Bailliere's Clinical Neurology: International Practice and Research, 1*(3), 583–609.

Nestor, P., & Hodges, J. R. (2001). The clinical approach to assessing patients with early-onset dementia. In J. R. Hodges (Ed.), *Early-onset dementia: A multidisciplinary approach* (pp. 23–46). Oxford, UK: Oxford University Press.

Pick's Disease Support Group. (2007). *The Pick's Disease Support Group: Welcome.* Retrieved 31 January 2007 from http://www.pdsg.org.uk/.

Randwick City Council. (2007). *Demographic profile: Education, Employment and income.* Retrieved 30th January 2007 from http://www.randwick.nsw.gov.au/default.php?id=18.

Ripich, D. N., Ziol, E., Fritsch, T., & Durand, E. J. (1999). Training Alzheimer's disease caregivers for successful communication. *Clinical Gerontologist, 21,* 37–56.

Rogers, M. A., & Alarcon, N. B. (1999). Characteristics and management of primary progressive aphasia. *ASHA Special Interest Division Neurophysiology and Neurogenic Speech and Language Disorders, 9*(4), 12–26.

Rogers, M. A., King, J. M., & Alarcon, N. B. (2000). Proactive management of primary progressive aphasia. In D. R. Beukelman, K. Yorkston, & J. Reichle (Eds.), *Augmentative communication for adults with neurogenic and neuromuscular disabilities* (pp. 305–337). Baltimore, MD: Brookes.

Royal College of Speech Language Therapists. (RCSLT). (2005a). *Clinical guidelines.* Oxford, UK: Speechmark.

Royal College of Speech and Language Therapists. (2005b). *Position paper: Speech and language therapy provision for people with dementia.* Retrieved 25 January 2007, from www.rcslt.org/resources/publications/dementia_paper.pdf.

Schneider, S. L., Thompson, C. K., & Luring, B. (1996). Effects of verbal plus gestural matrix training on sentence production in a patient with primary progressive aphasia. *Aphasiology, 10*(3), 297–317.

Schwartz, M. F., Marin, O. S. M., & Saffran, E. M. (1979). Dissociations of language functions in dementia: A case study. *Brain and Language, 7,* 277–306.

Shulman, M. D., & Mandel, E. (1988). Communication training of relatives and friends of institutionalized elderly persons. *The Gerontologist, 28,* 797–799.

Warrington, E. K. (1975). Selective impairment of semantic memory. *Quarterly Journal of Experimental Psychology, 27,* 635–657.

Weintraub, S., Rubin, N. P., & Mesulam, M. M. (1990). Primary progressive aphasia: Longitudinal course, neurological profile, and language features. *Archives of Neurology, 47*(12), 1329–1335.

Westbury, C., & Bub, D. (1997). Primary progressive aphasia: A review of 112 cases. *Brain and Language, 60*(3), 381–406.

APPENDIX: SURVEY QUESTIONS

1. What type of facility do you work in (e.g., acute hospital, community health team, rehab centre, etc.)?
2. What region of NSW do you work in (area health service or geographical location)?
3. Were you referred a client with confirmed or queried primary progressive aphasia in last year (June 30 2004 – July 1 2005)?
4. If so, how many clients, in this period?
5. How many females?   males?
6. Who referred the clients to the speech pathology service? (tick a box)

The tables accompanying the next four questions allow for responses regarding up to ten clients. If you are able to provide information on more than this number please record the extra data in a similar manner on the back of the questionnaire.

Referral source	Client 1	Client 2	Client 3	Client 4	Client 5	Client 6	Client 7	Client 8	Client 9	Client 10
Local medical officer										
Geriatrician										
Neurologist										
Other medical specialist										
Community nurse										
Other speech pathology service										
Other allied health professional										
Carer										
Self-referred										
Other										

7. Do you consider your clinical findings were used, by the specialist, to confirm or discard a diagnosis of PPA? How many cases did this apply to? *(Please give answer as a percentage)*

8. Was the patient made aware, by their medical officer, of their diagnosis of primary progressive aphasia?

	Client 1	Client 2	Client 3	Client 4	Client 5	Client 6	Client 7	Client 8	Client 9	Client 10
Yes										
No										

8b. If the clients was not made aware of the diagnosis, what other terms / labels were used by the medical officer to describe the condition?

9. Was the primary carer made aware, by the medical officer, of the diagnosis of primary progressive aphasia?

	Client 1	Client 2	Client 3	Client 4	Client 5	Client 6	Client 7	Client 8	Client 9	Client 10
Yes										
No										

10. What speech pathology service did you provide?

	Client 1	Client 2	Client 3	Client 4	Client 5	Client 6	Client 7	Client 8	Client 9	Client 10
Assessment Was this case referred to you as a queried (Q) or confirmed(C) case of PPA										
Individual Treatment (< 5 sessions)										
Individual Treatment (> 5 sessions)										
Group treatment session (< 5 sessions)										
Group treatment session (> 5 sessions)										
Review (< 5 sessions)										
Review (> 5 sessions)										
Education to patient										
Education to carer										
Referral to other speech pathology service										
Referral to other service										

11. If you have provided intervention to clients with PPA, could you please describe the types of intervention that were provided? (e.g., naming therapy, life books, AAC, conversation groups, etc.)

12. Do you refer PPA clients to stroke support groups or post-stroke aphasia groups?
13. Can you comment on appropriate existing support groups for patients with PPA and their carers, in your area?
14. Would you like to make any other comments about speech pathology service delivery to clients with PPA and their carers?

APHASIOLOGY, 2009, 23 (2), 175–191

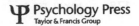

Relearning lost vocabulary in nonfluent progressive aphasia with MossTalk Words®

R. Jokel

University of Toronto, and Kunin-Lunenfeld Applied Research Unit, Toronto, Canada

J. Cupit

University of Toronto, Canada

E. Rochon

University of Toronto, and Toronto Rehabilitation Institute, Canada

C. Leonard

University of Toronto, and University of Ottawa, Canada

Background: The literature on aphasia has been growing rapidly, with reports of different therapeutic approaches for a post-stroke anomia. While individuals with post-stroke anomia frequently recover to some extent, the other end of the aphasia recovery continuum is occupied by those who experience relentless language dissolution as a result of progressive disorders such as primary progressive aphasia. One of the most recent additions to the field of aphasia rehabilitation is therapy whereby either part of or the entire therapy is administered via computer-based programmes. There have been few treatment studies investigating the rehabilitation of language abilities in people with primary progressive aphasia (PPA).

Aims: The objectives of this investigation were to examine the ability of PPA individuals to relearn lost words and to determine the extent of benefits derived from MossTalk Words®, a computer-based treatment for anomia.

Methods and Procedures: Using a multiple baseline across behaviours design, we explored treatment-specific effects, maintenance, and generalisation of improvements derived from this therapy programme. Two participants with nonfluent PPA were treated, each on three lists of words for which low and stable baselines were first established. Sessions occurred two to three times a week. Treatment involved the presentation of a picture on the computer screen, with the participants being required to name it. Success in treatment was measured by probing list naming every second session. Once a participant attained 80% accuracy over two consecutive probes, or participated in 12 sessions (whichever occurred first), treatment of a list was terminated and the next

Address correspondence to: Elizabeth Rochon, Department of Speech-Language Pathology, Rehabilitation Sciences Building, Room 160, University of Toronto, 500 University Ave., Toronto, Ontario, Canada M5G 1V7. E-mail: elizabeth.rochon@utoronto.ca

We are indebted to both participants for their cooperation and tenacity, and to our talented research assistants Eleanor Arabia and Lyndsay White. We also thank Ruth Fink for making the MossTalk Words® available to us. This study was supported by a CIHR IA Fellowship to R. Jokel, and a CIHR Doctoral Award to J. Cupit. The authors acknowledge the support of the Toronto Rehabilitation Institute, which receives funding under the Provincial Rehabilitation Research Program from the Ministry of Health and Long Term Care in Ontario, Canada.

http://www.psypress.com/aphasiology   DOI: 10.1080/02687030801943005

list was started. Each participant was tested on all items immediately after therapy, and again 1 month later.

Outcomes and Results: Both participants improved their naming skills with the MossTalk Words®. P1 required only four sessions to reach the proposed criterion of 80% (up to 100%) correct on each list. The effects of treatment were maintained immediately and, to a lesser degree, 4 weeks later. P2 required all 12 sessions for each of the three lists. Results were variable immediately after testing, but seemingly maintained 4 weeks later.

Conclusions: The results demonstrate that both participants with primary progressive aphasia benefited (although to a different extent) from a computer-based treatment for anomia. These results are encouraging and suggest that such a treatment may be a viable therapy approach for patients who suffer from PPA in the absence of a generalised cognitive impairment.

Keywords: Language therapy; Non-fluent progressive aphasia; Anomia; Computer-based therapy.

ANOMIA IN NONFLUENT PROGRESSIVE APHASIA

Aphasia is the inability to produce and/or understand language. Whereas most cases of aphasia occur as a result of a stroke (Gagnon, Schwartz, Martin, Dell, & Saffran, 1997; Nickels & Howard, 1995; Schwartz, Saffran, Bloch, & Dell, 1994), there are some conditions in which aphasia is seen as a manifestation of neurodegenerative changes in the fronto-temporal lobes of the brain (Mesulam, 1982; Mesulam & Weintraub, 1992; Rogers & Alarcon, 1998). Two types of progressive aphasia have been identified: the fluent variant known as semantic dementia (SD: Hodges, Patterson, Oxbury, & Funnell, 1992; Snowden, Goulding, & Neary, 1989) and the nonfluent variant referred to as nonfluent progressive aphasia (NPA: Croot, Patterson, & Hodges, 1998, 1999). NPA is characterised by dissolution of phonology and syntax, in the absence of cognitive and semantic deficits at the time of onset (Mesulam, 1982; Rogers & Alarcon, 1998; Thompson, Ballard, Tait, Weintraub & Mesulam, 1997). Deficits in reading (surface dyslexia) and writing (surface dysgraphia), in addition to predominantly phonological (formal) errors, are also seen in NPA (Mesulam & Weintraub, 1992; Watt, Jokel, & Behrmann, 1997).

A dominant symptom of aphasia is often anomia; a difficulty in naming or producing words. The language rehabilitation literature presents an abundance of studies on anomia therapy after stroke (e.g., Boyle, 2004; Ellis, 1985; Greenwald, Raymer, Richardson, & Rothi, 1995; Kiran & Thompson, 2003; Nickels & Best, 1996a; 1996b; and Nickels' review, 2002), but there are only a handful of reports on a structured approach to re-teaching lost vocabulary in progressive language disorders.

Recently some single case studies of relearning words or of treatment for naming deficits for individuals with SD have appeared in the literature. For instance, Frattali (2003) successfully utilised an errorless learning approach to re-teach words to an individual who showed between-class (verbs better than nouns) and within-class (living better than non-living things, biological motion better than tool motion verbs) dissociation due to SD. She concluded that the approach she used might be a useful technique for other individuals with progressive aphasia. Graham and colleagues (Graham, Patterson, Pratt, & Hodges, 1999, 2001) investigated the benefit of repeated home practice on the naming abilities of DM, an anomic individual with SD. DM kept notebooks containing lists of written words for practicing categorised words that he had difficulty retrieving spontaneously. Repeated practice led to better word retrieval for practised words than for words that were not practised. DM's performance declined when practice was stopped. Graham et al. (2001) compared the performance of DM (Graham et al., 1999) with that of another individual (AM) with SD, who practised naming words grouped alphabetically. The authors found that, unlike DM, AM did not benefit from repeated practice (Graham & Hodges, 1997). It was suggested that such factors as a difference in the severity of the naming impairment and the extent of semantic loss may have been responsible for the lack of gains found with AM as compared to DM.

Using a repeated exposure paradigm, Snowden and Neary (2002) demonstrated the importance of retained semantic knowledge for the relearning of words in KB, an individual with SD. In a second individual, CR, the same authors demonstrated the importance of personal "meaningfulness" on the individual's ability to recall defining information of names she had practised.

We (Jokel, Rochon & Leonard, 2006) designed a treatment approach for AK, a woman with SD who was able to relearn an impressive number of self-selected words via home practice. Paired with picture stimuli, AK used orthographic, phonological, and semantic information to facilitate the learning process. Effects of practice did not generalise to untrained items, but they were maintained 1 month and, to some extent, 6 months post treatment.

Reports of treatment for anomia in NPA are equally scarce. McNeil, Small, Masterson, and Fossett (1995) used a combination of pharmacological (dextramphetamine) and behavioural approaches in an individual with NPA. The behavioural approach consisted of hierarchical cueing of adjectives, contrasting synonyms and antonyms. The language intervention had a limited effect, while the pharmacological treatment appeared to be completely ineffective. Schneider, Thompson, and Luring (1996) trained the acquisition of past and future verb tenses in a woman with a 2½-year history of NPA. The treatment involved modelling production of target sentences with a target verb (e.g., *kiss*) supported with gestures. The treatment was found to be effective and some generalisation to untreated verbs occurred.

In addition to these impairment-focused studies, a more functional approach was described by Cress and King (1999). They present the cases of two individuals with NPA where an augmentative and alternative communication intervention was implemented. Upon completion of a communication needs assessment, their two participants were equipped with communication boards or books, and received training in the use of gestures. With the assistance of facilitators, both participants learned to use these alternative means of communication and became generators of their own gestures.

As is obvious from the above review, there is a clear need for continued investigation of the feasibility and effectiveness of treatment for naming deficits in individuals with progressive aphasia, with the goals of slowing the progression of lexical decline and/or maintaining current vocabulary.

COMPUTER-BASED TREATMENT STUDIES

For almost two decades computer-based therapies have been available as treatment options for language disorders. They have been administered under different regimes, such as with full guidance of clinicians, by the individuals themselves at home after a training period, or as a combination of the two. There is some evidence that individuals with chronic aphasia benefit from the computer-based approach and show some maintenance and generalisation of treatment gains (e.g., Deloche, Dordain, & Kremin 1993; cf. Van Mourik & Van de Sandt-Koenderman, 1992).

One of the first computer-based interventions for aphasia was introduced by Bruce and Howard (1987) in the form of self-generated cues via letter-to-sound conversions. All five individuals involved in the study responded well to both the initial letter and initial sound cues, with one individual no longer requiring cueing at the end of therapy. Improvements were observed for both the treated items and the untreated items. Best, Howard, Bruce, and Gatehouse (1997) used the same procedure for a person with a severe word retrieval impairment who improved after 5 weeks of therapy and maintained gains for an impressive 15-month period. Unlike many therapies reported in the literature, the treatment effect generalised to untreated items and spontaneous speech.

While clinician-supervised treatments have shown benefits for people with language disorders, so too have self-guided programmes. For instance, Pedersen, Vinter, and Olson (2001) demonstrated positive results for written naming when individuals were able to select from semantic, phonological, and written cues. Interestingly, Laganaro, Di Pietro, and Schnider (2003) demonstrated that participants in the outpatient phase of treatment benefited to a greater extent than those in the acute phase of their illness.

More recently, some therapy programmes have become Internet-based. Egan, Worrall, and Oxenham (2004) introduced such a treatment to 20 people with aphasia. The goal of the study was to facilitate Internet access for individuals with aphasia. At the end, all participants reported improved Internet skills. A more language-focused programme was designed by Mortley, Wade, and Enderby (2004) who addressed word retrieval monitored remotely with minimal input from clinicians. Seven people with word-finding problems resulting from post-stroke aphasia participated in two treatment sessions using StepByStep© a software developed specifically for the study. The therapy programme comprised semantic association, naming, reading, spelling, and spoken and written word–picture matching tasks. All of the participants improved on object and action naming post-treatment. Three individuals showed some generalisation to untreated items. Maintenance effects were seen in some individuals 6 weeks after completion of the study. The value/benefit of this treatment programme may be measured in both language-related improvements as well as clinician efficiency in the sense that no face-to-face intervention was required by the clinician.

Doesborgh et al. (2004) investigated the effects of a newly developed program called Multicue© on naming and verbal communication in 18 individuals with aphasia. Participants were randomly assigned to treatment or no-treatment groups. Those in the treatment group guided themselves through the most effective cues. Only those who were treated with the Multicue© program improved their naming, but the mean improvement failed to reach significance and there was no maintenance or generalisation.

MOSSTALK WORDS®

Description of the program

Another new computer-based therapy is MossTalk Words®, a program for individuals with receptive and expressive language impairments (Fink, Brecher,

Montgomery, & Schwartz, 2001; Fink, Brecher, Schwartz, & Robey 2002a; Fink, Brecher, Sobel, & Schwartz, 2005; Fink, Lowery, & Sobel 2002b). The system comprises a large array of words with corresponding pictures and cues (both spoken and written). There are three modules in the program: (1) Core-Vocabulary module: designed for individuals with severe anomia containing high-frequency items in a set of matching and naming exercises; (2) Multiple-Choice Matching module: with both naming and comprehension tasks in written and oral input; and (3) Cued Naming module: utilising a cueing hierarchy to facilitate single word production. Users can access either pre-programmed exercises or prepare custom-made tasks tailored to the needs of individual participants. A more detailed description of the program can be found in the above listed publications by Fink and her colleagues and on the Internet under *www.mosstalk.com*.

Treatment studies utilising MossTalk Words®

Fink et al. (2002a) tested their new software on six participants with a phonologically based naming disorder. Three participants with chronic aphasia received three sessions per week with a clinician guiding them through all of the steps of the Cued Naming module with multiple auditory and visual cues. The three remaining participants took part in a partially self-guided treatment, which included one clinician-guided session followed by two self-directed sessions per week. Individuals were trained for a maximum of 4 weeks on a 20-item list. The results showed that although there were item-specific gains in each condition for two out of three participants in each group, the acquisition and maintenance effects were greater for individuals in the clinician-guided group. For two individuals the benefits of treatment generalised to other untrained words and other production tasks. This study served to show that the treatment was effective and that it could be accomplished independently of a clinician's involvement. In addition, one of the individuals trained in this study showed subsequent gains in verb and sentence production in another study (Fink et al., 2002b). Other investigators have addressed questions of treatment effectiveness and intensity using MossTalk Words®.

Ramsberger and Basem (2005) treated four participants on two 40-word lists with both phonological and semantic spoken and/or written cues from the Cued Naming module. In Phase 1 they were randomly assigned to receive 20 sessions of treatment in either intense (5 sessions/week) or a non-intense (2 sessions/week) programme. In Phase 2 they received the same treatment with the alternate intensity. There was strong evidence for improvement regardless of treatment intensity. However, greater intensity was associated with better maintenance of gains when the treatment was removed. No generalisation to untreated items was observed in any of the four participants. Interestingly, all individuals found the non-intensive treatment more enjoyable.

Raymer, Kohen, and Saffell (2006) administered another MossTalk Words® module, Multi-Mode Matching Exercises, to five people with aphasia in two treatment schedules (1–2 times per week and 3–4 times per week). Two individuals worked on word comprehension skills and the other three worked on phonologically based naming tasks. They used spoken and written word–picture matching exercises paired with spoken production. All five participants improved in picture naming with the greater intensity of treatment but only two out of five improved with the lesser intensity schedule. Some generalisation to untreated items took place but naming of the lists was back to baseline at 1-month post treatment, regardless of the treatment intensity.

In summary, computer-based therapies appear to hold promise for the treatment of aphasia both in terms of their effectiveness in promoting treatment gains and in the flexibility of administration that they afford. The studies that have employed MossTalk Words® as a treatment programme for anomia have shown very good to excellent gains and, less frequently, some maintenance of those gains and/or generalisation to other stimuli. Thus far, only individuals recovering from a post-stroke aphasia have been targeted. In our study we chose to use MossTalk Words® to treat anomia in participants with nonfluent progressive aphasia.

THE PRESENT STUDY

In this study we investigated treatment-specific effects, maintenance, and generalisation of improvements using MossTalk Words® (Fink et al., 2001) with two individuals diagnosed with NPA. With our investigation we hoped to examine the effectiveness and feasibility of providing anomia treatment to individuals with this disorder, as well as to add to the growing body of evidence on the effectiveness of the MossTalk Words® program. Based on Fink et al.'s (2005) summary of findings from various studies utilising MossTalk Words® we judged individuals with non-fluent progressive aphasia to be good candidates for this treatment programme. Importantly, Fink et al. (2002a) successfully treated individuals with a phonologically based anomia in their study, and the naming impairments of patients with NPA are typically phonologically based (Watt et al., 1997). Fink et al. (2005) note that home practice with occasional clinician guidance and volunteer support has been found to be a cost-effective way of delivering therapy with MossTalk Words®. As we were introducing the program to a new population, namely individuals with NPA, and since findings from Fink et al. (2002a) seemed more robust in the clinician-guided condition, we chose to administer clinician-guided treatment in the clinic. Based on the supporting evidence from the literature on the effectiveness of cueing (e.g., Drew & Thompson, 1999; Wambaugh et al., 2001) we selected the Cued Naming module for our participants. In particular, we constructed a cueing hierarchy consisting of written initial letter, written whole word cues, and repetition (when necessary) based on the evidence that orthographic cues (Basso, Marangolo, Piras, & Galluzzi, 2001) and a combination of orthographic and phonological cues (e.g., Best, Herbert, Hickin, Osborne, & Howard, 2002; Drew & Thompson, 1999; Hickin, Best, Herbert, Howard, & Osborne, 2002; Jokel & Rochon, 1996; Kiran, Thompson, & Hashimoto, 2001) can be used successfully to treat (phonologically based) naming disorders.

Based on the available literature to date, we expected to see improvements in treatment with possible maintenance and generalisation to untreated items.

METHOD

Design

Examination of the effects of the therapy proceeded using a single-subject multiple baseline across behaviours design. The key advantage to this design is that it allows one to examine change and variability within an individual while effecting good experimental control (e.g., McReynolds & Kearns, 1983; Millard, 1998).

Participants

Two participants diagnosed with NPA were recruited for this study. The presence of a naming impairment was documented by their performance on the *Philadelphia Naming Test* (Roach, Schwartz, Martin, Grewal, & Brecher, 1996). Temporal atrophy in the left hemisphere was revealed in neuroimaging reports. Neither of the participants had a history of drug or alcohol abuse, a history of major psychiatric illness, and/or other neurological illness. Both participants were right-handed native speakers of English. Both had intact visual perception as measured by the minimal feature match subtest of the *Birmingham Object Recognition Battery* (Riddoch & Humphreys, 1993), and adequate single word reading abilities as measured by the single word reading subtest of the *Psycholinguistic Assessments of Language Processing in Aphasia (PALPA*; Kay, Lesser, & Coltheart, 1992). With the exception of age, they were well matched on all measures administered prior to the study (see Table 1).

Case presentation

At the beginning of the study, in May 2005, P1 was a 58-year-old retired teacher. She reported experiencing progressive difficulties in word retrieval and maths for 3–4 years. She had become less organised and did not read as much as before, which was out of keeping with her life-long habits and interests. Working for many years as a teacher-librarian she always had great facility with language and was able to verbally direct students to the correct shelf in search of a particular book. More recently, while still working, she noticed that more and more frequently she had to retrieve books herself, because she was no longer capable of describing their location to the students. On her neurologist's advice, P1 began taking Reminyl (cognitive enhancer) in 2003. She underwent several neuroimaging studies, the most recent of which was a SPECT scan that showed abnormality in the left temporal lobe. During this study P1 continued to live independently, and in her free time frequented the gym, and enjoyed going to movies and the theatre.

P2 was a 75-year-old retired pharmacist. Her presenting complaints included a mild memory impairment (for words) and depression. A SPECT scan of the brain carried out at the time of her initial referral in early 2005 showed mild hypoperfusion bilaterally in the temporal lobes, which was interpreted by the radiologist as a non-significant finding. At the time of the study P2 was taking a number of medications including an antidepressant (Celexa), and a cognitive enhancer (Aricept). She came to all sessions unaccompanied and followed her daily routines and hobbies. She continued to sing with a local choir. At the beginning of therapy, she lived alone in her own home. Towards the end of therapy she moved to an assisted-living accommodation on her family's insistence after a recent fall that had led to hospitalisation.

Table 1 reflects the language profile of each participant. The results of all pre-therapy tests allowed for a characterisation of the type and the level of severity of the language impairment and ensured that each participant was able to read and repeat single words. Their ability to follow visual cues on a computer screen was tested with practice items from the MossTalk Words® program. Both P1 and P2 appeared to have relatively spared comprehension in the face of prominent naming deficits. Their

TABLE 1
Results of pre-experimental language testing for P1 and P2

TASK (TEST)	P1	P2
Verbal Expression		
Spontaneous Speech	Slow & anomic	Hesitant & anomic
Picture Description (BDAE)	Slow, uncertain	Slow, uncertain
Confrontation Naming (BNT, $N = 60$)	43%	48%
Responsive Naming (BDAE, $N = 20$)	85%	100%
Repetition of Words (BDAE, $N = 10$)	90%	80%
Repetition of Sentences (BDAE, $N = 10$)	70%	100%
Auditory Comprehension		
Word Comprehension (PPVT, $N = 204$)	66th percentile	66th percentile
Following commands (BDAE, $N = 15$)	87%	90%
Sentence Comprehension (TROG, $N = 20$)	47th percentile	47th percentile
Paragraphs (BDAE, $N = 4$)	87%	100%
Reading		
Regular word reading (PALPA, $N = 20$)	100%	100%
Irregular word reading (PALPA, $N = 20$)	93%	93%
Paragraph reading ("Grandfather")	Slow but accurate	Accurate
Sentence Comprehension (BDAE, $N = 10$)	100%	100%
Spelling		
Regular words (PALPA, $N = 20$)	100%	90%
Irregular words (PALPA, $N = 20$)	80%	85%
Semantic Knowledge		
High Imageability Words (PALPA 51)	13/15, ($M = 13.43$, $SD = 1.26$)	12/15
Low Imageability Words (PALPA 51)	15/15, ($M = 12.25$, $SD = 1.86$)	12/15
Visual Lexical Decision (PALPA 25)	100%	97%
Visual Lexical Decision (PALPA 27)	100%	93%
Access to sem. from pictures (PPTT, $N = 52$)	98%	96%
Cognitive Screening		
Orientation	Intact	Intact
Memory (story retell – ABCD, $N = 17$)	14 imm., 14 del. (N)	11 imm., 10 del. (N)
Semantic Fluency (Animal names)	< 10th percentile	< 10th percentile
Phonemic Fluency (FAS)	< 10th percentile	< 10th percentile
Other		
Motor Speech Exam	Normal	Normal
Visual object matching (BORB, $N = 25$)	100%	96%

Sem. = semantic, imm. = immediate recall, del. = delayed recall, BDAE = Boston Diagnostic Aphasia Examination (Goodglass, Kaplan, & Barresi, 2001), BNT = Boston Naming Test (Goodglass et al., 2001), PALPA = Psycholinguistic Assessments of Language Processing in Aphasia (Kay et al., 1992), PPTT = Pyramids and Palm Trees Test (Howard & Patterson, 1992); PNT = Philadelphia naming Test (Roach et al., 1996), PPVT = Peabody Picture Vocabulary Test (Dunn & Dunn, 1997), TROG = Test for the Reception of Grammar-2 (Bishop, 2003), ABCD = Arizona Battery for Communication in Dementia Bayles & Tomoeda, 1997), BORB = Birmingham Object Recognition Battery (Riddoch & Humphreys, 1993).

semantic knowledge accessed verbally and nonverbally appeared to be intact. Their difficulties appeared to be in retrieving the phonological representations of words that were otherwise well understood in the auditory and written modalities.

Procedure

To obtain a list of words to be treated and ensure a stable baseline, participants were first shown all pictures available from the MossTalk Words® software package

($n = 420$) and asked to name them in three consecutive sessions. No cueing or feedback was provided. Responses were scored as correct only if the target word was produced completely accurately. Of the words that were in error in *each* session, three lists of words to be treated were constructed for each participant. For P1, this resulted in three lists of 14 items each. For P2, this resulted in two lists of 15 items each and one of 14 items. The three lists were equated as much as possible by frequency, length, and semantic category. They comprised words that were deemed useful by the two participants in their daily life (e.g., toast, robe, computer, hamburger). In addition, items that the participants knew well and could name consistently were added to each treatment list such that the resulting number of items in each treatment list was 20.

Clinician-supervised sessions lasting approximately 1 hour occurred three times a week for P1 and twice a week for P2 due to scheduling availability. Regularly scheduled probe testing of the three lists occurred. During probe testing, no cues were provided. The treated list was probed every two sessions and the untreated lists were probed every three sessions. The general treatment schedule for both participants was as follows. First, after having established a stable baseline of zero percent correct over three consecutive sessions, treatment of List 1 words began. The criterion for moving to treatment on a subsequent list was 80% correct over two consecutive probes or a maximum of 12 sessions (whichever occurred first). Once treatment on a new list was initiated, accuracy of response to previously treated items was probed every three sessions in order to examine maintenance effects. Training of treated items followed the procedure outlined in the manual of the MossTalk Words® program. The Cued Naming module with written initial letter and written whole word cues was used. Pictures were randomly presented on a screen and no corrective feedback was provided. When the participant failed to name the picture an initial letter cue was provided. If the participant still did not produce a response, the whole word cue was presented. If the participant was still unable to say the word, the clinician produced a model that the participant was to repeat. In all trials the participant was required to repeat the word after all the cues had been provided. Regardless of the patient's success in naming the picture, both cues were provided for each item. The effects of therapy were established if treated items improved during treatment while items on the untreated lists remained at baseline. The execution of the entire program was fully supervised and administered by a clinician and/or student clinician.

Generalisation of treatment gains to untrained stimuli was measured using the Philadelphia Naming Test (PNT, Roach et al., 1996). Generalisation of treatment effects to sentence production was measured using a task designed by Caplan and Hanna (1998). This task requires production of a grammatically correct sentence describing a picture, after the verb has been given and the sentence's desired structure (e.g., passive vs. active) has been indicated with arrows pointing to appropriate components of the picture. Post testing occurred immediately after completion of treatment of List 3, and maintenance effects were tested 1 month and 6 months after the completion of treatment.

RESULTS

Figure 1 shows the results of probe testing for P1. A visual analysis of the data clearly demonstrates the impact of the therapy on naming performance. P1 required

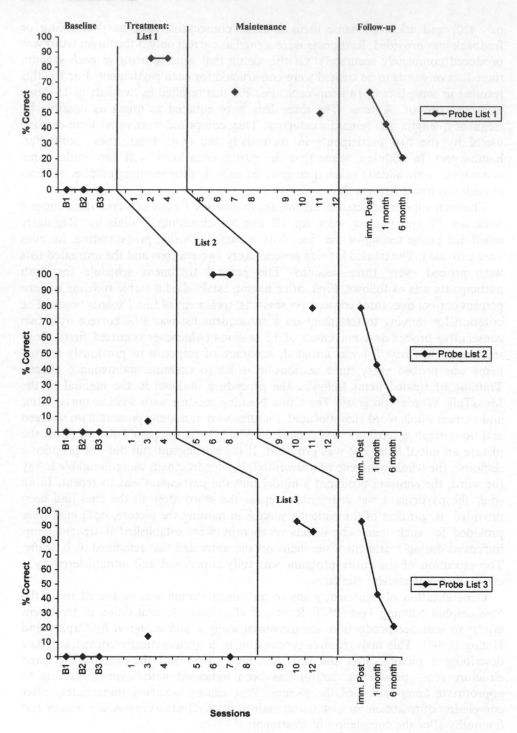

Figure 1. Results of treatment and maintenance for P1.

only four sessions to reach the criterion of 80% correct on two consecutive sessions (up to 100%) for each list. Good experimental control was evidenced by the fact that naming accuracy on untreated lists remained between 0–14% correct at all times. In

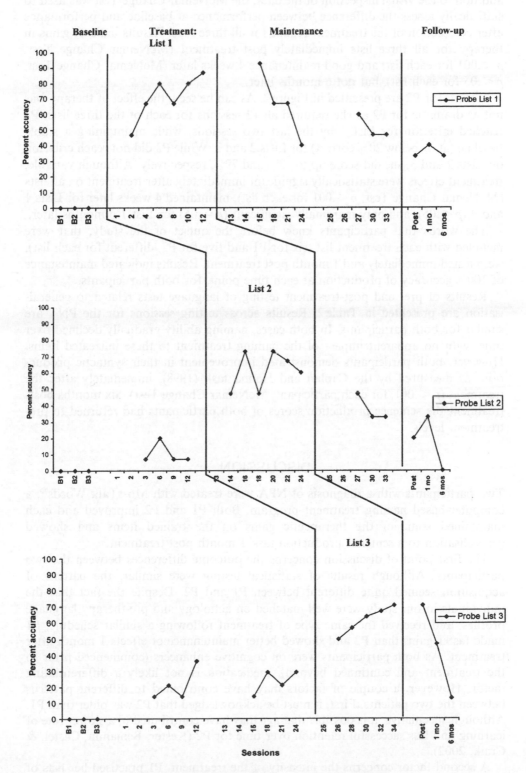

Figure 2. Results of treatment and maintenance for P2.

addition to the visual inspection of the data, the McNemar Change Test was used to statistically assess the difference between performance at baseline and performance after completion of the treatment regime for all three lists. Results indicate gains in therapy for all three lists immediately post treatment (McNemar Change Test, $p < .001$ for each list) and good maintenance 4 weeks later (McNemar Change Test, $p < .05$ for each list), but not 6 months later.

Results for P2 are presented in Figure 2. As can be seen, the effect of therapy was not as dramatic for P2 as she required all 12 sessions for each of the three lists. P2 reached criterion for List 1 by the last two sessions, while maintaining a stable baseline (at or below 20% correct) for Lists 2 and 3. While P2 did not reach criterion on Lists 2 and 3, she did score up to 73% and 79%, respectively. Although variable, treatment effects were statistically significant immediately after treatment on all lists (McNemar Change Test, $p < .001$ for each list), maintained 4 weeks later for Lists 1 and 3 ($p < .05$), and only marginally significant ($p = .06$) for List 1 6 months later.

The words that participants knew before the outset of the study, that were included with each treatment list (six for P1 and five for P2, different for each list), were tested immediately and 1 month post treatment. Results indicated maintenance of 100% accuracy of production at each time point, for both participants.

Results of pre- and post-treatment testing of language tests related to generalisation are presented in Table 2. Results across testing sessions for the PNT are similar for both participants. In both cases, naming ability gradually declined over time, with no apparent impact of the naming treatment to these untreated items. However, both participants demonstrated improvement in their syntactic production, as measured by the Caplan and Hanna task (1998), immediately after the treatment ($p < .001$, for each participant, McNemar Change Test). Six months posttreatment the sentence production scores of both participants had returned to pretreatment levels.

DISCUSSION

Two participants with a diagnosis of NPA were treated with MossTalk Words®, a computer-based naming treatment program. Both P1 and P2 improved and each maintained some of the therapeutic gains on the trained items and showed generalisation to a sentence production task 1 month post treatment.

The first point of discussion concerns the outcome differences between the two participants. Although results of statistical testing were similar, the pattern of acquisition seemed quite different between P1 and P2. Despite the fact that the individuals in our study were well matched on aetiology and pre-therapy language profiles, and received the same type of treatment following a similar schedule, P1 made faster gains than P2 and showed better maintenance of effects 1 month after treatment. As both participants were on cognitive enhancers (commenced prior to the treatment and continued beyond), medication is not likely a differentiating factor. However, a couple of factors may have contributed to different patterns between the two patients. First, it must be acknowledged that P2 was older than P1. Although speculative, it is possible that age may have contributed to a slower rate of learning and less successful retention over time for P2 (Kester, Benjamin, Castel, & Craik, 2002).

A second factor concerns the intensity of the treatment. P1 practised her lists of words three times a week with remarkable consistency. In contrast, P2 requested a

TABLE 2
Results of pre- and post-experimental testing for generalisation for P1 and P2

	P1			P2		
	Pre	Post	6	Pre	Post	6
PNT (N = 175)	132	124	121	143	132	110
SPT (N = 135)	95	120	92	94	107	95

6 = 6 months post treatment, PNT = Philadelphia naming Test (Roach et al., 1996), SPT = Sentence Production Test (Caplan & Hanna, 1998).

reduction in the frequency of her treatment sessions and could commit to only two visits per week. Although the literature on treatment intensity remains inconclusive at present, our results are consistent with those of Raymer et al. (2006), who reported that all five of their participants improved with a greater intensity of treatment (3–4 times per week), whereas only two out of five improved when the intensity was limited to 1–2 times per week. In line with the present findings, Ramsberger and Basem (2005) found that although a significant treatment effect was demonstrated in all four of their participants treated with MossTalk Words® regardless of intensity, maintenance of gains was associated with greater intensity (five versus two sessions/ week).

An important issue addressed by the present study relates to the utility and effectiveness of treatment for anomia in progressive aphasia. Clinicians working with individuals affected by neurodegenerative disorders are constantly question-ing whether it is worthwhile to rehabilitate these individuals. The data from this study and our previous work (Jokel et al., 2006) certainly suggest that it is. In both studies, not only did the participants improve on treated items that they could not name prior to treatment, they also maintained correct production of items they could name prior to treatment. The latter finding suggests that one possible benefit to treating progressive aphasia is in the maintenance of residual skills. This is a promising proposal and certainly warrants further systematic investigation.

It is also encouraging to note that the results of the present study are comparable to treatment effects using the MossTalk Words® program for individuals with anomia as a result of a stroke (Fink et al., 2002a; Raymer et al., 2006). Surprisingly, the maintenance of the treatment effects in the present study is better than that found in Raymer et al. (2006). In that study, naming performance of some of the participants returned to baseline only 1 month post treatment, whereas both P1 and P2 in our study maintained their naming accuracy above baseline performance at 3 and 6 months post treatment. A couple of possible reasons to account for this favourable finding include the use of different MossTalk Words® modules and the targeted modality (i.e., production vs comprehension). Raymer and her colleagues used the Multimodality Matching module to treat either comprehension or naming. By definition, matching requires pairing related or identical stimuli in the same or different modalities without an active retrieval of the stimulus itself or the act of oral production. We used the Cued Naming module with orthographic cues that required active retrieval. It has been suggested by Hickin et al. (2002) that a more active engagement on the part of the individual being treated is important in stimulating deeper processing of the therapy task, perhaps with the result of a longer-lasting improvement in word retrieval. In addition, the participants in the present study were required to repeat each word out loud. Just as accessing phonology has been found to be important for treatment gains (LeDorze & Pitts, 1995), it is possible that requiring the oral production of each word also facilitates a better maintenance of treatment effects.

Consistent with most therapy studies of word retrieval in aphasia, generalisation to untreated items did not occur in our participants, as no improvement was noted on the PNT. In fact, both P1 and P2 have lost some of the words that have not been trained but were intact prior to the study. However, both of the participants showed improvement in the accuracy of their syntactic production, as measured by the Caplan and Hanna (1998) task. One possible explanation for this finding may be linked to the work of Thompson et al. (1997) whereby two distinct subtypes of nonfluent progressive aphasia are described: anomic and agrammatic. It may be possible that our two participants presented with the anomic type of NPA and their post-treatment improvement in word retrieval resulted in improved sentence production. While the exact nature of the relationship between lexical retrieval and sentence production needs to be explored further, these results are consistent with some studies in the literature that have found a correlation between noun retrieval (Bird & Franklin, 1999) or verb retrieval (Berndt, Haendiges, Mitchum, & Sandson, 1997) and measures of sentence structure (cf. Butterworth & Howard, 1987; Edwards & Bastiaanse, 1998).

Before concluding, one drawback of the present investigation relating to the administration of the therapy should be noted. Although the MossTalk Words® program has been known to benefit patients with anomia as a result of a post-stroke aphasia in a self-guided approach, our two participants were treated with a clinician-guided programme. Neither of the two patients had a home computer that could accommodate the system requirements of the MossTalk Words® software. In addition, although both individuals used computers in their professional life, they were reluctant to learn the new program and be responsible for practice without guidance. This is consistent with the attitudes towards MossTalk Words® published by Fink and colleagues in their brief update on the program (Fink et al., 2005). So, while the results of the present study are encouraging with respect to the effectiveness of a computer-based therapy for individuals with progressive aphasia, they do not address the issue of independence in therapy usually promoted by the use of computers.

In conclusion, the present investigation is significant for a couple of reasons. First, it represents a very thorough and rigorous examination of the effectiveness of a promising, theoretically motivated computer-based treatment of naming deficits— MossTalk Words®. Given that computer-based treatments have only recently begun to gain momentum in the rehabilitation field (Katz & Wertz, 1997; Linebarger, Schwartz, & Kohn, 2001; Wertz & Katz, 2004), this study can be viewed as supporting the use of this new treatment tool. Second, and perhaps more importantly, as a result of this investigation two individuals with NPA improved their naming of words, which in turn may have been helpful in their daily conversations. These results are encouraging and suggest that a treatment such as MossTalk Words® may be a viable therapy approach for individuals who suffer from progressive aphasia in the absence of generalised cognitive impairment.

REFERENCES

Basso, A., Marangolo, P., Piras, F., & Galluzzi, C. (2001). Acquisition of new "words" in normal subjects: A suggestion for the treatment of anomia. *Brain and Language, 77,* 45–59.

Bayles, K. A., & Tomoeda, C. K. (1993). *Arizona Battery for Communication in Dementia.* Tucson, AZ: Canyonlands Publishing Inc.

Berndt, R. S., Haendiges, A. N., Mitchum, C. C., & Sandson, J. (1997). Verb Retrieval: 2 Relationship to sentence processing. *Brain and Language, 56,* 107–137.

Best, W., Herbert, R., Hickin, J., Osborne, F., & Howard, D. (2002). Phonological and Orthographic facilitation or word-retrieval in aphasia: Immediate and delayed effects. *Aphasiology, 16,* 151–168.

Best, W. M., Howard, D., Bruce, C., & Gatehouse, C. (1997). A treatment for anomia: Combining semantics, phonology and orthography. In S. Chiat, J. Marshall, & J. Law (Eds.), *Making new connections.* London: Whurr.

Bird, H., & Franklin, S. (1999). Cinderella revisited: A comparison of fluent and non fluent aphasia speech. *Aphasiology, 13,* 187–206.

Bishop, D. (2003). *Test for Reception of Grammar – Version 2 (TROG-2).* San Antonio, TX: Harcourt Assessment.

Boyle, M. (2004). Semantic feature analysis treatment for anomia in two fluent aphasia syndromes. *American Journal of Speech-Language Pathology, 13,* 236–249.

Bruce, C., & Howard, D. (1987). Computer-generated phonemic cues: An effective aid for naming in aphasia, *British Journal of Disorders of Communication, 22,* 191–201.

Butterworth, B., & Howard, D. (1987). Paragrammatisms. *Cognition, 26,* 1–37.

Caplan, D., & Hanna, J. E. (1998). Sentence production by aphasic patients in a constrained task. *Brain and Language, 63,* 184–218.

Cress, C., & King, J. (1999). AAC strategies for people with primary progressive aphasia without dementia: Two case studies. *Augmentative and Alternative Communication, 15,* 248–259.

Croot, K., Patterson, K., & Hodges, J. R. (1998). Single word production in nonfluent progressive aphasia. *Brain & Language, 61,* 226–273.

Croot, K., Patterson, K., & Hodges, J. R. (1999). Familial progressive aphasia: Insights into the nature and deterioration of single word processing. *Cognitive Neuropsychology, 16,* 705–747.

Deloche, G., Dordain, M., & Kremin, H. (1993). Rehabilitation of confrontation naming in aphasia: Relations between oral and written modalities. *Aphasiology, 7,* 201–216.

Doesborgh, S. J. C., van de Sandt-Koenderman, M. W. M. E., Dippel, D. W. J., van Harskamp, F., Koudstaal, P. J., & Visch-Brink, E. G. (2004). Cues on request: The efficacy of Multicue, a computer program for word-finding therapy. *Aphasiology, 18,* 213–222.

Drew, R. L., & Thompson, C. K. (1999). Model-based semantic treatment for naming deficits in aphasia. *Journal of Speech, Language, and Hearing Research, 42,* 972–989.

Dunn, L. M., & Dunn, L. M. (1997). *Peabody Picture Vocabulary Test* (3rd ed.). Circle Pines, MN: American Guidance Service.

Edwards, S., & Bastiaanse, R. (1998). Diversity in the lexical and syntactic abilities of fluent aphasic speakers. *Aphasiology, 12,* 99–117.

Egan, J., Worrall, L., & Oxenham, D. (2004). Accessible Internet training package helps people with aphasia cross the digital divide. *Aphasiology, 18,* 265–280.

Ellis, A. W. (1985). The production of spoken words: A cognitive neuropsychological perspective. In A. W. Ellis (Ed.), *Progress in the psychology of language, 2.* Hove, UK: Lawrence Erlbaum Associates Ltd.

Fink, R. B., Brecher, A., Montgomery, M., & Schwartz, M. F. (2001). *MossTalk Words* [computer software manual]. Philadelphia: Albert Einstein Healthcare Network.

Fink, R. B., Brecher, A., Schwartz, M. F., & Robey, R. R. (2002a). A computer-implemented protocol for treatment of naming disorders: Evaluation of clinician-guided and partially self-guided instruction. *Aphasiology, 16,* 1061–1086.

Fink, R. B., Brecher, A., Sobel, P., & Schwartz, M. F. (2005). Computer-assisted treatment of word retrieval deficits in aphasia. *Aphasiology, 19,* 943–954.

Fink, R. B., Lowery, J., & Sobel, P. (2002b). Clinical narrative. *Perspectives on Neurophysiology and Neurogenic Speech and Language Disorder, American Speech-Language Hearing Association Newsletter: Special Interest Division 2, 12,* 25–29.

Frattali, C. (2003). An errorless learning approach to treating dysnomia in frontotemporal dementia. *Journal of Medical Speech-Language Pathology, 12,* XI–XXIV.

Gagnon, D. A., Schwartz, M. F., Martin, N., Dell, G. S., & Saffran, E. M. (1997). The origins of formal paraphasias in aphasics' picture naming. *Brain & Language, 59*, 450–472.

Goodglass, H., Kaplan, E., & Barresi, B. (2001). *Boston Diagnostic Aphasia Examination – 3rd Edition.* New York: Lippincott, Williams & Williams.

Graham, K. S., & Hodges, J. R. (1997). Differentiating the roles of the hippocampal complex and the neocortex in long-term memory storage: Evidence from the study of semantic dementia and Alzheimer's disease. *Neuropsychology, 11*, 77–89.

Graham, K. S., Patterson, K., Pratt, K. H., & Hodges, J. R. (1999). Relearning and subsequent forgetting of semantic category exemplars in a case of semantic dementia. *Neuropsychology, 13*, 359–380.

Graham, K. S., Patterson, K., Pratt, K. H., & Hodges, J. R. (2001). Can repeated exposure to "forgotten" vocabulary help alleviate word-finding difficulties in semantic dementia? An illustrative case study. *Neuropsychological Rehabilitation, 11*, 429–454.

Greenwald, M. L., Raymer, A. M., Richardson, M. E., & Rothi, L. (1995). Contrasting treatments for severe impairments of picture naming. *Neuropsychological Rehabilitation, 5*, 17–49.

Hickin, J., Best, W., Herbert, R., Howard, D., & Osborne, F. (2002). Phonological therapy for word-finding difficulties: A re-evaluation. *Aphasiology, 16*, 981–999.

Hodges, J. R., Patterson, K., Oxbury, S., & Funnell, E. (1992). Semantic dementia: Progressive fluent aphasia with temporal lobe atrophy. *Brain, 115*, 1783–1806.

Howard, D., & Patterson, K. E. (1992). *The Pyramids and Palm Trees Test.* Bury St Edmunds, UK: Thames Valley Test Company.

Jokel, R., & Rochon, E. (1996). Treatment for an aphasic naming impairment: When phonology met orthography. *Brain and Cognition, 32*, 299–301.

Jokel, R., Rochon, E. A., & Leonard, C. (2006). Treatment for anomia in semantic dementia: Improvement, maintenance or both? *Neuropsychological Rehabilitation, 16*, 241–256.

Katz, R., & Wertz, R. (1997). The efficacy of computer-provided reading treatment for chronic aphasic adults. *Journal of Speech, Language and Hearing Research, 40*, 493–507.

Kay, J., Lesser, R., & Coltheart, M. (1992). *Psycholinguistic assessments of language processing in aphasia (PALPA).* Hove, UK: Lawrence Erlbaum Associates Ltd.

Kester, J. D., Benjamin, A. S., Castel, A. D., & Craik, F. I. M. (2002). Memory in elderly people. In A. D. Baddeley, M. D. Kopelman, & B. A. Wilson (Eds.), *Handbook of memory disorders.* Chichester, UK: John Wiley & Sons Ltd.

Kiran, S., & Thompson, C. K. (2003). The role of semantic complexity in treatment of naming deficits: Training semantic categories in fluent aphasia by controlling exemplar typicality. *Journal of Speech, Language and Hearing Research, 46*(4), 773–787.

Kiran, S., Thompson, C. K., & Hashimoto, N. (2001). Training grapheme-phoneme conversion in patients with oral reading and naming deficits: A model-based approach. *Aphasiology, 15*, 855–876.

Laganaro, M., Di Pietro, M., & Schnider, A. (2003). Computerised treatment of anomia in chronic and acute aphasia: An exploratory study. *Aphasiology, 17*, 709–721.

Le Dorze, G., & Pitts, C. (1995). A case study evaluation of the effects of different techniques for the treatment of anomia. *Neuropsychological Rehabilitation, 5*, 51–65.

Linebarger, M. C., Schwartz, M. F., & Kohn, S. E. (2001). Computer-based training of language production: An exploratory study. *Neuropsychological Rehabilitation, 11*, 57–96.

McNeil, M. R., Small, S. L., Masterson, R. J., & Fossett, T. R. D. (1995). Behavioral and pharmacological treatment of lexical semantic deficits in a single patient with primary progressive aphasia. *American Journal of Speech-Language Pathology, 4*, 76–87.

McReynolds, L. V., & Kearns, K. P. (1983). *Single-subject experimental design in communicative disorders.* Baltimore, MD: University Park Press.

Mesulam, M. M. (1982). Slowly progressive aphasia without generalised dementia. *Annals of Neurology, 11*, 592–598.

Mesulam, M. M., & Weintraub, S. (1992). Spectrum of primary progressive aphasia. *Bailiere's Clinical Neurology: International Practice and Research, 1*, 583–609.

Millard, S. K. (1998). The value of single-case research. *International Journal of Language and Communication Disorders, 33*, 370–373.

Mortley, J., Wade, J., & Enderby, P. (2004). Superhighway to promoting a client–therapist partnership? Using the Internet to deliver word-retrieval computer therapy, monitored remotely with minimal speech and language therapy input. *Aphasiology, 18*, 193–211.

Nickels, L. (2002). Therapy for naming disorders: Revisiting, revising, and reviewing. *Aphasiology, 16*, 935–980.

Nickels, L., & Best, W. (1996a). Therapy for naming disorders (Part 1): Principles, puzzles and progress. *Aphasiology, 10*, 21–47.

Nickels, L., & Best, W. (1996b). Therapy for naming disorders (Part 2): Specifics, surprises and suggestions. *Aphasiology, 10*, 109–136.

Nickels, L., & Howard, D. (1995). Phonological errors in aphasic naming: Comprehension, monitoring and lexicality. *Cortex, 31*, 209–237.

Pedersen, P. M., Vinter, K., & Olson, T. S. (2001). Improvement of oral naming by unsupervised computerized rehabilitation. *Aphasiology, 15*, 151–169.

Ramsberger, G., & Basem, M. (2005). *Partially self-administered computer-based cued naming therapy: A single subject study comparing treatment intensity replicated in four cases.* Poster presentation at the Academy of Aphasia, Amsterdam, Netherlands.

Raymer, A. M., Kohen, F. P., & Saffell, D. (2006). Computerized training for impairments of word comprehension and retrieval in aphasia. *Aphasiology, 20*, 257–268.

Riddoch, M. J., & Humphreys, G. W. (1993). *Birmingham Object Recognition Battery.* Hove, UK: Lawrence Erlbaum Associates Ltd.

Roach, A., Schwartz, M. F., Martin, N., Grewal, R. S., & Brecher, A. (1996). The Philadelphia Naming Test: Scoring and rationale. *Clinical Aphasiology, 24*, 121–133.

Rogers, M. A., & Alarcon, N. B. (1998). Dissolution of spoken language in primary progressive aphasia. *Aphasiology, 12*, 635–650.

Schneider, S. L., Thompson, C. K., & Luring, B. (1996). Effects of verbal plus gestural matrix training on sentence production in a patient with primary progressive aphasia. *Aphasiology, 10*, 297–317.

Schwartz, M. F., Saffran, E. M., Bloch, D. E., & Dell, G. S. (1994). Disordered speech production in aphasic and normal speakers. *Brain and Language, 47*, 52–88.

Snowden, J. S., Goulding, P. J., & Neary, D. (1989). Semantic dementia: A form of circumscribed cerebral atrophy. *Behavioral Neurology, 2*, 167–182.

Snowden, J. S., & Neary, D. (2002). Relearning of verbal labels in semantic dementia. *Neuropsychologia, 40*, 1715–1728.

Thompson, C. K., Ballard, K. J., Tait, M. E., Weintraub, S., & Mesulam, M-M. (1997). Patterns of language decline in nonfluent primary progressive aphasia. *Aphasiology, 11*, 297–331.

Van Mourik, M., & Van de Sandt-Koenderman, W. M. (1992). Multicue. *Aphasiology, 6*, 179–183.

Wambaugh, J., Linebaugh, C., Doyle, P., Martinez, Z., Kalinyak-Fliszar, M., & Spencer, K. (2001). Effects of two cueing treatments on lexical retrieval in aphasic speakers with different levels of deficit. *Aphasiology, 15*, 933–950.

Watt, S., Jokel, R., & Behrmann, M. (1997). Surface dysgraphia in nonfluent progressive aphasia. *Brain & Language, 56*, 211–233.

Wertz, R., & Katz, R. (2004). Outcomes of computer-provided treatment for aphasia. *Aphasiology, 18*, 229–244.

APHASIOLOGY, 2009, 23 (2), 192–209

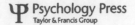

Psychology Press
Taylor & Francis Group

Relearning and retention of verbal labels in a case of semantic dementia

Cristina Green Heredia

Universidad de Málaga, Spain

Karen Sage and Matthew A. Lambon Ralph

University of Manchester, UK

Marcelo L. Berthier

Universidad de Málaga, Spain

Background: Previous studies looking at relearning and retention of word labels in people with semantic dementia have shown some improvement in naming immediately after the period of learning but this has not usually been maintained. Studies have also shown rigid learning of names, in the order of presentation and to the picture exemplars only, with no generalisation of learning.

Aims: This study aimed to explore relearning of a small vocabulary set in a person with semantic dementia (CUB) and to examine her ability to generalise this learning. In addition, it aimed to find out how long the learning persisted after therapy was completed given that semantic dementia is a progressive disorder.

Methods & Procedures: A single-case design was used where CUB was asked to learn 28 words while a further 28 were left as controls. A "look and say" method was used daily for 1 month. As well as examining learning of the therapy and control set, CUB was asked to name 168 other exemplars of the learning set to see whether there had been any transfer of her learning from the therapy set.

Outcomes & Results: CUB not only relearned a set of picture names but retained these without deliberate practice over a 6-month period. She was also able to generalise this learning to other visually similar exemplars in testing and in daily use. The maintenance of relearning was achieved despite severe deterioration in her semantic memory.

Conclusions: Possible reasons are explored as to why CUB was able to relearn and retain these words and why this may differ from all previously reported cases. Differences in amount of time spent relearning, number of items learned, therapy methods, the severity of semantic memory impairment, the degree of atrophy, and the behavioural profiles of people with semantic dementia do not provide adequate explanations for our individual's differential ability to retain her learning over 6 months. The most plausible explanation is that the person with semantic dementia generalised her learning to her everyday speech and this provided the source of maintenance for the relearned names.

Keywords: Semantic dementia; Anomia; Relearning; Generalisation; Maintenance.

Address correspondence to: Dr Karen Sage, Neuroscience and Aphasia Research Unit, School of Psychological Sciences, Zochonis Building, T15, University of Manchester, Oxford Road, Manchester M13 9PL, UK. E-mail: karen.sage@manchester.ac.uk

This work was supported by a Royal Society Travel Fellowship awarded to K. Sage. We are grateful to Dr Tomás Ojea from the Hospital Carlos Haya, Málaga for referring CUB to us, and most importantly to CUB and her family for their collaboration throughout.

http://www.psypress.com/aphasiology   DOI: 10.1080/02687030801942999

Semantic dementia is the temporal lobe variant of fronto-temporal dementia in which there is progressive but circumscribed bilateral atrophy of the anterior, inferolateral temporal lobes. This damage produces a gradual and eventually profound deterioration in semantic memory (Hodges, Patterson, Oxbury, & Funnel, 1992). The impairment affects both receptive and expressive skills and verbal as well as nonverbal modalities (Bozeat, Lambon Ralph, Patterson, Garrard, & Hodges, 2000b; Lambon Ralph & Howard, 2000). The syndrome is relatively homogeneous, with variations dependent on the relative atrophy of the left and right temporal lobes (Lambon Ralph, McClelland, Patterson, Galton, & Hodges, 2001; Snowden, Thompson, & Neary, 2004). A number of characteristics have been shown to be constant within semantic dementia (Rogers et al., 2004). For example, frequency and familiarity determine which concepts are better retained. General attributes (e.g., the legs of a zebra) are retained better, while item-specific information is more vulnerable (e.g., the stripes of the zebra), so that distinguishing between similar concepts becomes harder.

The amodal semantic impairment found in semantic dementia results in a profound anomia (Lambon Ralph et al., 2001). Indeed this is the most common presenting symptom in this patient group and causes considerable anxiety. Even people with extremely mild comprehension impairments tend to have significant word-finding difficulties, which accelerate over the early course of the disease (Lambon Ralph et al., 2001). Both clinically and academically, therefore, it is imperative to explore methods and techniques designed to restore, or at least maintain, a core activities of daily living (ADL) vocabulary in this patient group.

Despite the extensive literature dedicated to establishing the nature of the deficits in semantic dementia, studies looking specifically at interventions for these word-finding difficulties number only six to date (Frattali, 2004; Graham, Patterson, Pratt, & Hodges, 1999, 2001; Jokel, Rochon, & Leonard, 2002, 2006; Snowden & Neary, 2002). A summary of cases in each of these papers is provided in Table 1, along with scan details and background information. In each study, people with semantic dementia have benefited in the short-term from mass practice of selected concrete concept names. However, the retention of this learning over the longer term (measured between 2 weeks and 6 months after learning) without continued practice has been minimal or non-existent. Furthermore, the ability to retain words has been shown to rely on the degree of semantic degradation present at the start of the therapy programme (Snowden & Neary, 2002). If some meaning remains, then retention of the re-learnt word is longer but this partial conceptual knowledge does not prevent its eventual loss (Jokel et al., 2002, 2006). Where little meaning remains, it is very hard for the person with semantic dementia to relearn the corresponding label, let alone retain it without practice. Some specific details about the five existing case studies are reviewed below.

Graham et al. (1999) described the case of DM, a 59-year-old surgeon who had developed a method of note-keeping to retain words that he knew were disappearing from his vocabulary. He was meticulous in this method and would practise the lists he had made for himself over several hours a day. At the time of the study, DM's semantic abilities and naming skills were still relatively unimpaired. He scored 49/52 on the three-picture version of the Pyramids and Palm Trees Test (PPT, Howard & Patterson, 1992) and 71% on the Cambridge picture-naming test (Hodges et al., 1992). DM was given 100 words from four different categories to relearn while

TABLE 1
Summary of cases with semantic dementia where relearning has been undertaken, method used, and short- and long-term effects

Case	Reference	Age	Background	Scan	Semantic impairment[1]	Method	S T effects	LT effects
DM	Graham et al., 1999 (& 2001)	59	Surgeon	L temporal lobe atrophy, involving the pole and to smaller extent inferior region of mid and posterior temporal pole.	Mild 49/52 (PPT)	List learning within categories.	√	x
KB	Snowden & Neary, 2002	64	NR	Severe atrophy of temporal lobes R > L. Lesser involvement of medial temporal lobes.	Moderate to severe 25/52 (PPT)	Picture/spoken and written word labels.	x	x
CR	Snowden & Neary, 2002	57	NR	Selective atrophy L temporal lobe (MRI) L > R.	Moderate to severe 29/52 (PPT)	Picture/spoken and written word labels with autobiographical linking.	√	partial
AK	Jokel et al., 2002 & 206	63	Arts officer	Bitemporal atrophy, L > R. Some atrophy of L ventral frontal regions.	Moderate 37/52 (PPT)	Picture/spoken and written word labels.	partial	x
	Fratali, 2004	66	Military	Focal atrophy inferior medial aspect of L temp lobe relative sparing of hippocampus.	Moderate to severe	Pictures in conversation.	partial	x

[1] As measured using Palm Trees and Pyramids (Howard & Patterson, 1992) or equivalent. ST = short term (immediately post-therapy and up to 1 month post-therapy). LT = long term (6 months). NR = not recorded. Partial: indicates that the participant was able to learn the verbal labels for some of the items.

another four categories were kept as controls. He was asked to read and say the target words aloud for 30 minutes each day, for a total of 2 weeks. He was then re-assessed by generating as many items as he could for each of the four therapy categories and for the four control categories. Although DM showed immediate benefits from this learning method, in that he was able to generate significantly more category items than at baseline, he was not able to generate any new exemplars for that category. He also provided the list in almost exactly the same order as he had learnt it during therapy. DM showed a surprising improvement in one of the control categories (makes of car) and when this was investigated further, it transpired that he had been looking at these in a book over the 2 weeks and so, in effect, had also been relearning these items without the examiners' knowledge. After 8 weeks without practice, DM's performance returned to baseline levels. A follow-up study (Graham et al., 2001) of DM's retention of the learned categories was carried out 2 years later. DM had practised the lists during the 2 years and was able to recall these, despite deterioration on tests of semantic knowledge. These studies highlighted four characteristics that have been repeated across other investigations (see below): (1) persistent and regular practice seems to allow relearning to occur in semantic dementia; (2) maintenance of the relearning requires constant practice; (3) performance rigidly reflects item order; (4) there is little evidence of generalisation from target items to other concepts or exemplars.

Snowden and Neary (2002) studied two cases whose semantic and anomic difficulties were more severe than DM. KB was a 64-year-old woman who scored 25/52 on the three-picture version of the PPT (i.e., her performance was at chance) and was unable to name any pictures in the Boston Naming Test (BNT; Kaplan, Goodglass, & Weintraub, 1983). Information on KB's semantic knowledge of 60 line drawings from the Snodgrass and Vanderwart corpus was collected by asking her to name the picture and provide definitions both to the picture and the spoken word, and spoken word-to-picture matching. From these 60 items, 20 pictures that she failed to name were selected. KB was unable to demonstrate knowledge of 10 of the selected items and showed partial knowledge for the remainder. The learning procedure consisted of a baseline assessment of the 20 items during which KB attempted to name the pictures. KB was then shown each picture and its written label and was asked to read the word aloud while concentrating on the picture. The examiner then repeated the word aloud. All 20 pictures were then retested. This procedure was carried out three times in total. KB was then given a 2-week break during which she did not look at the materials and then two further learning sessions. She was retested 4 months later. KB learned a few words after the 2-week break, though not sufficient to show increase in naming accuracy over baseline. It is noteworthy, however, that items that were learnt came from the set for which she had shown partial semantic knowledge at the start.

Snowden and Neary (2002) contrasted this case with CR, a 57-year-old woman whose semantic and anomic difficulties were also severe. She scored 29/52 on the three-picture version of the PPT (again at chance) and 4/60 on the BNT. A similar procedure to that used for KB was used to establish a learning set of 20 items, although this time CR showed no knowledge on measures of naming, definition, and word-to-picture match for any of the 20 items. The learning trials were similar to those of KB in that she was shown the picture and written label, and asked to read the word aloud. The learning procedure was augmented in two ways: she was asked to provide descriptive information about the meaning of the word and to make links between the picture and objects in her own home/environment. CR then looked again at the picture and written label, this time with a spoken commentary from the experimenter about the item, using the definition and home environment information provided earlier. For example, for the item "duck", she was reminded that she had an ornamental duck on her wall and that there were ducks in the pond. Following this learning session, CR was provided with a self-study booklet for the 20 items that she had to look at, read, and say. CR practised for 20 minutes each day for 3 weeks and was faithful to the practice regime. When she was unable to remember a name she asked her husband for the semantic link, which he would then provide. CR's naming ability was perfect (20/20) both immediately and 60 days later. Her score dropped to 13/20 when tested 6 months later. At the 60-day assessment and at 6 months, the 20 pictures were also tested using random presentation order and with a different colour background. These changes produced a drop in CR's performance (15/20 and 8/20 respectively). These results imply a strongly context-dependent learning mechanism underlies these gains.

Jokel et al. (2002, 2006) described the case of AK, a 63-year-old woman who was an arts officer and a keen musician. Her semantic abilities and naming skills were moderately severe (she scored 37/52 on the PPT and 5/60 on the BNT). AK was asked to name, on two occasions, the 230-picture set from the Peabody Collection (Dunn & Dunn, 1997). Her comprehension of the items was tested using word-to-picture matching of the items. A set of 180 items was established, subdivided into three sets: 60 that she named and comprehended (+N+C), 60 that she did not name but did comprehend (–N+C), and 60 that she neither named or comprehended (–N–C). These sets were then further divided into treatment and control sets. The 30 pictures of each subset were placed on card with the written label and a brief description of the item (previously provided by AK) on the reverse. AK looked at the picture and read aloud the label and description of the item. She carried this out at home, practising for half an hour per day for 6 days. On the seventh day she was tested on the 30 items intermingled with 30 control items. Each of the three subgroups was treated for 1 week (a total of 3 weeks) in a specific order: first +N+C; then –N+C and finally –N–C. Retest of all therapy and control items was carried out 1 month after the end of the last treated set and 6 months later. Three important results arose from this study. First, items that were practised were retained better at all stages than items which were not. Second, best results were achieved with those items where AK retained some semantic knowledge. Lastly, even with practice, some items were lost over time in the +N+C set.

Finally, Frattali (2004) described a 66-year-old retired military man who was asked to relearn 20 nouns and 20 verbs using an errorless (but effortful) paradigm in which the therapist and the gentleman engaged in conversation about pictures in which target items were displayed. Therapy lasted for 2 hours a week over a period of 12 weeks. Some improvement, particularly in noun naming, was evident immediately after the therapy but this was not maintained at the 3-month follow-up assessment.

In summary, the reported cases to date have generally shown some improvement in naming immediately after the period of learning but this has not usually been maintained. Where it has been maintained (Snowden & Neary, 2002) the apparent gains diminish if the testing order and/or the appearance of the test items is altered, suggesting that some gains reflect rote learning. Given the paucity of previous studies, this study chose to replicate what had been carried out in previous studies so that comparison with other findings would be possible, and to extend previous findings by further post-therapy testing. In this study, various parameters that might influence relearning were explored with a person with semantic dementia, CUB. In striking contrast to the previously reported cases, CUB not only learned a set of picture names but retained these without deliberate practice over a 6-month period. She was also able to generalise this relearning to other visually similar exemplars in testing and in daily use.

CASE HISTORY

This study was approved by the local ethics committee of the University of Málaga. CUB was a 53-year-old married Spanish woman who had previously worked as a civil servant in the Justice Department until the onset of her illness. In 2002 she was signed off from work with depression. It was around this time that she began to have word-finding difficulties. She was first seen by our research group at the end of 2004, when her language was fluent with a tendency to talk garrulously such that, at times, it was difficult to interrupt her. Her speech was empty, with marked anomia, perseverations and the use of filler words such as "anyway", "simply", "precisely", "do you understand me?", "the topic is", "I know about this". She occasionally swore —something she had never previously been in the habit of doing. She complained of intrusive words that would come into her mind but for which she had forgotten their meaning (for example "níspero" [a soft fruit somewhat like a peach], "melocotón" [peach]). When this happened she would write them down. Her husband reported that she would then use them for a few days and then they would disappear again from her speech. Her husband also reported that she had some difficulty recognising old friends (although this was not the case with her immediate family). CUB had some insight into her problems, in particular, her progressive anomia. Comprehension deficits were apparent on examination; for example, when asked if she had a good appetite, she replied; "Appetite? I have forgotten. What is appetite?" An MRI scan from 2004 showed focal, bilateral temporal atrophy with a marked knife-edged shape in the left middle and inferior temporal gyri, but only mild atrophic changes in the right temporal lobe (Figure 1).

NEUROPSYCHOLOGICAL TESTING

Behavioural examination

CUB underwent a battery of neurological and neuropsychological tests at the end of 2004 and start of 2005. Her Mini-Mental Test score (Folstein, Folstein, & McHugh, 1975: Peña-Casanova, Gramunt, & Gich Fullà, 2004) was 24/30, failing the word recall and naming elements. General behaviour was examined via the Frontal Behavioral Inventory (Kertesz, Davidson, & Fox, 1997). She scored 21 (range: 0–36) on the negative behaviour scale and 15 (range: 0–27) on the disinhibition score, displaying apathy, inflexibility, loss of insight, semantic dementia, perseverations, irritability, inappropriateness, hyper-orality, and hyper-sexuality. The Leyton Obsessional Inventory (LOI: Cooper, 1970) was completed by her husband rather than CUB and so the interference and resistance scales could not be completed. The scores were very high (LOI symptoms: 45/46; LOI traits: 20/23) showing a number of

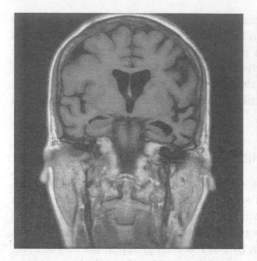 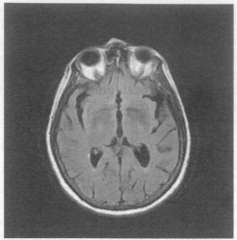

Figure 1. CUB: MRI coronal and axial slices. Note that the left hemisphere is shown on the right of the MR images.

obsessions (e.g., fear that her family would come to harm, distaste of any physical contact with people she did not know) and compulsions (e.g., the need to continuously check the gas, wash her hands). She also showed obsessional traits (e.g., the need to stick to a rigid timetable, sorting, ironing, and re-sorting her clothes continuously). The history provided by her husband suggested that some of the behaviours might well have been related to premorbid obsessive-compulsive personality traits. Other features are consistent with those found in semantic dementia and frontotemporal dementia more generally (e.g., clock-watching etc., Bozeat, Gregory, Lambon Ralph, & Hodges, 2000a; Snowden et al., 2001). CUB also reported that words would come into her mind unheeded. Some of these words were specific to her previous lifestyle (for example, administration, finance, and judicial vocabulary) while the rest were names of body parts and bodily functions as well as food and household items. There were also some animal names.

Cognitive testing

On the Raven's Coloured Progressive Matrices (Raven, 1985) CUB scored a total of 28/36, which placed her in the Grade II intelligence category (75th %ile). Her copy of the Rey figure (Osterreith, 1995) was perfect (36/36), an exact copy, while her immediate recall was severely impoverished (10/36, 3rd %ile), suggesting good visuospatial skills but severely impaired visual memory. On the Wechsler Memory Scale (Wechsler, 1976) she showed severe problems with logical memory (1/23), paired associate learning (3.5/21), and reproducing diagrams from memory (7/14). She showed severe difficulties with both semantic and letter fluency. She gave three animals in a category fluency task, plus one intrusion (a fruit "melón"). On the FAS (Borkowsky, Benton, & Spreen, 1967) she provided 11 correct responses. In addition, she gave three responses that were linked, not to the letter as required, but semantically ("sábana" [sheet], "cama" [bed], "manta" [blanket]). Her forward digit span (measured using EPLA/PALPA, Kay, Lesser, & Coltheart, 1992; Valle &

Cuetos, 1995) was 4. CUB retained her ability to read aloud and to spell accurately, as expected for languages with transparent orthography (Patterson, Okada, Suzuki, Ijuin, & Tatsum, 1998).

Face processing

Benton's Facial Recognition Test (Benton, Hamsher, Varney, & Spreen, 1978) assesses ability to match unfamiliar faces across different views. CUB scored 22 on the shortened form, which is equivalent to 46 on the full test version. Control performance is between 41–54 indicating that CUB had no difficulty with this task. In contrast, her ability to recognise and name famous faces was impaired. On this test, recognition is credited when the participant names the famous person or provides identifying information (for example, Juan Carlos Ferrero – "He's a tennis player"). CUB's recognition (12/56) and naming scores (2/56) were very poor in comparison to age-matched controls (naming: mean = 43.9/56, range 33–53).

Background language testing

On the Western Aphasia Battery (Kertesz, 1982), she gained an Aphasia Quotient of 66.2, which placed her in the category of anomic aphasia with particular difficulty in the naming subtest (1/20). In both spontaneous speech and picture description task, her speech was fluent but with a paucity of content words.

Phonological skills. Auditory discrimination was assessed using minimal word and nonword pairs from EPLA/PALPA (Kay et al., 1992; Valle & Cuetos, 1995). CUB showed a tendency to accept pairs as sounding the same (word test 28/28 same trials; 22/28 different trials, controls 27.68, $SD = 0.76$, nonword test 28/28 same trials, 23/28 different trials, controls 27.09, $SD=1.24$). On both these tests of auditory discrimination, therefore, CUB showed a mild to moderate impairment. Although CUB's hearing was not formally tested, this performance is unlikely to reflect a deficit in hearing acuity but is in line with other studies showing phonological difficulties in this client group, which are attributed to their semantic impairment (Jefferies, Jones, Bateman, & Lambon Ralph, 2005; Patterson, Graham, & Hodges, 1994; Patterson et al., 2006). On an assessment of auditory lexical decision from EPLA/PALPA, CUB performed at chance 48/160. CUB's single word repetition was at ceiling for verbs (50/50), adjectives (50/50), and functors (40/40), and close to ceiling for nouns (119/120) and nonwords (77/80). This pattern of excellent repetition yet impoverished word recognition is typical of semantic dementia (Jefferies et al., 2005; Patterson et al., 1994, 2006). CUB was able to read aloud all the words and nonwords that she had been asked to repeat. This retained reading ability reflects the nature of Spanish orthography, which is transparent in the translation of orthography to phonology (i.e., there are no irregular words in reading, at least at the level of phonology, although some inconsistency is present for stress assignment).

Semantic memory. On the Pyramids and Palm Tree Test (Howard & Patterson, 1992) CUB scored 33/52 on the three-picture and 31/52 on the three written word version of the test, showing a severe difficulty in identifying semantic associations, irrespective of modality of testing (English-speaking controls made up to a maximum of three errors on this test, Spanish controls made a maximum of two errors). On the spoken-word-to-picture matching task from EPLA/PALPA (Kay et al., 1992; Valle & Cuetos, 1995) she scored 15/40, making 11 close semantic, 8 distant semantic, 3 visual, and 3 unrelated errors (Spanish control mean 39.45, $SD = 1.67$).

CUB's semantic memory was reassessed 6 months after the end of the therapy programme (December 2005) when she scored 18/52 on the three-pictures version of PPT (Howard & Patterson, 1992), a performance that is at chance and significantly worse than at the start of the study when she scored 33/52 (McNemar, exact $p = .003$). By this time, her conversational speech had also deteriorated to stereotypical phrases and repetitive topics (such as her illness, her desire for a medicine that would help, etc.). She had begun to have behavioural difficulties such as wandering from home and kleptomania.

Naming skills. On the EPLA/PALPA naming by frequency test, CUB scored 13/60, 10 of which were high-frequency and 3 low-frequency items (which were, however, familiar and important everyday items for CUB).

Therapy method

From the 64 pictures that CUB failed to name in the Western Aphasia Battery and the EPLA/PALPA Naming by Frequency test, 56 were selected and divided into two sets of 28, one set for therapy and one set as a control. A list of these items and their translations are available in the Appendix. Both sets were matched on frequency, syllable, and phoneme length using BuscaPalabras (Davis & Perea, 2005). The mean values for both sets are set out in Table 2.

CUB's naming of the 56 items was re-measured prior to the start of therapy (baseline 2) when she was able to name 6 of the items in the control set and 2 in the therapy set (see Table 3).

CUB's errors at baseline were divided between no-response errors (60%) which she indicated in a number of ways ("I don't know this", "I have forgotten this", "I

TABLE 2
Mean frequency and length values for the therapy and control items

		Frequency	Syllable length	Phoneme length
Therapy items	Mean	36.26	2.61	5.86
	SD	57.92	0.69	1.69
Control items	Mean	36.31	2.50	5.50
	SD	52.14	0.69	1.35

TABLE 3
Naming accuracy for two baselines: Immediate post-therapy and at 1 and 6 months post-therapy

	Baseline 1	Baseline 2	Immediately post-therapy	1 month post-therapy	6 months post-therapy
Therapy items	0/28	2/28	28/28	27/28	23/28
Control items	0/28	6/28	5/28	6/28	0/28

used to know this"); descriptive information (25%), for example to the target "pram" she replied; "where you put children"; and superordinate errors (15%), for example to the target "pear" she replied; "it's a fruit". These errors are consistent with those shown by other people with semantic dementia (Jefferies & Lambon Ralph, 2006; Rogers et al., 2004).

A PowerPoint presentation was used for the 28 items, with each item pictured first, followed by the picture paired with its written label. In therapy, CUB tried to name the picture first but if she was unable to name it, she was then asked to move on to the page where the picture and written label were displayed together and to read aloud the name. The items were placed on a CD-ROM, which CUB looked at every day for 1 month, practising the items in the same order each day. During this self-practice, her husband reported that occasionally CUB would come and ask him what a word meant and he would show her the item or explain its meaning.

RESULTS

CUB's naming of the 56 items was tested immediately after the month-long, self-directed home therapy and again at 1 month and 6 months post therapy. Following the month's self-directed learning, CUB returned the CD-ROM to the researcher and did not continue to practise these words. During those 6 months CUB continued to take part in relearning other words selected by her husband and son.

In order to test her naming skills without the potential support of the original therapy order (see the introduction), the items were presented in a different order from that used in therapy and with the control items interleaved. Her last response was used to evaluate her answer. This was chosen as she would sometimes make a comment before naming—such as "this was on the computer", "you didn't put that on the computer"—and there were two items for which she produced "conduite d'approche" behaviour before naming the item (for example, to the picture of "hacha" [axe], she said "bacha, hacha" and "hucha, hacha" at 1 month and 6 months respectively). For two items "bañera" [bath] and "mesa" [table], she used a set phrase (which her husband had provided for her early in therapy when she had asked him for help). In order to access "bañera" [bath], she said "baño, bañera" [bathroom, bath] while for "mesa" [table], she said "mesa y silla" [table and chair]. The results of these assessments are shown in Table 3.

These results showed excellent relearning of the items immediately post therapy when she was able to name all the items. A comparison of scores at each of the three retest times (immediately post therapy, at 1 month follow-up, and at 6 months follow-up) showed a significant difference between the learned and control sets (immediately post therapy $\chi^2 = 35.07$, $df = 1$, $p < .001$, 1 month post therapy $\chi^2 = 28.99$, $df = 1$, $p < .001$, and at 6 months follow-up $\chi^2 = 35.07$, $df = 1$, $p < .001$). Naming improved significantly on the therapy set from baseline to immediate post therapy (McNemar, one-tailed, $p < .001$) and this significant difference was maintained at 1-month and at 6-month follow-up. A similar comparison of control items showed no significant difference (comparison of baseline with immediate post-therapy performance, McNemar, one-tailed, $p > .05$).

After 1 month without therapy, CUB named all but one item ("botón" [button]) although she recognised it as having been part of her therapy set. At 6 months follow-up, there were five items that she could no longer name (Table 4). Four of her five errors were the names of other items within the therapy set and related to the

TABLE 4
Targets and errors within the therapy set at 6 months follow-up, with error type

Spanish target	English translation	Spanish error	English translation	Error type
cama	bed	cubo	bucket	Within therapy set
globo	balloon	vaya	go	Phonologically related to another word in therapy set (vela – candle)
piano	piano	peine	comb	Within therapy set and phonologically related
sombrero	hat	botón	button	Within therapy set and semantically related
vaca	cow	dromodario	dromedary	Within therapy set and semantically related

target either semantically ("sombrero" [hat], – "botón" [button],) or phonologically ("peine" [comb] for "piano"). Although one error ("vaya" for "globo" [balloon],) was not in the therapy set, it was phonologically related to another therapy item ("vela" [candle]).

One important feature of conceptual knowledge is that it allows information about one stimulus to be appropriately generalised to other examples (McClelland & Rogers, 2003; Rogers et al., 2004). There is already some evidence to suggest that breakdown in conceptual knowledge produces under-generalisation in semantic dementia. Snowden, Griffiths, and Neary (1995) found that remaining conceptual knowledge (e.g., dog licence) did not generalise appropriately (e.g., to licences in general). Likewise in object use, Bozeat, Lambon Ralph, Patterson, and Hodges (2002) found that retained use for individuals' own everyday objects only generalised to another example if the two were visually similar. For visually dissimilar objects, people with semantic dementia often failed to recognise that they were the same type of object. In an attempt to evaluate this possibility in the context of name relearning, CUB was given a further naming test in which six different examples of each of the 28 therapy items were presented. For example she was shown a single banana, a bunch of bananas hanging from a tree, diced bananas, etc. (Figure 2).

This assessment was carried out immediately after the therapy when CUB scored 155/168 (92%). Her excellent naming performance on these alternative exemplars indicates that her relearning did generalise. Inevitably, however, many of the

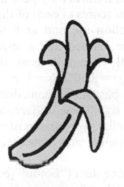
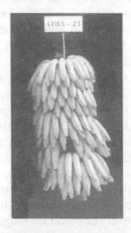
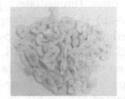

Figure 2. An example ("banana") of the different exemplars of a therapy item used in 168-item test.

pictured alternatives were visually similar to the original pictures and thus (as Bozeat et al., 2002 found) the generalisation may have been based on visual similarity. In order to test this possibility, the 168 items were rated for typicality by 17 controls to obtain a mean typicality measure for each item. The typicality of the named and unnamed items was compared and CUB showed a significant effect of typicality, $t(166) = 3.349$, $p = .001$. For example, CUB made errors on the more atypically represented items, such as the cut bananas from Figure 2.

GENERAL DISCUSSION

Previous reports of relearning in cases of semantic dementia have shown poor retention of learning in both the short and longer term. Where learning has taken place, performance deteriorates when test items are presented in a different order or with different backgrounds (Snowden & Neary, 2002). We presented a case of semantic dementia, CUB, who had moderately severe anomia and semantic difficulties at the time of testing, which declined significantly during the therapy study. CUB was able to relearn and retain, over time, 28 names for common objects. Unlike previously reported people, she was still able to name these when they were presented in a different order from that used in therapy and when presented among control items she had not learned. Despite her excellent learning, there was some evidence of "rote" learning. Two items ("bañera" [bath] and "mesa" [table]) were learned as set phrases "baño, bañera" [bathroom, bath] and "mesa y silla" [table and chair] respectively. When CUB made an error she used the name of another item from within the therapy set, which may provide some additional indications of rigidity within the relearning—as has been found in previous relearning studies. When she was asked to name six other exemplars of each item she scored 155/168 (92%), making errors on those items that were not visually similar to the learned target. One of the most remarkable aspects of CUB's abilities in relearning was the retention 6 months after relearning when, in all other respects, she had deteriorated severely. At that time, CUB's performance on semantic tasks was at chance, her speech was empty and repetitive, she was unable to name items in the control set that she had previously been able to name, and she had begun to show behavioural problems such as kleptomania and wandering. Yet, without continued practice, she named 23/28 (88%) of the therapy set. This aspect of her performance contrasts with the previous studies. There are a number of possible explanations for such a striking difference and these are considered below.

Amount of therapy

The amount of time CUB was asked to spend on relearning was longer than in the three other cases. CUB was asked to look at the CD-ROM every day for a month. The other cases varied from 2 weeks (Graham et al., 1999) to 3 weeks (Jokel et al., 2002, 2006; Snowden & Neary, 2002). CUB's husband reported that she did make an effort to look at the CD-ROM each day and, by day 3 of the month, she was able to recall the words without recourse to the written help on the next page. This suggests that she may have performed equally as well if she had been tested at 2 or 3 weeks after the start of her self-learning. It might equally be the case that the continued rehearsal of the items over the month, with the picture and written feedback, was critical in the successful maintenance of her learning. This study cannot distinguish between these two possibilities.

Number of items

The number of items that CUB was asked to learn (28) differed from other studies, which varied from a maximum 100 words from within five different categories (Graham et al., 1999) to 20 autobiographical items (Snowden & Neary, 2002). The closest in set size to CUB's 28 items was AK (Jokel et al., 2002, 2006) who, although asked to learn 90 items in total, was given these in three sets of 30 items at a time. AK's results at 1 month on the –N+C set was 13/30, a significantly poorer result than CUB's 27/28 ($\chi^2 = 16.39$, $df = 1$, $p < .001$) while at 6 months she retained 9/30 compared to CUB's 23/28 ($\chi^2 = 11.13$, $df = 1$, $p < .001$). However, the exact influence of the number of items is hard to gauge since there are too few studies with enough variation in set size to enable clear conclusions to be drawn.

Therapy method and item selection

There was remarkable similarity in the way each participant was taught the correct phonology for the items they were learning, each being a version of picture–name paired learning. In Frattali's study (2004), if the participant was unable to name a picture, then he was given the correct phonology for the word (either by reading aloud or repeating) before learning. Three cases (Graham et al., 1999; Jokel et al., 2002; Snowden & Neary, 2002) used a "look, attempt to name, repeat after me/read aloud if unable to say" method which was also used in this study. Thus, each participant appeared to undergo remarkably similar treatment protocols.

There were differences in the way items were selected and how the items were supported within the therapy programme. In one of the experiments for example, DM (Graham et al., 1999) generated his own words using a category fluency paradigm, whereas in a later experiment and in the other studies, controlled, researcher-generated word lists were used. CR (Snowden & Neary, 2002) used self-study in a similar way to CUB but via a booklet rather than CD-ROM and links were made to her own environment. Both CR (Snowden & Neary, 2002) and AK (Jokel et al., 2002, 2006) made use of biographical information to expand the information provided during relearning. CR made explicit links between her word relearning and her environment, while AK provided her own definitions for the words in her learning set which were then used during relearning. CUB was able to relearn using a simplified therapy format, without reference to autobiographical information. When CUB did ask for assistance from her husband (for example to name the chair), she learned the word in the context of the phrase he provided for her, "table and chair", suggesting that she learned how to pair the picture to the phonology provided. Thus, it would appear that variations in therapy method and item selection do not account for CUB's therapy results.

Severity of semantic memory

Differences in severity have been suggested for the different patterns between DM (Graham et al., 1999, 2001) and CR (Snowden & Neary, 2002). DM's semantic impairment was mild while all the other cases showed moderate to severe semantic impairment and anomia (see Table 1). If degree of semantic impairment and anomia were indicators of relearning ability, then CUB would be expected to perform in line with CR (Snowden & Neary, 2002), AK (Jokel et al., 2002, 2006) and Frattali's case (2004). Yet her relearning was superior and more resistant to loss across time than any of these. This is all the more perplexing given that, by the end of the study, CUB had the worst score on PPT (18/52).

Degree of atrophy

Table 1 sets out the scan reports for each case and from these it would be difficult to build a case for suggesting that differences in the location and extent of atrophy could account for the difference in relearning and retention. It may be that the relative sparing of other anatomical areas (such as the hippocampus and other medial temporal lobe structures) determines whether relearning can occur (assuming these structures underpin new learning: McClelland, McNaughton, & O'Reilly, 1995). However, reports based on visual inspection of the scans do not allow any formal exploration of any fine anatomical differences between the cases.

Premorbid experience and behavioural differences

There is little to suggest that premorbid differences could account for CUB's differential relearning. The occupations of KB and CK are not reported. However, DM was a retired surgeon, AK an arts organiser, and Frattali's (2004) case was a retired army officer. CUB was a high-functioning civil servant and so it would appear that all four were relatively well educated and motivated to retain and relearn. DM (Graham et al., 1999, 2001) and AK (Jokel et al., 2006) are both reported to have been fixated on the words they were losing, noting them down in a book, finding definitions in a dictionary, and devising their own ways to relearn them. CUB was similar to both of these in that she was obsessed by the loss of words and motivated to relearn them. It is interesting to note that the few therapy studies reported to date have been carried out with people who were fixated on their vocabulary loss. Consequently, there is a need to look across a more unselected group of people with semantic dementia to see whether others, who do not show this tendency, are also able to relearn.

Functional use/spontaneous speech

CUB's husband reported that, during and following therapy, she was able to use words she had learned at home appropriately. This functional use of therapy items in her spontaneous speech suggests that generalisation may have enabled a kind of "informal" practice, which allowed the words to be maintained for longer. This result is consistent with observations from other studies showing that everyday use and autobiographical knowledge enables longer-term retention of specific vocabulary as well as nonverbal activities such as object use (Bozeat et al., 2002; Snowden et al., 1994). The only aspect of her performance that does not seem to fit perfectly with this hypothesis is the (few) items that she named incorrectly at the 6-month follow-up (see Table 4). A number of these seem to relate more directly to everyday experience (bed, balloon, piano, hat, and cow) than some of the retained names (e.g., dromedary). Given this observation and the small number of unnamed items, future studies are required that incorporate a deliberate manipulation and careful testing within the functional framework of the participant's life.

In summary, it would appear that generalisation to spontaneous speech may be the most likely cause of CUB's excellent learning and maintenance of learnt names despite no formal practice. Other factors may be important in the success of relearning in semantic dementia too, but these possibilities will need further exploration in future studies that allow direct comparisons across cases.

We finish with a brief note on the relearning mechanisms that are harnessed in these patients. In this regard the complementary learning systems (McClelland et al., 1995) are a useful framework in which to think about learning both for normal participants and patient groups. Using an implemented PDP model, McClelland et al. argued that learning is supported by two interactive mechanisms each with different characteristics. Hippocampal/medial temporal lobe structures allow for rapid learning of novel associations across modalities but do so at the cost of rigid representations that permit limited generalisation from one example to another. The counter-combination (slow learning that licenses generalisation) is afforded by neocortical structures including those in more lateral temporal lobe structures (which bear the brunt of the atrophy in semantic dementia). Learning in the normal, intact system involves the two learning mechanisms working in tandem, thereby allowing rapid initial representation of the experienced events/stimuli and then the gradual formation of representations that allow generalisation across examples. In patients with amnesia following medial temporal lobe damage, the rapid learning system is impaired but slow learning and subsequent generalisation are possible via the neocortical learning system.

Patients with semantic dementia can be considered as a reversal of this pattern; while they do have medial as well as inferolateral temporal lobe damage, the neural circuits underlying new learning have good metabolism (Nestor, Fryer, & Hodges, 2006)—thus allowing the rapid yet rigid medial temporal lobe system to function. In contrast, the inferolateral regions are often severely atrophied and have a corresponding hypometabolism (Nestor et al., 2006). This aligns clearly with the notion that these regions are involved in long-term semantic representations that allow for appropriate generalisations (Rogers et al., 2004). It is possible, therefore, that the picture name learning observed in CUB and other patients with semantic dementia primarily reflects the functioning of the medial temporal lobe system. In this context, one can view name learning as the novel association of a picture (visual representation) with a name (phonological representation). The medial temporal lobe system can rapidly learn to associate the two over a small number of learning trials but this learning is inevitably rigid in nature—thus the patients often reproduce the information in exactly the same way (e.g., preserving the learning order, cues and build-up information that was presented at the time of learning, etc.). With impoverished long-term semantic representations, the patients are then unable to generalise this learning appropriately and can only do so when the novel stimulus is very similar (visually for pictures or phonologically for words). Accordingly, the learning tends to be limited to the exact stimulus used in the learning trials and cannot be generalised to another example of the same type (e.g., CUB did not generalise the name "banana" from a standard picture to slices of banana, but did to visually similar depictions). Information encoded in medial temporal lobe structures needs to be actively maintained through continued re-exposure—i.e., by continuous, repeated deliberate practice or, as would appear to be the most likely explanation for CUB's good retention, through generalisation to everyday use.

REFERENCES

Benton, A. L., Hamsher, K., Varney, N. R., & Spreen, O. (1978). *Contributions to neuropsychological assessment: Facial recognition*. New York: Oxford University Press.

Borkowsky, J. G., Benton, A. L., & Spreen, O. (1967). Word fluency and brain damage. *Neuropsychologia, 5*, 135–140.

Bozeat, S., Gregory, C. A., Ralph, M. A. L., & Hodges, J. R. (2000a). Which neuropsychiatric and behavioural features distinguish frontal and temporal variants of frontotemporal dementia from Alzheimer's disease? *Journal of Neurology Neurosurgery and Psychiatry, 69*, 178–186.

Bozeat, S., Ralph, M. A. L., Patterson, K., Garrard, P., & Hodges, J. R. (2000b). Non-verbal semantic impairment in semantic dementia. *Neuropsychologia, 38*, 1207–1215.

Bozeat, S., Ralph, M. A. L., Patterson, K., & Hodges, J. R. (2002). The influence of personal familiarity and context on object use in semantic dementia. *Neurocase, 8*, 127–134.

Cooper, J. E. (1970). The Leyton Obsessional Inventory. *Psychological Medicine, 1*, 48–64.

Davis, C., & Perea, M. (2005). BuscaPalabras: A program for deriving orthographic and phonological neighbourhood statistics and other psycholinguistic indices in Spanish. *Behavior Research, Methods, Instruments and Computers, 37*, 665–671.

Dunn, L. M., & Dunn, L. M. (1997). *Peabody Picture Vocabulary Test*. Circle Pines, MN: American Guidance Service.

Folstein, M. F., Folstein, S. E., & McHugh, P. R. (1975). Mini-Mental State Examination (MMSE). *Journal of Psychiatric Research, 12*, 189–198.

Frattali, C. (2004). An errorless learning approach to treating dysnomia in frontotemporal dementia. *Journal of Medical Speech-Language Pathology, 12*, XI XXIV.

Graham, K., Patterson, K., Pratt, K., & Hodges, J. (1999). Relearning and subsequent forgetting of semantic category exemplars in a case of semantic dementia. *Neuropsychology, 13*, 359–380.

Graham, K., Patterson, K., Pratt, K., & Hodges, J. (2001). Can repeated exposure to 'forgotten' vocabulary help alleviate word-finding difficulties in semantic dementia? An illustrative case study. *Neuropsychological Rehabilitation, 11*, 429–454.

Hodges, J. R., Patterson, K., Oxbury, S., & Funnel, E. (1992). Progressive fluent aphasia with temporal lobe atrophy. *Brain, 115*, 1783–1806.

Howard, D., & Patterson, K. (1992). *Palm Trees and Pyramids*. Bury St Edmunds, UK: Thames Valley Test Company.

Jefferies, E., Jones, R. W., Bateman, D., & Lambon Ralph, M. A. (2005). A semantic contribution to nonwords recall? Evidence for intact phonological processes in semantic dementia. *Cognitive Neuropsychology, 22*, 183–212.

Jefferies, E., & Lambon Ralph, M. A. (2006). Semantic impairment in stroke aphasia vs. semantic dementia: A case-series comparison. *Brain, 129*, 2132–2147.

Jokel, R., Rochon, E., & Leonard, C. (2002). Therapy for anomia in semantic dementia. *Brain and Cognition, 49*, 241–244.

Jokel, R., Rochon, E., & Leonard, C. (2006). Treating anomia in semantic dementia: Improvement, maintenance, or both? *Neuropsychological Rehabilitation, 16*, 241–256.

Kaplan, E., Goodglass, H., & Weintraub, S. (1983). *Boston Naming Test*. Philadelphia, USA: Lea & Febiger.

Kay, J., Lesser, R., & Coltheart, M. (1992). *Psycholinguistic Assessments of Language Processing in Aphasia (PALPA)*. Hove, UK: Lawrence Erlbaum Associates Ltd.

Kertesz, A. (1982). *Western Aphasia Battery*. New York: Grune & Stratton.

Kertesz, A., Davidson, W., & Fox, H. (1997). Frontal behavioral inventory: Diagnostic criteria for frontal lobe dementia. *Canadian Journal of Neurological Sciences, 24*, 29–36.

Lambon Ralph, M. A., & Howard, D. (2000). Gogi aphasia or semantic dementia? Simulating and assessing poor verbal comprehension in a case of progressive fluent aphasia. *Cognitive Neuropsychology, 17*, 437–465.

Lambon Ralph, M. A., McClelland, J., Patterson, K., Galton, C. J., & Hodges, J. (2001). No right to speak? The relationship between object naming and semantic impairment: neuropsychological evidence and a computational model. *Journal of Cognitive Neuroscience, 13*, 341–356.

McClelland, J. L., McNaughton, B. L., & O'Reilly, R. (1995). Why there are complementary learning systems in the hippocampus and neocortex: Insights from the successes and failures of connectionist models of learning and memory. *Psychological Review, 102*, 419–457.

McClelland, J. L., & Rogers, T. T. (2003). The parallel distributed processing approach to semantic cognition. *Nature Reviews Neuroscience, 4*, 310–322.

Nestor, P. J., Fryer, T. D., & Hodges, J. R. (2006). Declarative memory impairments in Alzheimer's disease and semantic dementia. *Neuroimage, 30*, 1010–1020.

Osterreith, R. (1995). Complex figure of Rey. In M. Lezak (Ed.), *Neuropsychological assessment* (3rd ed.). Oxford, UK: Oxford University Press.

Peña Casanova, J., Gramunt, N., & Gich Fullà, J. (2004). *Tests neuropsicológicos*. Barcelona: Masson.

Patterson, K., Graham, N., & Hodges, J. (1994). The impact of semantic memory loss on phonological representations. *Journal of Cognitive Neuroscience, 6*, 57–69.

Patterson, K., Lambon Ralph, M. A., Jefferies, E., Woollams, A., Jones, R., & Hodges, J. et al. (2006). 'Pre-semantic' cognition in semantic dementia: Six deficits in search of an explanation. *Journal of Cognitive Neuroscience, 18*, 169–183.

Patterson, K., Okada, S., Suzuki, T., Ijuin, M., & Tatsum, I. (1998). Fragmented words: A case of late-stage progressive aphasia. *Neurocase, 4*, 219–230.

Raven, J. C. (1985). *Raven's Progressive Matrices* (23rd ed.). London: H. K. Lewis & Co.

Rogers, T., Lambon Ralph, M. A., Garrard, P., Bozeat, S., McClelland, J. L., & Hodges, J. R. et al. (2004). Structure and deterioration of semantic memory: A neuropsychological and computational investigation. *Psychological Review, 111*, 205–235.

Snowden, J. S., Bathgate, D., Varma, A., Blackshaw, A., Gibbons, Z. C., & Neary, D. (2001). Distinct behavioural profiles in frontotemporal dementia and semantic dementia. *Journal of Neurology Neurosurgery and Psychiatry, 70*, 323–332.

Snowden, J. S., Griffiths, H. L., & Neary, D. (1995). Autobiographical experience and word meaning. *Memory, 3*, 225–246.

Snowden, J. S., & Neary, D. (2002). Relearning of verbal labels in semantic dementia. *Neuropsychologia, 40*, 1715–1728.

Snowden, J. S., Thompson, J. C., & Neary, D. (2004). Knowledge of famous faces and names in semantic dementia. *Brain, 127*, 860–872.

Valle, F., & Cuetos, F. (1995). *EPLA: Evaluación del procesamiento lingüístico en la afasia. Spanish edition: PALPA*. Hove, UK: Lawrence Erlbaum associates Ltd.

Wechsler, D. (1976). *WAIS: Escala de Inteligencia de Wechsler para adultos. Adaptación Española*. Madrid: TEA Ediciones S.A.

APPENDIX

THERAPY AND CONTROL ITEMS WITH THEIR ENGLISH TRANSLATIONS

Therapy set	Translation	Control set	Translation
plátano	banana	ancla	anchor
cama	bed	flecha	arrow
campana	bell	cesta	basket
mariposa	butterfly	pájaro	bird
botón	button	hueso	bone
dromedario	dromedary	libro	book
vela	candle	cámara	camera
iglesia	church	queso	cheese
payaso	clown	cigarro	cigarette
peine	comb	reloj	watch
vaca	cow	corona	crown
tenedor	fork	perro	dog
guitarra	guitar	pato	duck
sombrero	hat	elefante	elephant
luna	moon	uva	grape
lápiz	pencil	corazón	heart
piano	piano	caballo	horse
tijeras	scissors	plancha	iron
zapato	shoe	cocina	kitchen
cuchara	spoon	ratón	mouse
sol	sun	nariz	nose
mesa	table	pera	pear
corbata	tie	pipa	pipe
hacha	axe	cochecito	pram
globo	balloon	radio	radio
bañera	bath	sandwich	sandwich
cinturón	belt	camisa	shirt
autobús	bus	paraguas	umbrella

APHASIOLOGY, 2009, 23 (2), 210–235

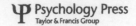

Known, lost, and recovered: Efficacy of formal-semantic therapy and spaced retrieval method in a case of semantic dementia

Nathalie Bier

Université de Sherbrooke, Canada

Joël Macoir

Université Laval, Canada

Lise Gagnon

Université de Sherbrooke, Canada

Martial Van der Linden

University of Geneva, Switzerland

Stéphanie Louveaux

Research Center on Aging, CSSS-Sherbrooke Geriatric University Institute, Canada

Johanne Desrosiers

Université de Sherbrooke, Canada

Background: Few studies have addressed rehabilitation in semantic dementia. A potentially promising method is formal-semantic therapy, which consists of tasks in which the names of concepts and their semantic characteristics are presented. It could also be enhanced by spaced retrieval, a learning method improving retention through recalling information after increasing recall intervals.
Aims: This study explores the efficacy of both a formal-semantic therapy and the spaced retrieval method to restore lost concepts in TBo, a woman with semantic dementia.
Methods & Procedures: The formal-semantic therapy consisted of giving TBo semantic feedback followed by a cueing technique to facilitate naming. Formal-semantic therapy with simple repetition was compared to formal-semantic therapy with spaced retrieval. TBo's performance was measured throughout the study with picture naming and

---

Address correspondence to: Nathalie Bier, Research Center on Aging, CSSS-IUSG, 1036, rue Belvédère Sud, Sherbrooke, Québec, Canada, J1H 4C4. E-mail: Nathalie.Bier@USherbrooke.ca

The first author was supported by PhD awards from the Quebec Rehabilitation Research Network, the Canadian Institutes of Health Research, the Interdisciplinary Training in Research on Health and Aging, and the Ordre des ergothérapeutes du Québec. The authors also wish to thank TBo for her enthusiastic participation in this study, as well as Lindsey Nickels, Karen Croot, Kim S. Graham and two anonymous reviewers for their invaluable comments on earlier drafts of this paper.

---

http://www.psypress.com/aphasiology   DOI: 10.1080/00207590801942906

generation of verbal attributes. Two untrained lists were also measured for generalisation effects.

Outcomes & Results: Results indicate that, after therapy, TBo could name 3/8 of the trained items, compared to no items on the untrained lists. She also showed an increase in performance for the evocation of specific semantic attributes of concepts, reaching 6/8 of correct responses. Moreover, she maintained her performance up to 5 weeks after the end of the study. Finally, when compared to simple repeated practice, spaced retrieval did not enhance learning and no generalisation was observed between trained and non-trained categories.

Conclusions: Along with recent results reported in the literature, TBo's results confirm that people with semantic dementia can improve their naming performance with training but that this is limited. However, formal-semantic therapy seems very promising for retraining specific semantic attributes. Instead of focusing on naming, we suggest that therapies used in semantic dementia should aim at restoring specific and functionally relevant concepts to enable the individuals to be more autonomous in daily living.

Keywords: Semantic dementia; Intervention; Learning; Aphasia; Formal-semantic therapy; Spaced retrieval.

Semantic dementia (SD) is a variant of frontotemporal dementia, characterised by progressive deterioration of semantic memory (Neary et al., 1998). Neuroradiological studies revealed that people with SD have focal atrophy of the temporal neocortex, generally more marked on the left side (Graham, Simons, Pratt, Patterson, & Hodges, 2000; Lambon Ralph, Graham, Ellis, & Hodges, 1998; Neary et al., 1998; Snowden, Goulding, & Neary, 1989). With respect to language, SD is responsible for word comprehension and naming deficits, whereas phonology and syntax are usually well preserved (Neary et al., 1998). Spelling impairment characterised by surface agraphia has also been reported in many cases of SD (e.g., Macoir & Bernier, 2002). On neuropsychological tests, these individuals often present with difficulties on any tasks requiring the activation of conceptual knowledge (Kertesz, Davidson, & McCabe, 1998; Papagno & Capitani, 2001; Schwarz, De Bleser, Poeck, & Weis, 1998). However, they show normal or near normal visuo-spatial capacities, perception, nonverbal reasoning, and problem-solving (Neary et al., 1998; Papagno & Capitani, 2001). People with SD also seem to have near normal episodic memory for perceptual information (Graham et al., 2000; Simons, Graham, Galton, Patterson, & Hodges, 2001) but episodic memory for verbal information is usually impaired (Graham, Patterson, Powis, Drake, & Hodges, 2002). With the progression of the disease, functional autonomy is progressively compromised since these individuals live in a world they can no longer understand. Consequently, cognitive intervention aimed at facilitating relearning of the lost knowledge necessary for everyday life function would appear to be of great interest in helping these people.

There have been very few studies aimed at relearning lost concepts in SD. According to some of these studies (Funnell, 2001; Graham, Patterson, Pratt, & Hodges, 2001; Jokel, Rochon, & Leonard, 2006; Snowden & Neary, 2002), people with SD can learn new verbal information. However, the new learning is generally modest and the participants show a rapid decline in performance after the end of the intervention. In fact, this learning seems to be dependent on many variables. First, the level of severity of the semantic deficit and, more specifically, the residual semantic knowledge could be a possible success factor (Graham, Patterson, Pratt, & Hodges, 1999; Jokel et al., 2006;

Snowden & Neary, 2002). For example, AK (Jokel et al., 2006) showed improved retrieval for 60% of concept names for which she showed residual knowledge on a word-to-picture matching task, as compared to a 37% improvement for concepts that she was unable to match correctly. Second, the presence of an episodic referent could also facilitate the relearning of concepts (Snowden & Neary, 2002). More specifically, new learning in people with SD could be tied to daily experiences that allow them to link the semantic information with a specific temporo-spatial context. For example, Snowden and Neary (2002) showed that CR remembered object names better when she frequently encountered those objects in her home environment.

Finally, as pointed out by Graham and colleagues (2001), the learning methods used by the participants to relearn lists of object names may also contribute to the modest performances observed. In fact, people with SD who participated in relearning studies (Funnell, 2001; Snowden & Neary, 2002) seemed to have learned the list of object names within a specific temporo-spatial context. For example, when they were required to name relearned objects presented in random order (Snowden & Neary, 2002), their performances decreased significantly. They also had a tendency to produce within-list errors instead of semantic errors (Graham et al., 1999; Snowden & Neary, 2002). Moreover, they presented specific improvement for trained items, without any generalisation to other tasks or modalities (Graham et al., 1999). These observations suggest that the type of learning method used, mainly rote learning, did not actually mobilise the semantic memory system.

In order to facilitate this mobilisation, and thus a more in-depth treatment of concepts, interventions might employ semantic therapies used in non-degenerative fluent aphasia (i.e., aphasia following stroke or traumatic brain injury). These therapies focus on restoring lost concepts and discriminating between these concepts (for a review, see Nickels, 2000). Even if they seem very relevant for people with SD, to our knowledge these therapies have never been used with this population. In semantic therapy, people with aphasia have to perform semantic processing when presented with a spoken or written word stimulus (e.g., semantic question: Is an apple a fruit?). These tasks are known as formal-semantic, in contrast to "pure" semantic tasks in which the target name is never produced, by the therapist or the participant (Nickels, 2000). Formal-semantic tasks have been used in aphasia, but not extensively, and have proven to be more effective with naming disorders than pure semantic tasks (de Partz, 2003; LeDorze, Boulay, Gaudreau, & Brassard, 1994).

The following types of improvement have been reported after formal-semantic treatment of aphasic naming disorders: (1) improvement specific to trained items (Behrmann & Lieberthal, 1989; LeDorze & Pitts, 1995; Marshall, Pound, White-Thompson, & Pring, 1990; Nettleton & Lesser, 1991; Wambaugh et al., 2001); (2) generalisation of improvement for trained items in tasks involving different modalities (Grayson, Hilton, & Franklin, 1997; Hillis, 1990)—for example, following a written naming task applied during treatment, HG (Hillis, 1990) showed improvement on treated items in tasks that recruit different input and output modalities such as auditory word–picture matching, spoken naming, repetition, and writing to dictation—(3) generalisation of treatment gains to untrained items belonging to the same categories as trained items (Behrmann & Lieberthal, 1989; Hillis, 1990). The study conducted with HG, a woman presenting with mixed aphasia following a traumatic brain injury (Hillis, 1990), illustrates an effective formal-semantic treatment. HG showed a semantic impairment leading to difficulties in differentiating between closely related concepts (e.g., tiger–lion). The purpose of the therapy was to help HG relearn semantic distinctions through a written naming task of drawings with semantic feedback. When an error was produced, the feedback consisted of emphasising the semantic attribute distinctions between the word produced and the target word. Results indicate that the semantic treatment was effective in improving HG's abilities to produce the trained names, not just in written picture naming but also in tasks performed in different modalities (e.g., oral naming, writing to dictation, reading).

As for formal-semantic therapies, the impact of methods on the efficacy of treatment has not yet been explored in SD. As already mentioned, participants involved in treatment studies are generally not exposed to specific learning methods (e.g., organising concepts by categories, increasing recall intervals). Learning methods, which optimise learning in normal learners by facilitating the encoding and retrieval of information (Baddeley, 1994), could be combined with a formal-semantic therapy to potentially enhance the effects of treatment and ensure long-term maintenance. In this respect, spaced retrieval could be of great interest since it combines the well-known effects of distributed practice (Hintzman, Summers, & Block, 1975; Russo, Mammarella, & Avons, 2002) with retrieval effects (Bjork, 1988; Landauer & Bjork, 1978; Wheeler, Ewers, & Buonanno, 2003). *Distributed practice* refers to the fact that training distributed in time is more effective than intensive training done over a short period of time (i.e., massed repetition). *Retrieval effects* refer to the long-term superiority of training done by successive recovery of information as compared to encoding carried out on several occasions. Operationally, in the spaced retrieval method, the participant is asked to recollect information after increasing time intervals, filled by a general spoken conversation or any other task. At the beginning of the treatment, time intervals are close enough to ensure learning (15 seconds, 30 seconds, 1 minute). Thereafter, the intervals are spaced according to the participant's performance: if the participant makes a mistake, the error is immediately corrected and the last successful interval is repeated, after which the time series continues (Camp, Foss, Stevens, & O'Hanlon, 1996). This method is very effective with normal learners to ensure learning and long-term retention (Landauer & Bjork, 1978), and has already been successfully used in Alzheimer's disease for relearning different kinds of information, such as face–name learning (Camp & Stevens, 1990), calendar use (Camp et al., 1996; McKitrick, Camp, & Black, 1992), and using a mobile phone (Lekeu, Wojtasik, Van der Linden, & Salmon, 2002). It has also been successfully used for the treatment of naming deficits in neurodegenerative diseases (Brush & Camp, 1998; McKitrick & Camp, 1993). Thus, this method may be promising to ensure learning and long-term retention in SD as well.

The general aim of the present study was to explore, in a woman suffering from SD, the efficacy of a formal-semantic therapy combined with a spaced retrieval method considered an optimisation factor. More specifically, the objectives were as follows: (1) to explore the efficacy of a formal-semantic therapy in relearning concepts (name and semantic attributes); (2) to assess the impact of the addition of the spaced retrieval method on this therapy compared to a simple repetition method; (3) to explore the long-term maintenance of the effects of the formal-semantic therapy with the spaced retrieval method compared to a simple repetition method; and, finally, (4) to explore possible effects of generalisation within trained categories and between trained and non-trained categories.

CASE REPORT

TBo is a 70-year-old, right-handed housewife, living with her husband in an apartment. She is a native French speaker and has a grade 9 education. In April 2004 she was referred to the Geriatric Program at the Quebec City Centre Hospitalier Universitaire because of word-finding and memory problems. At that time, TBo felt these problems had begun up to 5 years earlier, with progressive worsening. TBo essentially complained of difficulties in finding words during conversation. Her husband also noticed word-finding as well as spelling problems at home that often led to frustration and discouragement. Progressively, she stopped taking care of housekeeping (shopping, meal preparation, and domestic tasks). She maintained social contacts with friends and family, although she was sometimes confused about the names of her children and grandchildren as well as their occupations. A single photon emission computed tomography, as well as a magnetic resonance imaging (MRI) study including sagittal FLAIR and T2-weighted sequences and axial FLAIR, proton density, T1 and T2-weighted sequences were performed in November 2003. Both exams showed mild to moderate cortical atrophy, more marked around the left sylvian fissure and a left frontal hypoperfusion. There was no relevant medical history and all the biological and blood tests were normal. The neuropsychological and language examinations were conducted in September 2003 and March 2004 respectively. Testing was performed in French, with norms for the Quebec-French population.

Neuropsychological examination

Neuropsychological testing (see Table 1) showed no clinical signs of visuo-spatial deficits except for the object decision tasks of the Birmingham Object Recognition Battery (Riddoch & Humphreys, 1993). TBo's general nonverbal problem solving was between the 25th and the 50th percentile (Raven, 1938). For episodic memory, she performed within the normal range for tasks using perceptual information, except for part B of the Doors Test (Baddeley, Emslie, & Nimmo-Smith, 1994). She showed abnormal performance on some tasks measuring working memory, and particularly on the letter–number sequencing task (Wechsler, 1997), which measures the executive aspect of working memory. TBo also presented with difficulties in other executive functions, namely inhibition (Stroop test; Golden, 1978) and flexibility (Trail Making Test; Tombaugh, 2004).

Language examination

With regard to language (see Table 2), speech output was fluent, well-articulated, and grammatically correct but presented many signs of word-finding difficulties: aborted sentences, long response latencies, and occasional semantic paraphasias. Letter fluency was poor. Repetition was flawless for both words and nonwords. Reading was slightly impaired but within normal range, and marked by the presence of occasional regularisation errors. Written spelling of nonwords was flawless but TBo's performance on word writing to dictation for regular and irregular words was typical of surface agraphia, with the only errors being phonologically plausible errors and performance affected by orthographic regularity and lexical frequency. A similar pattern of error was also observed on a written picture-naming task. At the

TABLE 1
TBo's general neuropsychological evaluation

Neuropsychological testing	TBo
Visuo-spatial functions	
Benton Visual Form Discrimination (32)	29
Birmingham Object Recognition Battery (BORB):	
Length match task (30)	29
Size match task (30)	27
Minimal feature match (25)	24
Foreshortened match (25)	19
Object decision – easy (32)	30
Object decision – hard (32)	20*
General nonverbal problem solving	
Raven's Coloured Progressive Matrices (36)	25
Episodic memory	
DMS-48:	
Immediate recognition (48)	100% (276 s)
Delayed recognition – 1 hour (48)	98% (290 s)
Delayed recognition – 7 days (48)	94%
Warrington Face Recognition Test (50)	41
The Doors Test: Easy (12) – Hard (12)	10 – 4*
Spatial and temporal orientation (WAIS-III) (14)	12
Working memory	
Corsi block-tapping – forward	12*
Word span	3
Digit span – forward (WAIS-III)	3
Letter number sequencing	2*
Executive functions	
Stroop Test:	
Word reading	74
Colour naming	108*
Interference	250*
Trail Making Test – A	4 min*
Trail Making Test – B	_**

* Significantly impaired (more than 2 *SD* under scores of age- and education-matched control participants). ** Unable to complete the test. References for tests as follows: Benton visual form discrimination (Benton, Sivan, Hamsher, Varney, & Spreen, 1994); Birmingham Object Recognition Battery (Riddoch & Humphreys, 1993); Raven's Coloured Progressive Matrices (Raven, 1938); DMS-48 (Barbeau et al., 2004); The Doors Test (Baddeley et al., 1994); Spatial and temporal orientation (WAIS-III) (Wechsler, 1997); Corsi Block-Tapping Task (Kessels, van Zandvoort, Postma, Kappelle, & de Haan, 2000); Word span (Joanette et al., 1995); Forward digit span (WAIS-III) (Wechsler, 1997); Letter–number sequencing (WAIS-III) (Wechsler, 1997); Stroop Test (Golden, 1978); Trail Making Test (Tombaugh, 2004).

syntactico-semantic level, TBo performed normally in the spoken sentence–picture matching task. Her performance was slightly below the cutoff score for the written condition of the task, as well as for the shortened version of the Token Test (De Renzi & Faglioni, 1978). Finally, TBo was severely impaired in all tasks exploring semantic memory. Semantic category fluency (Joanette et al., 1995) was extremely poor and TBo encountered serious difficulties in confrontation naming investigated with the DO 80 (Deloche & Hannequin, 1997). In this task she mainly produced

TABLE 2
TBo's language investigation

Language testing	TBo
Lexical aspects of language	
Letter fluency (total PLT)	15*
Immediate and delayed repetition of words and nonwords	N
Reading	
Regular words (5)	5
Irregular words (15)	11
Nonwords (5)	3
Writing to dictation:	
Regular words (12)	11
Irregular words (15)	5*
Nonwords (5)	5
Written picture naming (15)	1*
Spoken word and sentence–picture matching (MT-86) (47)	37
Written word and sentence–picture matching (MT-86) (13)	8
Token Test (36)	25
Semantic memory	
Semantic Category Fluency (total)	11*
DO 80 (80) (picture-naming test)	57*
Pyramids and Palm Trees Test:	
Picture–picture (52)	37*
Word–word (52)	36*

*Comparison with control participants significantly different, with $p < .05$. Legend: N = normal performance according to norms. References for tests as follows: Letter Fluency (Joanette et al., 1995); MT-86 (Nespoulos et al., 1992); Token Test (De Renzi & Faglioni, 1978); Semantic Category Fluency (Joanette et al., 1995); D0 80 (Deloche & Hannequin, 1997); Pyramids and Palm Trees Test (Howard & Patterson, 1992).

semantic and visual-semantic paraphasias and showed problems of visual identification for two pictures. TBo also showed clear problems with semantic processing on the picture-to-picture association and the written word-to-written word association versions of the Pyramids and Palm Trees Test (Howard & Patterson, 1992).

Summary and diagnosis

Overall, TBo presented with deficits in all tests requiring semantic processing, whereas she performed almost normally on tests exploring visuo-perceptual abilities and visual episodic memory. Along with neuroimaging data, these results were suggestive of a clinical diagnosis of possible SD. TBo's semantic impairment as measured by the Pyramids and Palm Trees Tests was more marked than that of some other people with semantic dementia who have benefited from therapy (e.g., DM, reported by Graham et al., 1999), however her above-chance performance on a number of the additional semantic tests (see below) suggests that she had some remaining semantic knowledge about the sorts of items used in therapy. Since she also presented with difficulties in executive functions and working memory tests, the contribution of a frontal impairment to the clinical profile must also be considered. However, the presence of frontal impairment is not incompatible with a diagnosis of SD. Hypometabolism of the left frontal cortex has been observed in other individuals suffering from SD (Hodges, Patterson, Oxbury, & Funnell, 1992; Snowden et al., 1989).

A more detailed investigation of TBo's semantic impairments was conducted to assess her deficits regarding concrete and abstract concepts and attributes.

Investigation of the semantic deficit

We investigated the nature of TBo's semantic impairment through the administration of four semantic tasks: spoken word-to-picture matching, semantic similarity judgement, specific attribute-verification, and picture naming (see Table 3). In these tasks TBo's performance was compared to the results of five control participants by means of modified t tests (Crawford & Howell, 1998), which measure whether a single observation is significantly different from the mean of a small control sample. The five female controls had no cognitive impairment ($MMSE$ = 27.8; SD = 1.8) and were matched with TBo on age (mean = 71 ± 1.9) and years of education (mean = 7.2 ± 2.4). Modified t tests showed no differences between TBo and the control participants for age (t = .69, p = .53) or years of education (t = −.49, p = .33).

TABLE 3
TBo's performances on semantic tasks exploring her semantic deficits (mean performance)

Semantic task	TBo	Control participants
Specific attribute-verification task (156 items)	92*	130 ± 5.1
Living (76 items; critical value: 45)	42*	59.4 ± 3.21
Manufactured (48 items; critical value: 30)	32*	41.8 ± 1.3
Musical instruments (32 items; critical value: 21)	15*	28.8 ± 1.5
Perceptual attributes (78 items; critical value: 46)	47*	62.2 ± 1.8
Functional attributes (20 items; critical value: 14)	11*	17.4 ± 2.4
Encyclopaedic attributes (58 items; critical value: 35)	34*	51.6 ± 2.3
Picture naming (148 items)	88*	137 ± 9.17
Performance by categories:		
Living: (48 items)	20.7*	44.2 ± 4.4
Land animals (13 items)	9*	12 ± 1.2
Birds (9 items)	2*	8.8 ± .45
Insects (6 items)	.67*	5.6 ± .55
Fruits (10 items)	5*	9.2 ± 1.1
Vegetables (10 items)	4*	8.6 ± 1.67
Manufactured objects: (79 items)	55.7*	73 ± 5.1
Clothes (10 items)	6.7*	9.6 ± .55
Small manufactured objects (23 items)	15.3*	21 ± 1.41
Large manufactured objects (6 items)	3.7	5.6 ± .89
Tools (10 items)	6*	9.6 ± .55
Utensils and electric household appliances (11 items)	8.3*	10.4 ± 1.34
Furniture (9 items)	6.7	7.8 ± .84
Vehicles (10 items)	7*	9 ± .71
Musical instruments (11 items)	1.67*	10 ± .00
Body parts (10 items)	10	9.8 ± .45

*Comparison with control participants significantly different, with $p < .05$ (Crawford modified t tests).

Task 1: Spoken word-to-picture matching. TBo was given a spoken word–picture matching task (Caplan & Bub, 1992) in which she had to choose one of four pictures as a match to a spoken word. The picture set included the correct item and foils that were semantic, visuo-semantic, or unrelated. It comprised 20 pictures of living concepts (animals, fruits, vegetables) and 20 paired pictures of manufactured concepts (tools, household items) that were controlled for lexical frequency, familiarity, visual similarity, and word length. TBo's performance was below the mean of the control participants for living concepts only (14/20; 70%; $t = -10.2$; $p = .003$) and was at chance level (critical value = 14, $p = .50$ $\alpha = .95$). Her performance was much better than chance for manufactured concepts and was comparable to control participants (19/20; 95%; $t = -1.5$; $p = .11$).

Task 2: Semantic similarity judgement task. TBo was administered a semantic similarity judgement task on written words consisting of 40 concrete living triplets (e.g., *lapin – castor – lièvre*, "rabbit – beaver – hare") and 40 concrete manufactured triplets (e.g., *sofa – divan – tabouret*, "sofa – couch – stool") matched for lexical frequency, and familiarity. TBo was asked to point to the word that was least similar in meaning. Her performance was better than chance (critical value = 18, $p = .33$, $\alpha = .95$) but she was well below the mean of the control participants for both living (30/40; 75%; $t = -5.1$; $p = .003$) and manufactured concepts (34/40; 85%; $t = -4.7$; $p = .004$). The difference between living and manufactured concepts was not significant ($t = -1.11$; $p = .27$).

Task 3: Specific attribute-verification vask. In this task, we selected 19 living things, 12 manufactured objects, and 8 musical instruments from the black and white pictures of the Snodgrass and Vanderwart (1980) set and prepared a semantic questionnaire aimed at their specific attributes, i.e., attributes that were common to only some members of the category. For each stimulus, we created four statements, giving a total of 156 statements, aimed at perceptual, encyclopaedic, and functional attributes. Half of these statements were true and half were false. The contrast between true and false statements was designed to require fine-grained distinctions between close category coordinates. The 156 statements were presented three times and in random order.

As shown in Table 3, TBo was well below normal range for every type of statement (all observed p-values < .05). There were no significant differences between her performances on living things, manufactured objects and musical instruments (Kruskall-Wallis's $\chi^2 = 3.39$, $p = .184$). There were no significant differences in her performance between perceptual, encyclopaedic and functional attributes (Kruskal-Wallis's $\chi^2 = 0.014$, $p = .90$). Except for manufactured concepts and perceptual attributes, for which she was slightly above chance level, TBo was not better than chance for every type of statements (see Table 3).

Task 4: Picture naming. TBo's ability in picture naming was assessed through a list of stimuli composed of 148 black and white pictures (Snodgrass & Vanderwart, 1980). The experimental list was composed of 48 pictures of living concepts, 79 pictures of manufactured concepts, 11 pictures of musical instruments, and 10 pictures of body parts. Stimuli were presented three times in random order with no time limit. A picture was considered to be named accurately if TBo provided the correct target name or a possible alternative (e.g., cochon "pig"→ porc "pig").

As shown in Table 3, TBo was impaired for all semantic categories. The difference between TBo's and the controls' performance was significant (all observed p-values $< .01$). A significant difference between living, manufactured, musical instruments, and body parts was observed (Kruskal-Wallis's $\chi^2 = 32.9$, $p < .001$). TBo's performance was significantly lower for living concepts and musical instruments as compared to body parts and manufactured concepts (all observed p-values $< .001$). Her naming performance for musical instruments was particularly poor (15.2%; mean score for controls = 91%). In contrast, she presented with perfect performance for body parts (100%). Significant differences were observed between living subordinate categories (all observed p-values $< .02$). TBo's performance was particularly low for birds and insects (all observed p-values $< .01$). There was no significant difference in her performance between manufactured subordinate categories (Kruskal-Wallis's $\chi^2 = 3.9$; $p = .68$). Her performance was influenced by frequency and familiarity (frequency: Spearman's $r = .46$, $p < .0001$; familiarity: $r = .43$, $p < .0001$) as well as visual complexity ($r = -.32$, $p < .0001$). With respect to error analysis, TBo mainly produced semantic paraphasias (54%), followed by vague circumlocutions (19%) and "don't know" responses (16%). She also occasionally produced visual errors (3%; e.g., ball $\rightarrow$ moon) and sometimes indicated she did not recognise the depicted concept.

Summary and comments

To summarise, results from the four semantic tasks reveal that TBo presented with a semantic deficit affecting living and manufactured concepts. Results from the picture-naming task pointed to a more serious deficit for living objects and musical instruments than for manufactured objects, while naming abilities for body parts were intact. With respect to semantic attributes, results from the specific attribute-verification task also revealed that TBo presented with a general semantic deficit affecting specific attributes of concepts, whether they were of perceptual, encyclopaedic or functional types.

This profile suggested that the intervention should be oriented not only towards the retrieval of names but also include the relearning of specific semantic attributes of concepts. A specific intervention was planned to help TBo relearn object names and specific attributes with a formal-semantic therapy combined with the spaced retrieval method. The project was approved by the Research Ethics Committee of the Research Center on Aging in Sherbrooke, Canada. Informed written consent was obtained from TBo.

TREATMENT STUDY

Selection of treatment stimuli

Treatment stimuli were selected on the basis of TBo's performance on the picture-naming task and specific attribute-verification task. To choose items that were consistently failed, we searched for three consecutive failures on the same items in picture naming as well as for three consecutive failures on one or more of the four questions per item of the semantic questionnaire. In total, 41 items were consistently failed according to both criteria and were selected for treatment.

From TBo's performance on the neuropsychological evaluation, the semantic tasks and stimuli selection sessions, we observed that she became easily tired. To avoid fatigue and thus a possible floor effect, we limited the number of stimuli to 24 (see Appendix, Table A1). Three lists of eight stimuli were prepared based on their category membership and matched for familiarity, frequency, and visual complexity scores: a trained set (familiarity = 2.6 ± .64; frequency = 24 ± 27; visual complexity = 3.7 ± .79), a control set (familiarity = 2.5 ± .47; frequency = 12.5 ± 14.3; visual complexity = 4.0 ± .68), and a neutral set (familiarity = 2.6 ± .89; frequency = 14.2 ± 18.4; visual complexity = 3.1 ± .66). The trained set consisted of pictures and names belonging to the categories of fruits, birds, insects, and musical instruments. The control set consisted of pictures and names of the same categories and was prepared to assess possible generalisation across items from the same category. The neutral set was prepared to assess possible generalisation across different categories. It consisted of stimuli with no semantic relationships with stimuli from the target and control lists (vehicles, tools, miscellaneous objects, utensils, and kitchen appliances). All pictures were from the set of Snodgrass and Vanderwart (1980) pictures initially used to assess naming.

General design of the cognitive intervention

TBo was exposed to an alternating treatment design, ABCBCBCA, with multiple baselines (Ottenbacher, 1986; Wilson, 1987). The study comprised three general phases: the baseline phase (A), which consisted of measures taken before the interventions; the intervention phase (B and C); and the post-treatment phase consisting of measures taken after completion of the interventions (back to A). The intervention phase consisted of an alternation between intervention B,

TABLE 4
Treatment study design

Sessions	Intervention 1 (B) Spaced retrieval and semantic feedback	Intervention 2 (C) Repetition and semantic feedback
1	Baseline 1	Baseline 1
2	Baseline 2	Baseline 2
3	Baseline 3	Baseline 3
4	Picture naming – list 1	
5		Picture naming – list 2
6	Picture naming and generation of attributes – list 1	
7		Picture naming and generation of attributes – list 2
8	Picture naming and generation of attributes – list 1	
9		Picture naming and generation of attributes – list 2
10	Long-term retention measures (1 week)	Long-term retention measures (1 week)
11	Long-term retention measures (2 weeks)	Long-term retention measures (2 weeks)
12	Long-term retention measures (5 weeks)	Long-term retention measures (5 weeks)

formal-semantic therapy with a spaced retrieval method, and intervention C, formal-semantic therapy without specific learning method, which consisted of a simple repeated practice (see Table 4). The design consisted of measuring trained (target set) and untrained stimuli (control and neutral sets) during the entire study in order to assess the efficacy of the treatment and possible generalisation. TBo was exposed to three sessions of baseline testing, followed by six intervention sessions: three for intervention B and three for intervention C (two sessions per week). She was also exposed to three testing sessions for long-term retention, which took place 1, 3, and 5 weeks after the end of the intervention. The study took place over a period of 3 months. During the maintenance period, TBo did not have access to the material and we instructed her not to practise at home.

The simple repeated practice method was added to explore the possible superiority of spaced retrieval in terms of new learning and long-term retention. To compare the efficacy of the two learning methods, the eight treated items were divided into two lists of four items (see Appendix, Table A2), respectively assigned to intervention B (list 1) and intervention C (list 2). The two lists were matched in terms of familiarity (list 1 = 2.4; list 2 = 2.9), frequency (list 1 and list 2 < 50), and visual complexity (list 1 = 3.7; list 2 = 3.6). They comprise three different categories and were matched on two out of those three categories (list 1: birds, musical instruments, fruits, and vegetables; list 2: insects, musical instruments, fruits, and vegetables).

A: Baseline

The 24 selected stimuli were tested three times in the following two tasks during baseline sessions: picture naming and generation of verbal attributes from spoken words. The 24 stimuli were presented in random order to TBo. In the naming task, a picture was considered to be named accurately if TBo provided the correct target name only. Generation of verbal attributes consisted of asking TBo to give as many semantic attributes as possible for each of the 24 stimuli. General and specific attributes were accepted. General attributes were defined as attributes shared by all or most of the members of a category and specific attributes were defined as attributes only found for a few members of the category (Caramazza & Shelton, 1998).

For the two baseline tasks, TBo's performance was compared to the results of the same five female controls who took part in the semantic tasks investigating TBo's semantic impairments.

B and C: Intervention and measures

B: Formal-semantic therapy and spaced retrieval (sessions 4, 6, and 8). To summarise the procedure, each intervention session began with a presentation phase which consisted of presenting TBo with the four pictures (list 1) along with: (a) their corresponding spoken name, (b) a specific attribute (see Appendix), and (c) the written name of their category. This procedure was repeated twice altogether for the same four items, presented in random order. In session 4 the pictures were presented to TBo, who was asked to recall their corresponding names according to spaced retrieval with increasing time recall intervals. The instructions were: "Can you tell me the name of this object?" In the following sessions (6 and 8) she had to name the pictures and also give their attributes. The instructions were: "Can you tell me the name of this object and the things you know about it?" When the correct response was not produced (wrong answer or no answer), this was scored as an error and TBo was presented with the formal-semantic therapy procedure consisting of a semantic feedback and cueing technique.

Then, 15 minutes after the end of each session (4, 6, and 8), the complete list of 24 selected stimuli was presented to TBo for picture naming and generation of semantic attributes from spoken words.

Spaced retrieval: In session 4 the spaced retrieval method, based on Camp and colleagues' procedure (Camp et al., 1996), began after the presentation phase by showing TBo the first picture and asking her to recall its corresponding name (0-second recall interval). The picture was then hidden and presented for naming 15 seconds later. This procedure was repeated at increasing time recall intervals of 30 seconds, 1 minute, 1½ minutes, 2 minutes, 2½ minutes, 3 minutes, 3½ minutes, and so on, until the end of the session was reached. When TBo produced a semantic error, the experimenter used the semantic feedback and graded cueing technique described below. In the subsequent trial the experimenter returned to the last successful recall interval and, if successful, the series of recall intervals was continued. A new target was introduced when the preceding one reached its 1½-minute recall interval successfully, until all four targets were introduced. Each target then followed its own recall progression until the end of the session was reached. Thus, for the first item, gaps between each recall interval were initially filled with general conversation. When the first item reached its 1½-minute recall interval successfully, the second item was introduced. Thus, the gaps planned for the following intervals of the first item (2 minutes, 2½ minutes, 3 minutes, etc.) were first filled by the interval repetitions of the second item. When the second item reached its 1½-minute recall interval successfully, the third item was introduced and so on. Thus, the gaps of the remaining intervals of the first item were filled with recalls of the second, third, and then fourth items until the end of the session was reached. Consequently, during the spaced retrieval method condition, the number of times each item was presented was dependent on TBo's progression on each item.

In sessions 6 and 8, TBo had to give the corresponding name of each picture and also its specific semantic attributes. The recall intervals followed the same procedure as used for session 4.

Formal-semantic therapy: Semantic feedback and cueing technique. The goal of the formal-semantic therapy was to restore the link between the concept and its corresponding name through semantic feedback, directly based on Hillis's (1990) procedure. The feedback was introduced each time TBo made a semantic error when attempting to name a picture. It aimed at emphasising the differences between the object presented and the name given by TBo. For example, if TBo said "apple" when presented with the picture of a peach, the experimenter showed her the picture corresponding to the erroneous response and contrasted the different semantic attributes between it and the target item (e.g., "The apple has a smooth shiny skin and may be grown in Quebec, the peach has a soft textured skin and cannot be grown in Quebec"). When TBo was unable to give a response, a graded cueing technique was used, which consisted of giving the following cues one by one until a correct response was produced: (1) first the category membership of the item, (2) then a semantic cue (specific attribute) if she was still unable to produce the answer, and (3) finally a phonemic cue (first letter or first syllable) if the category membership and the specific attribute did not trigger the response. The correct response was provided if she was still unable to produce it after the third cue.

C: Formal-semantic therapy with simple repetition (sessions 5, 7, and 9). Each session of intervention C began with a presentation phase, identical to the intervention B presentation phase, after which the simple repetition method was introduced. In session 5 each picture was presented in random order to TBo and she was asked to recall their corresponding names. However, since there were many presentations per session and few items, it was obviously impossible to avoid repetition in the stimuli presentation order. In sessions 7 and 9 TBo had to name the pictures and give their attributes. If she produced an error she received semantic feedback and the cueing technique (formal-semantic therapy) following the same procedure as used for intervention B. When the four names were recalled once, the experimenter presented the list for a second time, and so on until the session ended. List 2 was repeated 20 times, which equalled the number of presentations achieved in session 4 with spaced retrieval. Each item was repeated eight times during session 7, and 11 times during session 9, which equalled the number of presentations achieved in sessions 6 and 8 with spaced retrieval. Then, 15 minutes after the end of each session (5, 7, and 9), the 24 selected stimuli were presented to TBo for picture naming and generation of semantic attributes.

Maintenance, generalisation, and specificity of intervention

At 1, 3, and 5 weeks after the end of the therapy, TBo's performance on the 24 items was evaluated with the same two tasks used during the baseline and interventions phases. To confirm a possible "within-category generalisation effect", a list of 21 further stimuli, belonging to similar semantic categories as the treated and control stimuli, was presented to TBo for picture naming at each of the maintenance testing sessions. The specificity of the semantic treatment was assessed through a letter fluency task (i.e., word generation in response to a cue letter), a task that did not require much semantic involvement. Some of the treated words began with the same letter used during letter fluency.

Statistical analyses

For the analyses, TBo's performance at baseline testing was compared to the performance of the control participants using modified *t* tests comparing data from a single participant with results from a small control group (Crawford & Howell, 1998). Since normality tests showed that most variables did not follow a normal distribution (Shapiro-Wilks, all observed *p*-values $< .02$), Kruskal-Wallis's χ^2, Friedman's χ^2, Mann-Whitney's *U*, and Wilcoxon's *Z* tests were used to analyse TBo's data.

RESULTS

A: Results of baseline testing

The performances of TBo and the control participants at baseline testing are presented in Table 5. TBo was unable to name any of the 24 pictures at the three

TABLE 5
TBo's baseline performances and comparison with normal controls

Baseline measures	TBo (mean of the three trials)	Control participants
Naming – 24 items	0*	20.6 ± 3.36
Generation of verbal attributes from spoken words	22.1*	59.6 ± 16.4
(total number of characteristics named)		
General attributes – total	17.7	35.6 ± 9.1
Target	6.7	13.8 ± 3.4
Control	6.3	12.6 ± 5.2
Neutral	4.7	9.2 ± 2.9
Specific attributes – total	4.4*	24 ± 7.7
Target	0*	11.2 ± 3
Control	1.7	5.6 ± 3.3
Neutral	2.7	7.2 ± 3

*Comparison with control participants significantly different, with $p < .05$.

testing sessions, therefore confirming the stability of her performance for these items. Her ability to generate general semantic attributes was lower than the performance of the control participants but the differences were not statistically significant (all observed p-values > .05). Her performance was, as a whole, stable across the three trials (Friedman's $\chi^2 = 0.80$; $p = .67$). On the general attributes generation task, her performance was slightly better for trained and control items (6.7 and 6.3) than neutral items (4.7). However, for specific semantic attributes TBo's performance was below the control participants' and stable across the three trials (Friedman's $\chi^2 = 0$; $p = 1.0$). She was better at generating general than specific attributes and the difference between the two types of attributes was significant (Wilcoxon's $Z = -2.4$; $p = .17$). On specific attributes, her performance was slightly better for neutral items (2.7) than trained (0) and control items (1.7).

B and C: Intervention

TBo's performances were analysed in two parts. First, the effect of the formal-semantic therapy was analysed by comparing her performances on picture naming and generation of attributes on the eight target items (lists 1 and 2 combined) with the other two sets (control and neutral) during baseline, intervention, and post measures. Second, the specific effect of the spaced retrieval method, compared to simple repetition, was analysed by comparing TBo's performances on lists 1 and 2 for picture naming and generation of attributes, during baseline, intervention, and post measures.

Efficacy of the formal-semantic therapy: Picture naming. Visual inspection of the graphed data (Figure 1a) showed that TBo presented with a limited but clear increase in performance between baseline and intervention phases on the trained items while the two other stimuli lists remained at baseline level. a mean of 38% of correct responses (3/8) was reached during the learning phases for the target items (0/8 for session 4, 3/8 for sessions 5, 7, and 9, and 2/8 for sessions 6 and 8). Visual inspection also showed maintenance of performance at post-intervention testing. Statistical analysis comparing TBo's mean performance on trained items over the

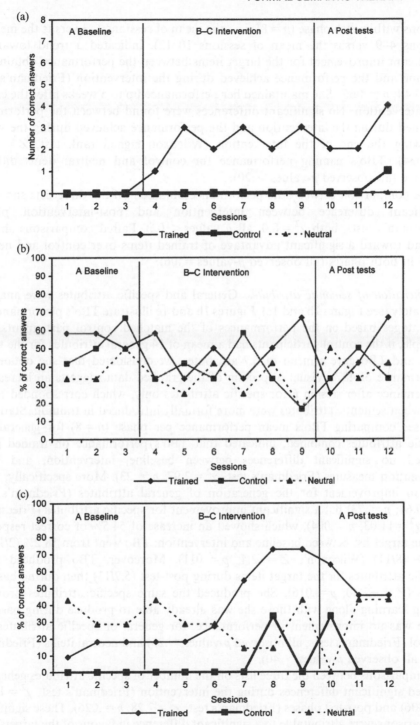

Figure 1. TBo's performances on naming and generation of semantic attributes. (a) TBo's performance on the three lists for confrontation naming (*n* = 8 items per list). (b) TBo's performances on the three lists for generation of general attributes (*n* = 8 items per list; each observation represents TBo's performance compared to control participants). (c) TBo's performances on the three lists for generation of specific attributes (*n* = 8 items per list; each observation represents TBo's performance compared to control participants).

sessions within each phase ($n = 8$) (i.e., the mean of sessions 1–3 versus the mean of sessions 4–9 versus the mean of sessions 10–12), indicated a trend towards a significant improvement for the target items between the performance obtained in baseline and the performance achieved during the intervention (Friedman's test, $\chi^2 = 5.44$; $p = .066$). She maintained her performance up to 5 weeks after the end of the intervention. No significant differences were found between the performance obtained during the intervention and the performance achieved during the weeks following the end of the intervention (Wilcoxon signed rank test, $Z = -.97$; $p = .334$). TBo's naming performance for control and neutral items did not improve (all observed p-values > .20).

The comparison between the performance obtained on the three lists showed a significant difference between intervention and post-intervention phases (Friedman's tests, both $\chi^2 = 8.0$; all p values < .02). Paired comparisons showed a trend toward a significant advantage of trained items over control and neutral items in both phases (all observed p-values = .06).

Generation of semantic attributes. General and specific attributes were analysed separately (see Figures 1b and 1c). Figures 1b and 1c illustrate TBo's performances in percentages based on the performances of the matched control participants. For example, if the control participants had a mean of 14 general attributes for the target items and TBo gave a mean of 6.7 attributes, we considered that she obtained a performance of 48%. Visual inspection of the graphed data suggests an increase in performance after session 6 for specific attributes only, which corresponded to the time when semantic attributes were more formally introduced in training. Statistical analyses comparing TBo's mean performance per phase ($n = 8$) for general and specific attributes combined, indicated that TBo's performance on trained items showed no significant differences between baseline, intervention, and post-intervention measures (Friedman's test, $\chi^2 = 2.97$; $p = .23$). More specifically, there was no improvement for the generation of general attributes (Friedman's test, $\chi^2 = 0.64$; $p = .73$) but a significant improvement for specific attributes (Friedman's test, $\chi^2 = 11.03$; $p = .004$), which showed an increase of 54.5% of correct responses for the target list between baseline and intervention: TBo went from 18.2% (2/11) to 72.7% (8/11) (Wilcoxon's $Z = -2.4$; $p = .011$). Moreover, TBo produced more specific attributes for the target items during post-test (5.7/11) then during baseline (2/11) ($Z = -2.40$; $p = .016$). She produced the same specific attributes provided during learning along with those she was already able to produce during baseline. There was no improvement in performance, for general or specific attributes, for control (Friedman's tests, all observed p-values > .25) and neutral items (Friedman's tests, all observed p-values > .40).

Comparisons between the three lists on the number of specific attributes generated showed significant differences during the intervention (Friedman's test, $\chi^2 = 10.08$; $p = .006$) and post-test phases (Friedman's test, $\chi^2 = 7.28$; $p = .026$). These significant comparisons were attributable to a significant difference in favour of the targets over the other two lists (Wilcoxon's tests, all observed p-values < .05), with the exception of the comparison between targets and neutrals during the intervention phase (Wilcoxon's $Z = -1.68$; $p = .093$). Furthermore, on post measures 2 and 3, target and control were almost equivalent. It is worth noting that TBo gave more specific attributes during baseline for neutral items than for target items.

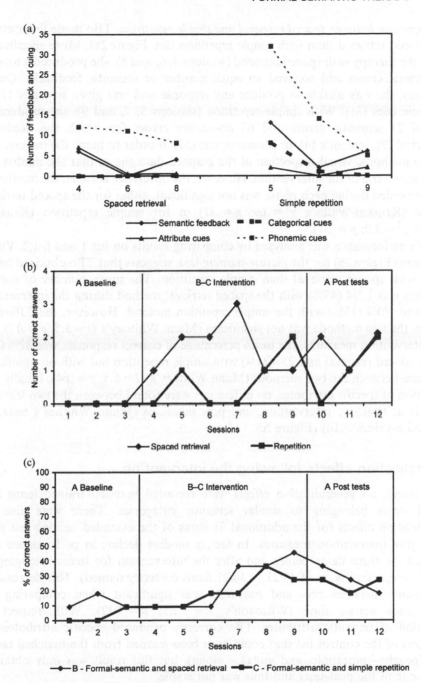

Figure 2. Comparison of TBo's performance with spaced retrieval and simple repetition. (a) Number of semantic feedbacks and cueings needed with spaced retrieval and simple repetition. (b) TBo's performance on naming with spaced retrieval and simple repetition (each observation represents TBo's performance on the four items of each list). (c) TBo's performance on generation of specific attributes with spaced retrieval and simple repetition ($n = 4$ items per condition; each observation represents TBo's performance compared to control participants).

Comparison between spaced retrieval and simple repetition. TBo made fewer errors with spaced retrieval than with simple repetition (see Figure 2a). More specifically, during the therapy with spaced retrieval (sessions 4, 6, and 8), she produced a total of 10 semantic errors and received an equal number of semantic feedbacks. On 38 occasions, she was unable to produce any response and was given semantic (7) or phonemic cues (31). With simple repetition (sessions 5, 7, and 9), she produced a total of 21 semantic errors and 64 no-answer errors for which she needed a categorical (9), semantic (4), or phonemic cue (51) in order to name the picture. For the two methods, visual inspection of the graphed data shows that she needed less cueing at the end of the intervention. However, the difference between the number of cueings needed during each phase was not significant, either for the spaced retrieval method (Kruskal-Wallis's $\chi^2 = .69$; $p = .71$) or for simple repetition (Kruskal-Wallis's $\chi^2 = 2.0$; $p = .37$).

TBo's performance was analysed by comparing results on list 1 and list 2. Visual inspection (Figure 2b) for the picture-naming task suggests that TBo obtained better results with spaced retrieval than simple repetition. The mean number of correct responses was 1.7/4 (46%) with the spaced retrieval method during the intervention phase and .70/4 (13%) with the simple repetition method. However, the difference between the two methods was not significant (Mann Whitney's $U = 3.5$; $p = .17$). On post-intervention measures, the mean percentage of correct responses was 42% (1.7/4) with spaced retrieval and 25% (1/4) with simple repetition but with no significant difference between the two methods (Mann Whitney's $U = 6.5$; $p = .64$). Finally, for generation of specific attributes, no differences were found between the two learning methods at baseline, intervention, and post measures (Mann Whitney's tests, all observed p-values $> .10$) (Figure 2c).

Generalisation effects following the intervention

For naming, no generalisation effects were recorded between trained items and control items belonging to similar semantic categories. There were also no generalisation effects for the additional 21 items of the extended naming test used during post-intervention measures. In fact, a modest decline in performance was observed for these items before and after the intervention for items belonging to trained categories (mean of 13/21 vs 10/21 items correctly named). This decrease in performance between pre- and post-tests was significant when comparing the performance across time (Wilcoxon's $Z = -2.1$; $p = .032$). With respect to generation of semantic attributes, TBo correctly produced specific attributes for two items of the control list that could have been learned from the matched target items (peach – pineapple, and guitar – violin), but this result was only obtained during one of the post-tests and thus was not stable.

Lexical access: Specificity of the intervention

The specificity of the intervention was assessed through a letter fluency task (P-L-T) performed before and after treatment in which TBo could have produced some of the names pertaining to the target list and control list. She never produced those items during the pre- and post-tests and a decrease in performance was observed (15 and 9 words produced before and after intervention, respectively).

GENERAL DISCUSSION

We have reported the case of TBo, a woman presenting with a general semantic deficit in a context of semantic dementia (SD). The general aim of this study was to explore the efficacy of a formal-semantic therapy combined with a spaced retrieval method to facilitate relearning of lost concepts and long-term retention. The study also explored possible generalisation gains obtained after the intervention.

Results suggest that the formal-semantic therapy led to better naming and generation of specific verbal attributes in TBo compared to baseline and the untrained lists. For the learning method, spaced retrieval was not statistically superior to the simple repetition condition. The beneficial effect of the formal-semantic therapy persisted and was maintained up to 5 weeks after the end of the intervention, with no difference between spaced retrieval and simple repetition. Finally, no generalisation within and between categories was observed. The intervention also appeared to be very specific since no improvement in the letter fluency task was observed.

In spite of these limitations, TBo's response to treatment was comparable to that obtained by other individuals with non-degenerative semantic deficits given formal-semantic therapy for naming. As a whole, participants obtain a 10% to 65% improvement in performance (Drew & Thompson, 1999; Grayson et al., 1997; LeDorze & Pitts, 1995; Marshall et al., 1990; Nettleton & Lesser, 1991; Wambaugh et al., 2001). TBo's performance was also comparable with that observed in previous studies with individuals with SD. For example, KB, the participant treated by Snowden and Neary (2002), correctly named 30% of the treated items with repeated rehearsal. Similarly, the participant reported by Funnell (2001) learned six new vegetable names with repeated practice. Our results thus confirm that people with SD can improve their naming performance with training, but that this improvement is limited. They also suggest that a formal-semantic therapy does not lead to better results in naming (this study) than does simple practice (other studies).

Formal-semantic therapy, however, seems promising for retraining specific semantic attributes in SD (at least in the short term, as TBo's performance decreased after several weeks with no treatment). In this respect, TBo showed a major increase in performance during the intervention phase, reaching 8/11 (73%) of correct responses by the end of the intervention. The better results obtained by TBo for generation of semantic attributes than for picture naming are noteworthy. It is generally suggested that techniques focusing on semantic attributes and promoting semantic processing may enhance naming (Nickels, 2002). Some authors hypothesised that this enhancement occurs by recreating the semantic network of the target concept. Re-establishing part of that network when trying to name a concept could facilitate the retrieval of the corresponding word in the output lexicon and could lead to its effective spoken production in naming (Coelho, McHugh, & Boyle, 2000). Since TBo's naming performance was worse than her capacity to generate specific attributes, one might think that the number of relearned semantic attributes was insufficient to restore the link between her semantic and phonological representations and increase her naming performance to the level of her generation of semantic attributes. This indicates the importance of further determining the amount of knowledge that has to be relearned in order to restore the link between a concept and its phonological representation in SD as well as in aphasia. As pointed out by Jokel and colleagues (2006), there could also be some kinds of semantic knowledge, like function or sensory experiences, which would be more useful in linking a concept with its name.

One of the aims of this study was also to explore the efficacy of two types of learning method to enhance performance in SD when combined with a formal-semantic therapy. In fact, our study was a first attempt to explore the impact of spaced retrieval on performance in SD. The analysis of TBo's performance indicates no statistical advantages of this method over simple repetition. Although the small number of items used in our study could explain the lack of significant results (due to a lack of statistical power), some authors have also recently reported that different repetition schedules are as effective as spaced retrieval with non-degenerative aphasia. Morrow and Fridriksson (2006) observed that individuals with aphasia showed similar success for naming with a strict spaced retrieval method as with random selection of four possible intervals (1, 2, 4, and 8 minutes). In fact Fillingham and collaborators (Fillingham, Sage, & Lambon Ralph, 2005), when comparing different repetition-based treatments, observed that the precise treatment method used does not seem to make a difference to the degree of improvement in naming performance. Rather, they showed that one of the most important factors for naming success in non-degenerative disease could be the number of production attempts during therapy. In the present study TBo performed the same number of naming attempts with the two treatment methods, which could explain the comparable efficacy of spaced retrieval and simple repetition. However, further studies should determine if the number of naming attempts is in fact an important factor in enhancing the efficacy of naming treatment in SD.

The question regarding which treatment method might be more effective in SD was also discussed by Graham and colleagues (2001). These authors suggested that DM, the participant they studied, benefited from learning by using an approach in which errors are kept to a minimum. Spaced retrieval is also hypothesised to be an errorless-learning method when applied in dementia (Camp et al., 1996), although recent evidence shows that some persons with dementia of the Alzheimer's type may produce as many errors with the spaced retrieval method as with other schedules of practice (Hochhalter, Bakke, Holub, & Overmier, 2004). In the present study TBo made fewer mistakes with the spaced retrieval method than with simple repetition, which was more like a trial-and-error approach in which the participant is encouraged to "guess" the answer at each trial. If the production of errors was an important contributing factor to the efficacy of treatment in SD, we would have observed better performance with spaced retrieval than with simple repetition. However, such a pattern was not observed in TBo. Future studies should explore this errorless hypothesis using more items and more sessions than we used in this exploratory study.

In addition to these aspects, Graham and colleagues (2001) also discussed DM's need to rehearse the list of treated names in a similar order to that used in the presentation. In fact, when this order was changed during testing, DM's performance declined significantly. The authors hypothesised that DM's learning was rote in nature and was highly dependent on the ordered link between the items in the list. In our study the items were, as much as possible, randomly presented to TBo during learning and testing. Although both random presentation (in our study) and rigid presentation order (Graham et al., 1999) led to a significant improvement in performance, it seems that random presentation of items should be used in SD interventions in order to reduce the participant's reliance on strict, context-dependent learning.

Like other individuals with SD (Graham et al., 2001; Snowden & Neary, 2002), TBo showed item-specific improvement only in naming and generation of verbal attributes. For example, DM, the participant reported by Graham and colleagues (2001), showed no generalisation to untrained items even after extensive practice. Contrary to these disappointing results, some participants with non-degenerative deficits showed generalisation to items pertaining to trained categories (Drew & Thompson, 1999; Grayson et al., 1997) as well as to other modalities (Hillis, 1990) following a formal-semantic therapy. Since no generalisation was observed in TBo, it is thus logical to think that the amount of relearned information was not sufficient to allow naming of the items with which the treated concepts share semantic attributes. Nevertheless, as suggested by Graham and colleagues (2001), generalisation may not be a realistic objective to pursue in SD.

In fact, new learning in SD could be typically bound to a specific spatial and temporal context (Bozeat, Lambon Ralph, Patterson, & Hodges, 2002; Funnell, 2001; Snowden & Neary, 2002; Snowden, Griffiths, & Neary, 1994), especially with the progression of the disease (Funnell, 2001). Thus, new learning could rely more on episodic memory than on semantic memory, and generalisation within the semantic system may not occur. In TBo's case, although she improved in her ability to produce some names, she was only able to produce them within the specific context of the therapy. For example, she could not produce any of the trained items during a letter fluency test. It may be that her new learning, as with participant DM (Graham et al., 2001), was simply an association, or a linking, of a name with a picture. The same episodic learning can be hypothesised for TBo's performance on the generation of semantic attributes, in which no generalisation effect was observed, and which may also reflect the simple linking between a verbal description and a name (or a picture). However, TBo's long-term performance indicates that she maintained her naming of 2/8 items over the 5-week maintenance period, especially on naming, even with no further practice. This may suggest that the training resulted in a consolidation of links within her semantic memory and that this recovered knowledge was then independent of the episodic scaffolding provided during training. Our results are not clear enough to support one hypothesis (semantic consolidation) over the other (episodic linking), but future studies should try to explore further the mechanism by which treatment has its effect in SD. For example, following Funnell's (2001) hypothesis that with the progression of the disease, new learning in SD becomes more and more dependent on episodic memory, long-term retention and generalisation of knowledge should be observed in people with early SD and not in more severe cases of SD.

In sum, TBo's results confirm that, in an experimental context, improved retrieval of object names in SD is possible but rather limited. They also suggest that for SD the use of a formal-semantic therapy could be more effective for enhancing relearning of semantic attributes than concept names, although long-term retention of specific semantic attributes decreased in our study. Such a therapeutic objective could thus be more promising in future clinical studies than the usual focus on naming. The use of a particular treatment method does not seem to influence the success of the treatment. Finally, generalisation may not be a realistic objective to pursue in SD. It should be noted that this study was exploratory. Consequently, our results should be interpreted with caution. In fact, significant differences between treatment methods or generalisation effects may not have been observed because there were too few items to detect small differences or because there were not enough treatment sessions. Other studies, perhaps using more items and more sessions, are necessary to confirm our results.

From a clinical point of view our results, and those reported in the literature, raise several questions regarding the best approach to use in SD. First, since therapy was more effective for relearning of semantic attributes than for improving naming abilities, in the short term, the general objective of treatment for people with SD should be reconsidered. Indeed, from a functional perspective there is less need to remember that an apple is called an apple, than to know that this object can be eaten and cooked. The formal-semantic therapy could thus focus on retraining functional attributes of concepts according to what the person needs to know in order to be more independent in daily living. In the context of a degenerative disease, this functional approach seems logical since the intervention should aim at a direct and rapid impact on the person's functional autonomy and quality of life (Van der Linden, Juillerat, & Adam, 2003). Moreover, as pointed out by Nickels (2002), item-specific learning of relevant functional knowledge, instead of generalisation, is a reasonable objective and seems logical in a context of degenerative disease.

Second, as shown in our study and that of Hillis (1990), semantic feedback seems important to facilitate learning of semantic attributes. However, since episodic memory is relatively well preserved in SD, the therapy could also rely on this preserved capacity. Some authors (Bozeat et al., 2002; Funnell, 2001; Snowden & Neary, 2002) have suggested that new learning in SD could be enhanced when tied to a specific spatial and temporal context that a person will encounter frequently in his/her daily routine. For example, the person could learn how to use the objects, in relation to other objects, in the specific environment where he/she will have to use them. The relearned concepts could thus be anchored in a rich temporo-spatial context. Moreover, if the person with SD can introduce these relearned concepts in his/her daily life, their frequent utilisation could also lead to long-term retention. Such an ecological therapy should lead to better performance in semantic processing of trained concepts and to long-lasting maintenance of the functional use of concepts in daily living.

REFERENCES

Baddeley, A., Emslie, H., & Nimmo-Smith, I. (1994). *The Doors and People Test*. Windsor, UK: Thames Valley Test Company.

Baddeley, A. D. (1994). *La mémoire humaine: théorie et pratique* [Human memory: Theory and practice]. *Grenoble: Presses Universitaires de Grenoble*.

Barbeau, E., Tramoni, E., Joubert, S., Mancini, J., Ceccaldi, J., & Poncet, M. (2004). Evaluation de la mémoire de reconnaissance visuelle: Normalisation d'une nouvelle épreuve en choix forcé (DMS48) et utilité en neuropsychologie clinique [Evaluation of visual recognition memory: Norms of a new forced-choice recognition test (DMS-48) used in clinical neuropsychology]. In M. Van der Linden, et les membres du (Eds.), *L'évaluation des troubles de la mémoire*. Marseille, France: Solal Éditeurs.

Behrmann, M., & Lieberthal, T. (1989). Category-specific treatment of a lexical-semantic deficit: A single case study of global aphasia. *British Journal of Disorders of Communication, 24, 281–299.*

Benton, A. R., Sivan, A. B., Hamsher, K., Varney, N. R., & Spreen, O. (1994). *Contributions to neuropsychological assessment – A clinical manual* (2nd ed.). Oxford, UK: Oxford University Press.

Bjork, R. A. (1988). Retrieval practice and the maintenance of knowledge. In M. M. Gruneberg, P. Morris, & R. Skykes (Eds.), *Practical aspects of memory* (Vol. 2, pp. 396–401). London: Academic Press.

Bozeat, S., Lambon Ralph, M. A., Patterson, K., & Hodges, J. R. (2002). When objects lose their meaning: What happens to their use? *Cognitive, Affective & Behavioral Neuroscience, 2*, 236–251.

Brush, J. A., & Camp, C. J. (1998). Spaced retrieval during dysphagia therapy: A case study. *Clinical Gerontologist, 19*, 96–99.

Camp, C. J., & Stevens, A. B. (1990). Spaced-retrieval: A memory intervention for dementia of the Alzheimer's type. *Clinical Gerontologist, 10*, 58–61.

Camp, J. C., Foss, J. W., Stevens, A. B., & O'Hanlon, A. M. (1996). Improving prospective memory task performance in persons with Alzheimer's disease. In M. Brandimonte, G. O. Einstein, & M. McDaniel (Eds.), *Prospective memory: Theory and applications* (pp. 351–367). Mahwah, NJ: Lawrence Erlbaum Associates Inc.

Caplan, D., & Bub, D. (1992). Psycholinguistic assessment of aphasia. In D. Caplan (Ed.), *Language: Structure, processing and disorders* (pp. 407–425). Cambridge, MA: MIT Press.

Caramazza, A., & Shelton, J. R. (1998). Domain-specific knowledge systems in the brain: The animate–inanimate distinction. *Journal of Cognitive Neurosciences, 10*, 1–34.

Coelho, C. A., McHugh, R. E., & Boyle, M. (2000). Semantic feature analysis as a treatment for aphasic dysnomia: A replication. *Aphasiology, 14*, 133–142.

Crawford, J. R., & Howell, D. C. (1998). Comparing an individual's test score against norms derived from small samples. *The Clinical Neuropsychologist, 12*, 482–486.

de Partz, M-P. (2003). Rééducation des troubles sémantiques. In T. Meulemans, B. Desgranges, S. Adam, & F. Eustache (Eds.), *Évaluation et prise en charge des troubles mnésiques* (pp. 315–332). Marseille, France: Solal Éditeurs.

De Renzi, E., & Faglioni, P. (1978). Development of a shortened version of the Token Test. *Cortex, 14*, 41–49.

Deloche, G., & Hannequin, D. (1997). *Test de dénomination orale d'images (DO 80)* [Picture naming test (DO 80)]. Paris: Les Éditions du Centre de Psychologie Appliquée.

Drew, R. L., & Thompson, C. K. (1999). Model-based semantic treatment for naming deficits in aphasia. *Journal of Speech, Language, and Hearing Research, 42*, 972–989.

Fillingham, J. K., Sage, K., & Lambon Ralph, M. (2005). Further exploration and an overview of errorless and errorful therapy for aphasic word-finding difficulties: The number of attempts during therapy affects outcome. *Aphasiology, 19*, 597–614.

Funnell, E. (2001). A case of forgotten knowledge. In R. Campbell & M. Conway (Eds.), *Broken memories* (pp. 225–236). Oxford, UK: Blackwell.

Golden, J. C. (1978). *Stroop color and word test*. Chicago, IL: Stoelting Co.

Graham, K. S., Patterson, K., Powis, J., Drake, J., & Hodges, J. R. (2002). Multiple inputs to episodic memory: Words tell another story. *Neuropsychology, 16*, 380–389.

Graham, K. S., Patterson, K., Pratt, K. H., & Hodges, J. R. (1999). Relearning and subsequent forgetting of semantic category exemplars in a case of semantic dementia. *Neuropsychology, 13*, 359–380.

Graham, K. S., Patterson, K., Pratt, K. H., & Hodges, J. R. (2001). Can repeated exposure to "forgotten" vocabulary help alleviate word-finding difficulties in semantic dementia? An illustrative case study. *Neuropsychological Rehabilitation, 11*, 429–454.

Graham, K. S., Simons, J. S., Pratt, K. H., Patterson, K., & Hodges, J. R. (2000). Insights from semantic dementia on the relationship between episodic and semantic memory. *Neuropsychologia, 38*, 313–324.

Grayson, E., Hilton, R., & Franklin, S. (1997). Early intervention in a case of jargon aphasia: Efficacy of language comprehension therapy. *European Journal of Disorders of Communication, 32*, 257–276.

Hillis, A. E. (1990). Effects of separate treatments for distinct impairments within the naming process. In T. Prescott (Ed.), *Clinical aphasiology: 19* (pp. 255–265). Austin, TX: Pro-Ed.

Hintzman, D. L., Summers, J. J., & Block, R. A. (1975). What causes the spacing effect? Some effects of repetition, duration, and spacing on memory for pictures. *Memory & Cognition, 3*, 287–294.

Hochhalter, A. K., Bakke, B. L., Holub, R. J., & Overmier, J. B. (2004). Adjusted spaced retrieval training: A demonstration and initial test of why it is effective. *Clinical Gerontologist, 27*, 159–168.

Hodges, J. R., Patterson, K., Oxbury, S., & Funnell, E. (1992). Semantic dementia: Progressive fluent aphasia with temporal lobe atrophy. *Brain, 115*, 1783–1806.

Howard, D., & Patterson, K. (1992). *The Pyramids and Palm Trees Test*. Bury St Edmunds, UK: Thames Valley Test Company.

Joanette, Y., Ska, B., Poissant, A., Belleville, S., Lecours, A. R., & Peretz, I. (1995). *Protocole d'évaluation optimale neuropsychologique (PENO)* [Protocol of Optimal Neuropsychological Evaluation (PONE)].

Université de Montréal: Centre de recherche en santé et vieillissement, Institut universitaire de gériatrie de Montréal (CAN).

Jokel, R., Rochon, E., & Leonard, C. (2006). Treating anomia in semantic dementia: Improvement, maintenance, or both? *Neuropsychological Rehabilitation, 16*, 241–256.

Kertesz, A., Davidson, W., & McCabe, P. (1998). Primary progressive semantic aphasia: A case study. *Journal of the International Neuropsychological Society, 4*, 388–398.

Kessels, R. P., van Zandvoort, M. J., Postma, A., Kappelle, L. J., & de Haan, E. H. (2000). The Corsi Block-Tapping Task: Standardization and normative data. *Applied Neuropsychology, 7*, 252–258.

Lambon Ralph, M. A., Graham, K., Ellis, A. W., & Hodges, J. R. (1998). Naming in semantic dementia – What matters? *Neuropsychologia, 36*, 775–784.

Landauer, T. K., & Bjork, R. A. (1978). Optimum rehearsal patterns and name learning. In M. M. Gruneberg, P. E. Morris, & R. N. Sykes (Eds.), *Practical aspects of memory* (pp. 625–632). London: Academic Press.

LeDorze, G., Boulay, N., Gaudreau, J., & Brassard, C. (1994). The contrasting effect of a semantic versus formal-semantic technique for the facilitation of naming in a case of anomia. *Aphasiology, 8*, 127–142.

LeDorze, G., & Pitts, C. (1995). A case study evaluation of the effects of different techniques for the treatment of anomia. *Neuropsychological Rehabilitation, 5*, 51–65.

Lekeu, F., Wojtasik, V., Van der Linden, M., & Salmon, E. (2002). Training early Alzheimer patients to use a mobile phone. *Acta Neurologica Belgica, 102*, 114–121.

Macoir, J., & Bernier, J. (2002). Is surface dysgraphia tied to semantic impairment? Evidence from a case of semantic dementia. *Brain & Cognition, 48*, 452–457.

Marshall, J., Pound, C., White-Thompson, M., & Pring, T. (1990). The use of picture/word matching task to assist word retrieval in aphasic patients. *Aphasiology, 4*, 167–184.

McKitrick, L. A., & Camp, C. J. (1993). Relearning the names of things: The spaced-retrieval intervention implemented by a caregiver. *Clinical Gerontologist, 14*, 60–62.

McKitrick, L. A., Camp, C. J., & Black, F. W. (1992). Prospective memory intervention in Alzheimer disease. *Journal of Gerontology: Psychological Sciences, 47*, 337–343.

Morrow, K. L., & Fridriksson, J. (2006). Comparing fixed- and randomized-interval spaced retrieval in anomia treatment. *Journal of Communication Disorders, 39*, 2–11.

Neary, D., Snowden, J. S., Gustafson, L., Passant, U., Stuss, D., & Black, S. et al. (1998). Frontotemporal lobar degeneration: A consensus on clinical diagnostic criteria. *Neurology, 51*, 1546–1554.

Nespoulous, J-L., Lecours, A. R., Lafond, D., Lemay, A., Puel, M., & Joanette, Y. et al. (1992). *Protocole Montréal-Toulouse d'examen linguistique de l'aphasie. MT-86 Module Standard Initial: M1 [Montréal-Toulouse Protocole of Linguistic Evaluation of Aphasia. MT-86 Initial Standard Module: M1]*. (2nd ed. revised by Renée Béland & Francine Giroux). Isbergues: L'Ortho-Édition.

Nettleton, I., & Lesser, R. C. (1991). Therapy for naming difficulties in aphasia: Application of a cognitive neuropsychological model. *Journal of Neurolinguistics, 6*, 139–157.

Nickels, L. (2000). Semantics and therapy in aphasia. In W. Best, K. Bryan, & J. Maxim (Eds.), *Semantic processing: Theory and practice* (pp. 108–124). London: Whurr Publishers.

Nickels, L. (2002). Therapy for naming disorders: Revisiting, revising, and reviewing. *Aphasiology, 16*, 935–979.

Ottenbacher, K. J. (1986). *Evaluating clinical change: Strategies for occupational and physical therapy.* Baltimore, MD: Williams & Wilkins.

Papagno, C., & Capitani, E. (2001). Slowly progressive aphasia: A four-year follow-up study. *Neuropsychologia, 39*, 678–686.

Raven, J. C. (1938). *Progressive matrices: A perceptual test of intelligence. Individual form.* Oxford, UK: Oxford Psychologists Press Ltd.

Riddoch, M. J., & Humphreys, G. W. (1993). *Birmingham Object Recognition Battery (BORB).* Hove, UK: Lawrence Erlbaum Associates Ltd.

Russo, R., Mammarella, N., & Avons, S. E. (2002). Toward a unified account of spacing effects in explicit cued-memory tasks. *Journal of Experimental Psychology: Learning, Memory, & Cognition, 28*, 819–829.

Schwarz, M., De Bleser, R., Poeck, K., & Weis, J. (1998). A case of primary progressive aphasia. A 14-year follow up study with neuropathological findings. *Brain, 121*, 115–126.

Simons, J. S., Graham, K. S., Galton, C. J., Patterson, K., & Hodges, J. R. (2001). Semantic knowledge and episodic memory for faces in semantic dementia. *Neuropsychology, 15*, 101–114.

Snodgrass, J., & Vanderwart, M. 1. (1980). A standardised set of 260 pictures: Norms for name agreement, familiarity, and visual complexity. *Journal of Experimental Psychology: Human Learning and Memory, 6*, 174–215.

Snowden, J. S., Goulding, P. J., & Neary, D. (1989). Semantic dementia: A form of circumscribed cerebral atrophy. *Behavioral Neurology, 2*, 167–182.

Snowden, J., Griffiths, H., & Neary, D. (1994). Semantic dementia: Autobiographical contribution to preservation of meaning. *Cognitive Neuropsychology, 11*, 265–288.

Snowden, J. S., & Neary, D. (2002). Relearning of verbal labels in semantic dementia. *Neuropsychologia, 40*, 1715–1728.

Tombaugh, T. N. (2004). Trail Making Test A and B: Normative data stratified by age and education. *Archives of Clinical Neuropsychology, 19*, 203–214.

Van der Linden, M., Juillerat, A. C., & Adam, S. (2003). Cognitive rehabilitation. In R. Mulligan, M. Van der Linden, & A. C. Juillerat (Eds.), *The clinical management of early Alzheimer's disease* (pp. 169–233). Mahwah, NJ: Lawrence Erlbaum Associates Inc.

Wambaugh, J. L., Linebaugh, C. W., Doyle, P. J., Martinez, A. L., Kalinyak-Fliszar, M., & Spencer, K. A. (2001). Effects of two cueing treatments on lexical retrieval in aphasic speakers with different levels of deficit. *Aphasiology, 15*, 933–950.

Wechsler, D. (1997). *Wechsler Adult Intelligence Scale-III (WAIS-III)*. New York: Psychological Corporation.

Wheeler, M. A., Ewers, M., & Buonanno, J. F. (2003). Different rates of forgetting following study versus test trials. *Memory, 11*, 571–580.

Wilson, B. A. (1987). Single-case experimental designs in neuropsychological rehabilitation. *Journal of Clinical and Experimental Neuropsychology, 9*, 527–544.

APPENDIX

TABLE A1
List of the 24 items used during the intervention

Target items list	Neutral items list	Control items list
Parrot	Peacock	Anchor
Owl	Eagle	Crown
Guitar	Violin	Toaster
Mushroom	Pepper	Chisel
Peach	Pineapple	Nut
Saxophone	Trombone	Sailing boat [in French "voilier"]
Bee	Fly	Helmet
Caterpillar	Beetle	Razor

TABLE A2
Specific attributes used for the target items and specific attributes spontaneously generated by TBo following the intervention (for target items only)

Target items list	Attributes used during the intervention phase
List 1:	
Parrot	Has bright colours
Owl	Lives during the night
Guitar	Is made of wood
Mushroom	Grows on the ground
List 2:	
Peach	Does not grow in Québec
Saxophone	Is made of metal
Bee	Lives in a hive
Caterpillar	Transforms itself into a butterfly

APHASIOLOGY, 2009, 23 (2), 236–265

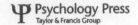

The benefits and protective effects of behavioural treatment for dysgraphia in a case of primary progressive aphasia

Brenda Rapp and Brian Glucroft

Johns Hopkins University, Baltimore, MD, USA

Background: Spoken and written language difficulties are the predominant symptoms in the progressive neurodegenerative disease referred to as primary progressive aphasia (PPA). There has been very little research on the effectiveness of intervention on spoken language impairments in this context and none directed specifically at progressive written language impairment.

Aims: To examine the effectiveness of behavioural intervention for dysgraphia in a case of primary progressive aphasia.

Methods & Procedures: We carried out a longitudinal single-case study that allowed us to examine the effectiveness of a non-intensive spell-study-spell intervention procedure. We did so by comparing performance on four sets of words: trained, repeated, homework, and control words at five evaluations: baseline, during intervention, after the intervention, and at 6- and 12-month follow-up.

Outcomes & Results: We find that: (1) at the end of the intervention, Trained words show a small but statistically significant improvement relative to baseline and an advantage in accuracy over Control, Homework, and Repeated word sets. (2) All word sets exhibited a decline in accuracy from the end of treatment to the 6-month follow-up evaluation, consistent with the degenerative nature of the illness. Nonetheless, accuracy on Trained words continued to be superior to that of Control words and not statistically different from pre-intervention baseline levels. (3) Repeated testing and practice at home yielded modest numerical advantages relative to Control words; but these differences were, for many comparisons, not statistically significant. (4) At 12 months post-intervention, all words sets had significantly declined relative to pre-intervention baselines and performance on the four sets was comparable.

Conclusions: This investigation documents—for the first time—that behavioural intervention can provide both immediate and short-term benefits for dysgraphia in the context of primary progressive aphasia.

Language difficulties may be the predominant symptom in progressive, neurodegenerative disease (Mesulam, 1982). In many of those cases, written language difficulties may accompany spoken language impairments, or may even be the primary presenting language deficit (Westbury & Bub, 1997). There has been very little research on the effectiveness of intervention (behavioural or pharmacological)

Address correspondence to: Brenda Rapp, 135 Krieger Hall, Johns Hopkins University, Baltimore, MD 21218, USA. E-mail: rapp@cogsci.jhu.edu

We are grateful for the support of NIH grant DC006740; to Alexis Kruczek and Joelle Urrutia for their hard work and dedication to this project; to Ranjan Maitra (University of Iowa, Department of Statistics) for his help with statistical analyses; and for CB's friendship and example of humour and humanity throughout difficult times.

http://www.psypress.com/aphasiology   DOI: 10.1080/02687030801943054

on spoken language impairments in progressive neurological disease and, to our knowledge, none directed specifically at progressive written language impairment. Here we report on a study of the effectiveness of behavioural intervention for dysgraphia in a case of primary progressive aphasia. We use a spell-study-spell training procedure that has been used with some success in a number of cases of acquired dysgraphia (Beeson, 1999; Rapp & Kane, 2002). The findings of this investigation indicate that the behavioural intervention yielded significant immediate gains as well as medium-term benefits for trained words relative to untrained control words.

PROGRESSIVE APHASIA AND DYSGRAPHIA

A decline in spoken language abilities is a common feature of a wide range of different neurodegenerative diseases and, in some cases, may be the predominant symptom in the initial stages or even throughout the course of the disease. Primary progressive aphasia (PPA) refers to specifically to those degenerative conditions in which spoken language represents the only, or salient, domain of cognitive decline for at least the first 2 years of the disease (Mesulam, 1982; Mesulam, Grossman, Hillis, Kertesz, & Weintraub, 2003; Weintraub, Rubin, & Mesulam, 1990). This investigation will focus on written language production which may be disrupted in a wide range of neurodegenerative diseases (see Graham, 2000, for a review) including Alzheimer's disease, frontal and/or temporal lobe atrophy, posterior cortical atrophy, and cortico-basal degeneration. Furthermore, Westbury and Bub (1997), in their review of published reports of 112 individuals diagnosed specifically with progressive aphasia, indicated that although written language abilities were not routinely evaluated in the context of PPA, in 8% of the cases in their total sample, written language difficulties (dysgraphia: 5%, dyslexia: 3%) were actually the presenting symptoms. There have also been a few reports of individuals in whom dysgraphia was not only the presenting, but also the predominant, symptom for an extended period of time (Graham, Patterson, & Hodges, 1997; Luzzi & Piccirilli, 2003), a condition referred to by Graham (2000) as "primary progressive dysgraphia". In contrast, it has also been reported that written language abilities may be relatively preserved throughout the course of the progressive spoken language deterioration or that written language abilities may be affected only in later stages (see Luzzatti, Iaiacona, & Agazzi, 2002, for a review). In fact, some researchers have commented that for a number of individuals with progressive aphasia, written language remains a relative strength and they sometimes rely on written language for their communication (Cress & King, 1999; Holland, McBurney, Moossy, & Reinmuth, 1985; Kertesz, Hudson, Mackenzie, & Munoz, 1994; Mesulam & Weintraub, 1992; Murray, 1998;Weintraub et al., 1990). Despite the relative paucity of data on written language in neurodegenerative disease, the picture that emerges is one in which written language impairment is a common symptom, often occurring alongside spoken language deterioration; however, written language may be either selectively affected or preserved for considerable periods of time during the course of the disease.

The specific dysgraphias that have been described in the context of neurodegenerative diseases are apparently similar, in terms of symptomatology and underlying functional deficits, to those observed in patients with non-progressive brain lesions that result from stroke, head injury, or surgery (Graham, 2000). For example, in neurodegenerative cases there are very frequent reports that include spelling impairments that primarily affect the retrieval of the spellings of familiar words that are stored in long-term memory (Ardila, Matute, & Inozemtseva, 2003; Croisile, Carmoi, Adeleine, & Trillet, 1995; Hillis et al., 2006; Platel, Lambert, Eustache, & Cadet, 1993; Rapcsak, Arthur, Bliklen, & Rubens, 1989). This memory system is often referred to as the *orthographic lexicon* (see Figure 1), and deficits to this system are sensitive to the frequency of words and typically result in the production of phonologically plausible spelling errors (e.g., spelling "yacht" as YOT) if the sublexical phonology-to-orthography conversion process remains relatively intact. The deficit pattern that emerges from damage to the orthographic lexicon (or the lexical system more generally) is referred to clinically as "surface dysgraphia". There are also reports of cases of neurogenerative disease in which the written language deficits especially affect the processes involved in using the knowledge of the sublexical, regular relationships between sounds and letters that are necessary for the spelling of unfamiliar words or pseudowords—the *phonology-to-orthography conversion system* (Luzzatti, Iaiacona, & Agazzi, 2003). This deficit is characterised by difficulties in spelling pseudowords and is often referred to as "phonological dysgraphia".

In addition, deficits specifically affecting the ability to hold letters in the *graphemic buffer* (i.e., orthographic working memory) during the serial process of producing a written or oral spelling have also been described in cases of progressive disease (O'Dowd & Zubicaray, 2003), as have been a range of peripheral impairments. The peripheral impairments arise at different stages of letter shape production, and include not only fairly commonly reported deficits of motor execution that result in poorly formed letters, but also deficits that are apparently due to such things as a failure to remember the shapes of letters (Graham, Zeman, Young, Patterson, & Hodges, 1999), difficulties with a specific case or font (e.g., Graham et al., 1997), difficulties with spacing of letters, and other spatial aspects of writing, and so forth. In many cases, and particularly with disease progression, multiple processing mechanisms within the spelling system are affected. It is a matter of debate whether or not there is a specific order in which deficits to the spelling system arise with disease progression. Some researchers have suggested that the norm is a progression from central (lexical) impairments to more peripheral deficits (Graham, 2000; Hughes, Graham, Patterson, & Hodges, 1997), while others have claimed that there is no fixed order and that the progression depends, for each individual, on the specific neuro-geography of the disease progression (e.g., Luzzatti et al., 2003).

INTERVENTION IN CASES OF PROGRESSIVE APHASIA

There have been only a few papers reporting the results of specific interventions in cases of PPA (Cress & King, 1999; McNeil, Small, Masterson, & Fossett, 1995; Murray, 1998; Pattee, von Berg, & Ghezzi, 2006; Schneider, Thompson, & Luring, 1996). These papers vary in the extent to which they include control conditions and/ or assessment measures that allow for a statistical evaluation of the effectiveness of the treatment approaches. Nonetheless, the existing literature consistently indicates promising outcomes for a range of treatment approaches.

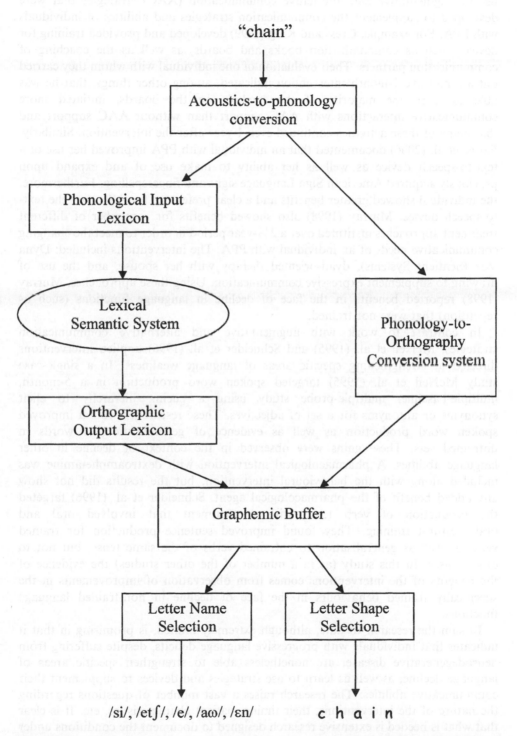

"chain"

Acoustics-to-phonology
conversion

Phonological Input
Lexicon

Lexical
Semantic System

Phonology-to-
Orthography
Conversion system

Orthographic
Output Lexicon

Graphemic Buffer

Letter Name
Selection

Letter Shape
Selection

/si/, /etʃ/, /e/, /aω/, /ɛn/   c h a i n

Figure 1. The cognitive mechanisms involved in written (or oral) spelling to dictation. Adapted from Buchwald and Rapp (2006).

Cress and King (1999), Pattee et al. (2006), and Murray (1998) all report on the use of augmentative and alternative communication (AAC) strategies that were developed to supplement the communication strategies and abilities of individuals with PPA. For example, Cress and King (1999) developed and provided training for devices such as communication books and boards, as well as the coaching of communication partners. Their evaluation of one individual with whom they carried out an intensive 1-month intervention indicated, among other things, that he was able to learn the majority of the symbols on the boards, initiated more communicative interactions with AAC support than without AAC support and that many of these activities continued even 1 year after the intervention. Similarly, Pattee et al. (2006) documented that an individual with PPA improved her use of a text-to-speech device as well as her ability to make use of and expand upon previously acquired American Sign Language signs and fingerspelling. Furthermore, the individual showed greater benefits and a clear preference for ASL over the text-to-speech device. Murray (1998) also showed benefits for a number of different treatment approaches instituted over a 2½-year period in order to meet the changing communicative needs of an individual with PPA. The interventions included: Dyna Vox (Sentient Systems), dyad-oriented therapy with her spouse, and the use of drawing to supplement expressive communication. Using these approaches, Murray (1998) reported benefits in the face of decline in language functions (such as repetition) that were not trained.

In contrast to work with augmentative and alternative communication strategies, McNeil et al. (1995) and Schneider et al. (1996) applied interventions directed at strengthening specific areas of language weakness. In a single-case study McNeil et al. (1995) targeted spoken word production in a 5-month, multiple-baseline, multiple-probe study using a cueing hierarchy to elicit synonyms or antonyms for a set of adjectives. These researchers found improved spoken word production as well as evidence of generalisation to words in untrained sets. These gains were observed in the context of decline in other language abilities. A pharmacological intervention with dextroamphetamine was included along with the behavioural intervention, but the results did not show any added benefit of the pharmacological agent. Schneider et al. (1996) targeted the production of verb tense with a treatment that involved oral and oral + gestural training. They found improved sentence production for trained verbs as well as generalisation to untrained verbs of the same tense, but not to other tenses. In this study (as in a number of the other studies) the evidence of the benefits of the interventions comes from observation of improvements in the specifically trained behaviours in the face of decline in non-trained language functions.

In sum the research to date, although extremely limited, is promising in that it indicates that individuals with progressive language deficits, despite suffering from neurodegenerative disease, are nonetheless able to strengthen specific areas of language decline, as well as learn to use strategies and devices to supplement their communicative abilities. The research raises a vast number of questions regarding the nature of the interventions, their timing, patient characteristics, etc. It is clear that what is needed is extensive research designed to document the conditions under which intervention benefits can be maximised in order to extend language use and effective communication skills for as long as possible.

TREATMENT OF ACQUIRED, NON-PROGRESSIVE DYSGRAPHIAS

The investigation described in this paper involves a single case study of an individual with progressive aphasia and dysgraphia in which intervention is targeted at strengthening the representations of words spellings (the orthographic lexicon). To our knowledge there has been no published research involving treatment of progressive dysgraphia, and even the literature regarding behavioural intervention in acquired dysgraphia is relatively small. The training procedures implemented in this study are similar to those that have been applied in various cases of acquired, non-progressive dysgraphias that resulted from stroke, infection, tumour resection, head injury, and other aetiologies. We briefly review these here.

A number of treatment studies have targeted specific components of the spelling process (see Figure 1), such as the semantic component (Hillis, 1991, 1992), the sublexical phonology-to-orthography conversion system (Carlomagno, Iavarone, & Colombo, 1994; de Partz, Seron, & Van der Linden, 1992; Hatfield, 1983; Luzzatti, Colombo, Frustaci, & Vitolo, 2000), the graphemic buffer (Hillis, 1989), or the orthographic lexicon (Aliminosa, McCloskey, Goodman-Schulman, & Sokol, 1993; Beeson, 1999; Beeson & Hirsch, 1998; Beeson, Hirsch, & Rewega, 2002; Behrmann, 1987; Behrmann & Byng, 1992; Carlomagno et al., 1994; Clausen & Beeson, 2003; de Partz et al., 1992; Hatfield & Weddel, 1976; Hillis & Caramazza, 1987; Rapp, 2005; Rapp & Kane, 2002; Raymer, Cudworth, & Haley, 2003; Schmalzl & Nickels, 2006; Scron, Deloche, Moulard, & Rousselle, 1980; Weekes & Coltheart, 1996). In addition, there have been some studies that have targeted the interaction between lexical and sublexical processes (Beeson, Rewega, Vail, & Rapcsak, 2000) and others that have focused on components that are specifically required for written as compared to oral spelling (Mortley, Enderby, & Petheram, 2001; Pound, 1996).

The majority of these treatment studies have been directed at strengthening the representations of word spellings stored in the orthographic lexicon. These studies have generally employed techniques in which the correct spellings of words are repeatedly presented for study and spelling and/or delayed copy. This general method is based on the assumption that neural injury has weakened/damaged the representations of words in long-term memory and that the repeated presentation of words will strengthen or facilitate retrieval of these representations. Various other techniques have also been used (for a review see Beeson & Rapcsak, 2002) for improving different aspects of the spelling process. For example, Hillis and Caramazza (1987) taught error detection and correction strategies to an individual with a deficit affecting graphemic buffering, and Hillis (1989) used a cueing hierarchy in another case. A number of the studies that have been directed at remediating deficits affecting the sublexical processes of the phonology-to-orthography conversion system have focused on re-teaching pho-neme–grapheme relationships, often by pairing each phoneme with a "key word" that the individual can spell (Carlomagno & Parlato, 1989; de Partz et al., 1992; Hatfield, 1983; Hillis Trupe, 1986; Luzzatti et al., 2000). There are also reports of studies that use computers and word processors to facilitate repetitive practice or to complement an intervention that targets specific cognitive processes (e.g., Mortley et al., 2001).

The treatment outcomes in these studies are generally positive with regard to improvement on treated items, although there is considerable variability with regard to generalisation and maintenance. Despite the relatively small number of controlled studies of treatment outcomes in non-progressive dysgraphia, it is clear that spelling deficits arising from impairments to different functional components are amenable to improvement even many years after the onset of the dysgraphia. Furthermore, in at least some cases, this improvement has been shown to have a functional impact on daily life (see Beeson & Rapscak, 2002, for discussion). Also important is the observation that in at least some individuals with both aphasia and dysgraphia, the dysgraphia has been shown to be more amenable to intervention than the aphasia (Beeson, 1999; Beeson et al., 2002; Beeson, Rising, & Volk, 2003; Robson, Marshall, Chiat, & Pring, 2001). That is, the effectiveness of dysgraphia treatment is not always dependent on the integrity of the spoken language system. This is consistent with other evidence of the relative independence of at least some of the cognitive components of written and spoken language processing (for a review see Rapp, Benzing, & Caramazza, 1997; Rapp & Caramazza, 2002). The independence of certain aspects of the written and spoken language systems may have implications for the role of dysgraphia treatment in the context of progressive spoken language impairment.

INTERVENTION IN A CASE OF PROGRESSIVE DYSGRAPHIA

It is important to determine whether or not treatment approaches that have been successful in cases of non-progressive dysgraphia can be applied in cases of neurodegenerative disease to either improve written language abilities or prolong skill levels in the face of the degenerative disease process: This is the aim of this paper. We report on a single case study of a woman diagnosed with primary progressive aphasia with dysgraphia, for whom dysgraphia was the initial symptom. The two behavioural interventions used in this study were a spell-study-spell type procedure implemented in the laboratory as well as a modified version of the same procedure that was carried out independently in the home. Two control conditions were included to determine treatment effectiveness and generalisation to untrained words. Finally, the maintenance of gains was assessed in follow-up evaluations at 6 and 12 months after the end of the intervention. In the General Discussion we consider, among other issues, the role of dysgraphia intervention in the context of spoken language deterioration and the similarities and differences between interventions in non-progressive versus progressive dysgraphia.

CASE STUDY

CB was a right-handed, college-educated, professional artist and illustrator of children's books, who was born in 1941. She was an avid reader and excellent speller, and had planned to begin writing professionally before her neurodegenerative illness made this impossible. She reports that a grandfather and an aunt suffered from dementia. CB recalled experiencing the earliest symptoms of language difficulties in 1996 at the age of 55. At that time she found that she was occasionally unable to spell common, irregular words (such as BELIEVE) and that she occasionally found reading for meaning to be more difficult and slower than it had been previously. She reported that in the subsequent 5 years she began to experience word-finding difficulties, and difficulties with calculation as well as with her artwork. In 2001 she sought evaluation, and clinical neuropsychological testing was carried out at that time and as well as in 2003 and 2004[1] (see Table 1 for a time-line). She was able to

---

[1] We are grateful to Drs Hillis and Selnes at Johns Hopkins Hospital for providing us with the results of the neuropsychological diagnostic testing that they carried out with CB.

TABLE 1
Timeline of the major events referred to in this investigation

Date	Evaluation/Observations
1996	Earliest symptoms of language difficulties
Dec 2001	*Neuropsychological Evaluation 1:* Mild cognitive impairment
Dec 2003	*Neuropsychological Evaluation 2:* Diagnosis of PPA
Jan–April 2004	*Pre-intervention Evaluation*
May–Aug. 2004	*INTERVENTION STUDY*
Sept 2004	*Neuropsychological Evaluation 3:* Further cognitive deterioration
Dec–Feb 2005	*Post-Intervention Evaluation and Follow-up 1*
July 2005	*Post Intervention Follow-up 2*

live alone and fairly independently with only some outside assistance until 2006, at which time family and friends began to make arrangements for a living situation in which she would receive more supervision.

Neuropsychological testing

A diagnosis of PPA was made on the basis of CB's performance on the 2001 and 2003 neuropsychological evaluations (Table 2). In 2001, CB was diagnosed as having moderately severe neurocognitive impairment of an undetermined aetiology. Her symptoms included mild dysnomia, marked dyscalculia, dysgraphia, mild-to-moderate deficits of attention and new learning, psychomotor slowing, and mild constructional difficulties. In contrast, delayed recall and verbal recognition memory and frontal lobe-type functions were within normal limits. MRI scanning at the time revealed asymmetric temporal parietal atrophy (see Figure 2). The 2003 evaluation revealed a continued anomia, with the written modality more impaired than the spoken, and a deterioration in language functions in the face of fairly stable performance in memory and non-language tasks. On this basis CB was diagnosed with primary progressive aphasia of a fluent-type, most likely due to frontotemporal lobar degeneration or Pick complex.

The dysgraphia intervention study reported in this paper began in 4/2004 shortly after the second cognitive neuropsychological evaluation (in 12/2003) and ended 4 months later in 8/2004, with follow-up evaluations 6 and 12 months after the end of the intervention. CB underwent a third cognitive neuropsychology evaluation in 9/2004, shortly after the intervention phase of the study. As indicated in Table 2, this third evaluation revealed an accelerating pace of language deterioration—e.g., Controlled Oral Word Association Test (Benton & Hamsher, 1976), a written noun/verb picture naming task (unpublished)) as well as impairment of verbal memory (Rey Auditory Verbal Learning Test; Schmidt, 1996), and general cognitive functions (Mini Mental Status Examination; Folstein, Folstein, & McHugh, 1975); Wechsler Memory Scale (Wechsler & Stone, 1973). However, visual perception remained relatively stable (Rey-Osterreith Complex Figure Test; Osterreith, 1944; Rey, 1942). Further information regarding patterns of spared and impaired abilities during the period of 2003–2005 will be reported below in the context of the intervention study.

TABLE 2

CB's performance on a set of neuropsychological tests at three time points

	12/2001	12/2003	9/2004
MMSE (Mini Mental Status Examination)			
[29 (1.3)]	26/30	26/30	20/30
	(Z = −2.31)	(Z = −2.31)	(Z = −6.92)
WMS (Wechsler Memory Scale)			
Information and Orientation	13/14	14/14	12/14
[13.5 (0.6)]	(Z = −0.83)	(Z = .83)	(Z = −2.5)
Grooved Pegboard Test			
Dominant	13%ile	< 1%ile	< 1%ile
Nondominant	12%ile	< 1%ile	< 1%ile
Trail making			
A [35.8 (11.9)]	53 sec	98 sec	93 sec
B [81.2 (38.5)]	166 sec	discont @ 300s	discont@ 200s
Rey Auditory Verbal Learning Test (RAVLT)			
Total [49.4 (7.5)]	28/75	27/75	12/75
	(Z = −2.85)	(Z = −2.98)	(Z = −4.98)
Delayed recall [10.2 (2.5)]	8/15	8/15	3/15
	(Z = −0.88)	(Z = −0.88)	(Z = −2.88)
WMS (Wechsler Memory Scale)			
Digits forward span [8.4 (1.9)]	7	7	5
Backward span [6.5 (2.0)]	4	3	2
Warrington Recognition Memory Test			
Words	68th %ile		
Faces	25th %ile		
Rey-Osterreith Complex Figure			
Direct [30 (4.21)]	33/36	27/36	26/36
	(Z = .71)	(Z = −.71)	(Z = −0.95)
Immediate [16.57 (7.53)]	11.5/36	12.5/	14/36
	(Z = −.67)	36(Z = −0.54)	(Z = −0.34)
Delayed [14.21 (7.5)]	–	12/36	15/36
		(Z = −0.29)	(Z = 0.11)
Stroop			
Color	Z = −4.39	Z = −104	–
Color word	Z = −4.61	Z = −4.34	–
Boston Naming Test [55.6 (3.5)]	25/30	48 /60 (−2.17)	
Controlled Oral Word Association Test (F-A-S)	37 words	22 words	5 words
[42 (12.1)]	(Z = −0.41)	(Z = −1.67)	(Z = −3.05)
Noun/verb picture naming			
spoken: N/V	–	87% / 90%	87% / 83%
written: N/V		53% / 47%	27% / 10%

Wherever possible scores are reported as Z scores or percentiles. Numbers in [ ] correspond to the mean score of normal subjects and their (SD). MMSE (Folstein et al., 1975); WMS (Wechsler & Stone, 1973); Grooved Pegboard (Trites, 1984); Trail making (Reitan, 1992); RAVLT (Schmidt, 1996); WMS (Wechsler et al., 1973); Warrington Recognition Memory Test (Warrington, 1984); Boston Naming Test (Kaplan et al., 1983); Rey-Osterreith Complex Figure (Osterreith, 1942; Rey, 1942); Controlled Oral Word Association Test (Benton & Hamsher, 1976); Stroop (adapted from Golden & Freshwater, 2002); Noun/verb picture naming (unpublished).

DYSGRAPHIA INTERVENTION STUDY

In addition to the clinical neuropsychological evaluations, a number of tasks were administered as part of the dysgraphia intervention study itself with the following

2001   2004

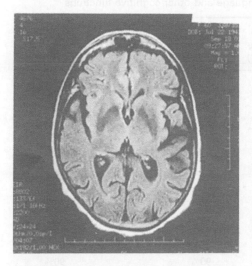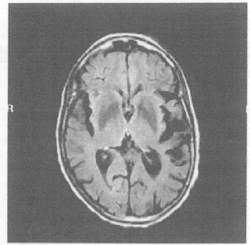

Figure 2. MRI scans taken of CB in 2001 and 2004, showing asymmetric temporal parietal atrophy.

two objectives: (a) to assess a range of cognitive and language abilities at three time points: prior to the onset of training, after the end of training and during the follow-up period, and (b) to determine the specific deficits affecting CB's spelling system.

General assessment

It was important to evaluate a range of skills in order to characterise the backdrop against which intervention-related changes might take place. That is, in order to attribute any significant changes specifically to the behavioural intervention it was important to evaluate if other skill domains were stable or deteriorating during the period of the intervention study.

As indicated in Table 3, at the onset of the investigation CB showed good visuo-spatial skills, as well as language comprehension. In language comprehension she showed fairly intact performance in both written and spoken domains. With regard to spoken language, her comprehension was adequate at both the single word and sentence level, as indicated in the tasks in Table 3 as well as in informal interactions. As concerns spoken language production, CB showed excellent abilities in word and nonword repetition as well as in sentence completion (completing sentence onsets such as: "John wanted to leave, but..."). These areas of fairly intact performance contrasted with her moderately impaired spoken picture (confrontation) naming. Errors in picture naming were semantic (ant → "mosquito"; 29%), phonological, including phonologically similar words (camel → "cannibal"; 14%) and nonwords (penguin → "kerwin";14%), circumlocutions and definitions (lettuce → "salad stuff, greens"; 43%). Anomia was also observed in her spontaneous speech, which was grammatical and fluent although slowed by occasional word-finding difficulties and circumlocutions. Her writing to dictation of both words and nonwords was severely impaired and will be discussed in greater detail below.

Although not all tasks were administered at all subsequent time points, the results (Table 3) indicate that throughout the entire period of this investigation CB's

TABLE 3
Results of additional assessment of language and other cognitive functions

	Pre-training (12/03-4/04)	Post-training (9/04-10/04)	6 month Follow-up 1 (12/04-2/05)	12 month Follow-up 2 (7/05-9/05)
Language comprehension				
Spoken				
-Word (PPVT) (*n* = 175)	68%ile	63%ile	68%ile	19%ile
-Sentence (JHU Screener) (*n* = 26)	96%	92%	–	77%
Written				
-Visual Lexical Decision (PALPA 25) (*n* = 120)	96%	85%	–	80%
Language Production (JHU Language Screeners)				
Spoken				
-Picture naming (*n* = 41)	83%	59%	–	–
-Oral reading (*n* = 35)	83%	71%	–	–
-Single word repetition (*n* = 15)	100%	93%	–	93%
-Sentence completion (*n* = 10)	100%	90%	–	90%
*Written**				
-Spelling to dictation				
-words (*n* = 79)	15%	13%	–	–
-nonwords (*n* = 33)	39%	15%	–	–
Visuo-spatial				
-BORB-length match (*n* = 30)	90%	93%	–	–
-BORB-object recognition (*n* = 62)	98%	100%	–	–
-BVRT (direct copy/15 sec delay) (*n* = 20)	–	100% / 20%	–	97% / 23%

PPVT = Peabody Picture Vocabulary Test (Dunn & Dunn, 1981); BORB = Birmingham Object Recognition Battery (Riddoch & Humphreys 1993). JHU = Johns Hopkins University Language Screeners (unpublished-different items are used in different modalities; lists include a range of word frequencies and lengths); PALPA = Psycholinguistic Assessment of Processing in Aphasia (Kay et al., 1992); BVRT = Benton Visual Retention Test (Benton Sivan, 1991). *Spelling accuracy is reported as: # of correct strings/total strings attempted (rather than as letters correct) so as to be more comparable to other word tasks in this table.

performance was stable for a range of visual abilities as measured by certain subtests of the BORB and the Benton Visual Retention Test. Spoken language was fairly stable from pre-training to post-training and through at least the first follow-up assessment in the following areas: single word auditory comprehension, single word repetition, and sentence completion. In contrast to these areas of stability, the testing documents significant deterioration during this same time period in spoken confrontation naming, $\chi^2(1) = 5.9$, $p < .01$, and in the spelling to dictation of nonwords, $\chi^2(1) = 4.9$, $p < .05$.

In sum, with respect to language, comprehension was better preserved than production, both in the written and spoken modalities, and written production was more affected than spoken production In contrast, visuo-spatial skills remained quite stable throughout the entire 18-month period of intervention and follow-up.

Dysgraphia assessment

The primary purpose of the dysgraphia assessment was to identify the components of the spelling system that were affected, focusing especially on those involved in writing words to dictation, as this was the task that was used in the intervention study. All spelling accuracies are reported as number of letters correct/letters in the stimuli. Each target letter was assigned a score of 0, 0.5, or 1; with a score of 1 assigned if the target letter was present and in the correct position, 0.5 if it was present but in the incorrect position, and 0 if the target letter was absent. Using this scoring method, for any given word set, percent correct equals the total score/total number of letters in all of the target words in the set. Although not reported, responses were also scored according to whether each word was correct or incorrect. The results obtained by considering letter or word accuracy revealed essentially the same pattern; however, we prefer letter accuracy as it is a far more sensitive measure.

According to Figure 1, writing to dictation of familiar words first requires understanding the dictated word. This is accomplished by identifying the word among the forms of familiar words stored in phonological long-term memory (the phonological lexicon) and then using this as a basis for accessing its stored meaning in the semantic system. CB's good performance on single word comprehension as measured by the PPVT (Table 3) through the first follow-up evaluation, allows us to be fairly certain that her spelling difficulties did not originate in her failure to understand the words dictated to her. Furthermore, for all spelling-to-dictation tasks, CB was asked to repeat every word before spelling it and on the rare occasion that she failed to repeat the stimulus correctly, it was repeated to her until she was able to produce it correctly.

Subsequent to auditory comprehension, the spelling-specific components involved in spelling to dictation include the orthographic lexicon, the graphemic buffer, letter shape selection, and motor execution. The orthographic lexicon is the long-term memory store of the spellings of familiar words. Once a representation has been accessed in the orthographic lexicon it is maintained active by the graphemic working memory process (graphemic buffer) while the form of each letter is selected by the letter-shape conversion process to be produced in serial manner by the motor system. The dysgraphia assessment evaluated the integrity of each of these spelling-related components.

We can infer that significant damage to post-buffering letter-shape selection and motor execution processes are unlikely to have been important contributors to CB's spelling difficulties on the basis of two sets of observations. First, there were no significant differences between CB's written and oral spelling accuracies on the same list of 27 words (approximately half low and half high frequency, half four-letter and half eight-letter words) letter accuracy: 62% (98/160) vs 59% (94/160); $\chi^2(1) = .21$, ns. This similarity indicates that there is no special difficulty in producing written spellings, and thus indicates that the spelling errors probably originated at a point in processing before written and oral spelling diverge. Consideration of Figure 1 indicates that either the orthographic lexicon and/or the graphemic buffer are likely deficit sites. Second, although, as indicated in Table 4, CB's performance in writing single letters to dictation (92% and 90% correct) and in transcribing from one case to another (89% to 92% correct) are not perfect, and indicate that some errors might have arisen in the course of letter-shape selection, the magnitude of such a deficit is not commensurate with the magnitude of her spelling difficulties.

There are specific findings indicating that both the orthographic lexicon and the graphemic buffer have been affected, and it is likely that both deficits contributed to CB's spelling difficulties. Damage to the orthographic lexicon is indicated by a significant difference in her combined oral and written spelling accuracy for high vs

TABLE 4
CB's performance across a range of single-letter tasks both pre and post intervention

Task	Upper/Lower Case	Pre-Training	Post-Training
Direct Copy	LC	100% (26/26)	100% (26/26)
	UC	100% (26/26)	100% (26/26)
Naming	LC	96% (25/26)	92% (48/52)
	UC	100% (26/26)	94% (49/52)
Direct Copy Transcoding	UC to LC	92% (48/52)	89% (23/26)
	LC to UC	90% (47/52)	89% (23/26)
Writing to Dictation	LC	92% (48/52)	90% (47/52)
	UC	98% (51/52)	98% (51/52)

UC = upper case; LC = lower case; $n = 26$ includes the 26 letters of the alphabet evaluated once; $n = 52$ includes the 26 letters evaluated twice.

low frequency words: 73% (166.5/229) vs 57% (138/241); $\chi^2(1) = 12.3$, $p < .001$. Damage to the graphemic buffering process is indicated by a significant effect of word length. CB was able to produce the letters of four-letter words significantly more accurately than those of eight-letter words: 71% (79/112) vs 54% (108.5/200); $\chi^2(1) = 7.9$, $p < .01$.

Although CB's nonword spelling abilities were not extensively examined, the data in Table 3 indicate significantly impaired performance in nonword spelling with errors such as "kittle" → CIKOL; "reash" → CHEACH; "bruth" → BURTH). Nonetheless, it is noteworthy that accuracy with nonwords was superior to her performance with words. Difficulties in nonword spelling are expected when there are graphemic buffering difficulties as the buffering process is required for both words and nonwords. For this reason it is difficult to know if CB's difficulties with nonwords can be accounted for solely by the buffering deficit or if there is an additional deficit to the sublexical system. Relevant to this question is the fact that in word spelling CB sometimes produced phonologically plausible errors ("candle" → CANDIL), an indication that, at least on some occasions, when retrieval from the orthographic lexicon failed, the sublexical conversion system successfully generated a plausible spelling.

Table 5 reports the distribution of error types that CB produced in spelling a number of words lists. Her overall letter accuracy was 68% on these lists and, with respect to error types, it is noteworthy that she did not produce semantic or

TABLE 5
Distribution of CB's error types in word lists administered for spelling to dictation during pre-training evaluations

	Pre-Training
Phonologically plausible	11% (5/44)
Visually Similar Word	14% (6/44)
Visually Similar Nonword	55% (24/44)
Semantic	0%
Morphological	0%
Other	21% (9/44)

morphological errors in spelling to dictation. Her errors included not only phonologically plausible errors ("mercy" → MIRCEY; "method" → METHED) but also visually similar word errors in which the word response contained at least 50% of the target's letters ("crown" → COW; "hook" → HONK), visually similar nonword errors in which the response contained at least 50% of the target letters ("shrug" → SHUG; "prison" → PRISTON), as well as nonword responses that differed from the target by more than 50% of letters ("schedule" → SHEN; "province" → PARVERIS; note that we did not distinguish between orthographically vs phonologically similar responses). These types of errors are certainly consistent with a system in which there are deficits to both the orthographic lexicon and graphemic buffering while the remaining components remain relatively intact.

In sum, at the onset of the investigation both auditory comprehension and the peripheral post-buffering spelling processes seemed to be quite intact and were almost certainly not the major cause of the spelling difficulties. Instead, these difficulties were apparently the consequence of deficits affecting the orthographic lexicon, graphemic buffer and, possibly, sublexical phonology-to-orthography conversion.

Training protocol

There were four phases: pre-training, training, post-training, and follow-up. All four stimulus sets were presented for spelling to dictation twice during pre- and post-training evaluations and at the first follow-up, and only once at the second follow-up. Subsequent to the two pre-training (baseline) evaluations, training was carried out typically in biweekly sessions of approximately 3 hours, for a total of 11 complete administrations of the Trained and Repeated word sets. At each training session, the Trained words and the Repeated words were administered in a blocked fashion, with the order of blocks alternating from session to session. Each word set was divided into halves, as it typically required two sessions to administer both sets of words. After baseline testing, the duration of the intervention was 15 weeks (there were some interruptions in the training due to CB's travel or illness). Therefore, each word of the Trained and Repeated word sets was presented for a total of 11 times over a 15-week period. The follow-up evaluations were administered at approximately 6 and 12 months following the end of the training phase.

Stimulus categories

Stimuli consisted of four word sets ($n = 20$ for each set) that were matched for lexical frequency, letter length, regularity, and concreteness: Trained, Repeated, Homework, and Control words. Table 6 reports on the mean values for these variables for each list. For the second follow-up evaluation, reduced word sets for all word categories were used in order to limit the amount of time needed for the evaluation. This was done to accommodate CB's deteriorating and increasingly slow spelling performance. Each reduced set consisted of a subset of 10 of the items from each original 20 word sets, selected so that: (a) the four lists were matched with one another (as well as to the original 20-word lists) with respect to frequency, length and concreteness and (b) each subset of 10 items was matched in accuracy with the accuracy of the list it was derived from at Follow-up 1.

TABLE 6

Average (Avg) and standard deviation (in parentheses) for length in letters, concreteness and frequency for words in the four experimental lists

	Avg Length	Avg Concreteness	Avg. PG probability	Avg Frequency
Trained	5.7 (1.34)	496.85 (112.3)	.69 (.18)	43.15 (60.7)
Repeated	5.7 (1.34)	509 (104.0)	.73 (.14)	42.9 (60.6)
Homework	5.7 (1.34)	491.1 (121.3)	.71 (.17)	44.85 (68.7)
Control	5.7 (1.34)	510.1 (107.4)	.70 (.13)	41.5 (53.9)

Avg. PG probability corresponds to average phoneme–grapheme probability computed as an average of every PG mapping in each list based on the values in Hanna et al. (1996).

Training procedures

A spell-study-spell procedure, similar to that used in a number of the studies described in the Introduction, was applied to the Trained words, such that, at every training session, CB was asked: (1) to spell each word to dictation, (2) to study the word presented on a written notecard while the experimenter repeated the word and orally named each of its letters and then, if the word had been spelled incorrectly, (3) to attempt to spell it again. This procedure was repeated until the word was correctly spelled (or for three repetitions). To be clear, when a word was spelled correctly on the first attempt, the word was still presented for CB to study and only then did the experimenter continue to the next word.

Repeated words were simply presented for spelling to dictation at each training session without feedback. Homework words were repeatedly copied and self-tested at home. Specifically, CB was given sheets of paper each with one of the target words written at the top. She was instructed to copy the word 10 times, turn the page, and then try to spell it from memory. She then was to turn back the page to check to see if it was correctly spelled and, finally, she was supposed to study the correctly spelled word. It is important to note that CB did not carry out homework with consistency and regularity and so it is not possible to consider this study to be an adequate test of the real efficacy of the homework condition. Nonetheless, we present the results for the Homework condition as it may reflect "real-world" limitations on the application of this type of treatment (especially with clients who live alone and don't have someone to help supervise their homework). Control words were presented for spelling to dictation only at the time of the pre and post-treatment evaluations and at the two follow-ups.

The protocol structure allowed us to evaluate the following four effect types: word-specific treatment effects, word-specific homework effects, generalised learning effects, word-specific repetition effects. The evaluation of these effects is influenced by the fact that we are considering a neurodegenerative disorder. In the case of relatively stable diseases and conditions, we assume that during the intervention period, performance will remain unchanged in the absence of treatment. In the case of degenerative disease, while stability is one possibility, another is that in the absence of treatment, performance will deteriorate. These two possibilities and their impact on data interpretation will be considered in the following discussion.

Word-specific treatment effects refer to treatment benefits that affect the Trained words themselves and cannot be attributed simply to repeated attempts to spell the word or to natural progression (improvement or deterioration). In cases of *non-progressive* deficits, a treatment effect is indicated if there is better spelling performance on Trained words at the end of treatment than at the beginning, accompanied by better spelling performance on Trained versus Repeated words at the end of treatment. The latter is necessary to show that it was not merely the repeated testing that was efficacious, but that the treatment procedure itself was beneficial. However, in the context of a neurodegenerative disease, to show the effectiveness of treatment it is not required that the treatment actually improves performance relative to pre-treatment baseline. Instead, it must be shown that the treatment provided some benefit relative to the possible deterioration that might otherwise have occurred during the same time period. Performance on the Repeated words provides both an index of degeneration and takes into account any possible benefits of repeated testing. Therefore, in degenerative cases all that is required to show word-specific treatment effects is a significant difference between Trained words and Repeated words at the end of treatment.

Word-specific homework benefits are also treatment effects and therefore are subject to the same logic as word-specific treatment effects. That is, to demonstrate the specific benefits of Homework, these words should either (a) be spelled better at post-treatment than at baseline, and also better than Repeated words at post-treatment; or (b) simply be spelled better than Repeated words at post-treatment.

Generalised learning effects, in the case of non-progressive deficits, would be manifested by improvement in accuracy levels for the Control words from the beginning to the end of treatment. This is because we assume that, in the absence of treatment, control words will be stable from pre to post treatment. In the case of neurodegenerative disease, if we were to find such an improvement for the Control words it would, of course, indicate generalisation. However, if we were to find that performance on Control words stayed the same, or deteriorated between pre and post intervention evaluations, we could not reject the possibility that there might have been generalisation. This is because we have no way of knowing the extent of deterioration in the absence of treatment, and so we cannot be sure that the observed deterioration is equal to or less than would have occurred without treatment. There doesn't seem to be any good way to resolve this ambiguity; therefore even in the absence of improvement for control words, generalisation cannot be ruled out.

Word specific repetition effects are manifested, in the case of non-progressive deficits, by better spelling performance on the Repeated words at the end of treatment compared to the beginning accompanied by either (a) no generalised learning effect, or (b) an effect of repetition beyond that of generalised learning (spelling performance with the Repeated words better than that of the Control words at the end of treatment). This is because a repetition effect can only be distinguished from a generalised learning effect if the benefit to repeated words is greater than any benefits that apply to all words. In degenerative cases either of these two patterns would, of course, also constitute evidence of word specific repetition effects. However, in the case of a degenerative disorder, if there are no clear generalisation effects, word-specific repetition effects would be indicated (whether or not performance on Repeated words improved from pre to post intervention) if there were better performance on Repeated versus Control words at the end of treatment (i.e., control words show greater deterioration in performance).

RESULTS

Pre to post treatment effects

Two sets of analyses were used to evaluate the effect types described above. The first set of analyses involves comparisons of the spelling accuracies of the four word sets at pre versus post treatment evaluations. For comparisons of the *same* word sets at different time points we used the Wilcoxon matched pairs (signed rank) test, and for comparisons of *different* word sets at the same time point we used the chi-square test. Two-tailed tests are reported unless otherwise noted. The second analysis involves a regression analysis comparing the trajectory of change for the Trained versus Repeated conditions from pre to post-treatment. This regression analysis considers not only performance at pre and post-treatment "endpoints" but also includes all of the intermediate accuracy scores. For Repeated words these intermediate scores correspond to the results of administering the Repeated words for spelling to dictation at each treatment session; for Trained words these scores correspond to CB's first response to each of the words during the training trials (before she went on to carry out the study-spell procedure). This regression analysis was only possible for Trained versus Repeated words as none of the other stimulus conditions involved acquiring accuracy data at points other than at pre and post-treatment (and follow-up).[2]

Analysis 1. Pre and post treatment letter accuracies for each list were combined (added) across the two evaluations carried out at each of these time points. This was done in order to reduce variability and increase power. A comparison of the accuracy levels between stimulus conditions at Pre intervention reveals no significant differences between Trained, Repeated, Homework, or Control words (chi square values for these comparisons ranged from .01 to .80), indicating that all word sets were starting from a comparable level.

First, visual inspection of changes in pre to post training accuracies (Figure 3) indicates a fairly clear overall pattern of results such that: Trained words increase in accuracy, Control words decrease in accuracy, and Homework and Repeated words remain fairly stable at an intermediate level of accuracy. Statistical evaluation reveals the following:

1. A *word-specific treatment effect* was indicated by a significant improvement in letter accuracy for Trained words from pre to post training evaluations, T = 1596 ($N = 91$) $p < .05$. This effect was not due simply to repeated evaluations, as the accuracy of Trained words was greater than that of Repeated words at post-treatment, $\chi^2(1) = 4.94$, $p < .05$. In order to provide a more concrete sense of the types of changes observed for the Trained words, Table 7 reports CB's responses for the first pre-training evaluation and the final post-training evaluation.

2. There was no significant improvement for Homework words from Pre to Post Treatment, T = 1411 ($N = 77$) $p < .65$, nonetheless, there was evidence of a *word-specific homework effect* given CB's superior performance with Homework vs

---

[2] We had hoped to acquire similar data for the Homework words but because CB did not do the homework consistently and because she had no one at home to supervise her work and help organise the materials, we couldn't be certain of the accuracy of the homework data, nor of the conditions under which they were obtained.

Training Effects

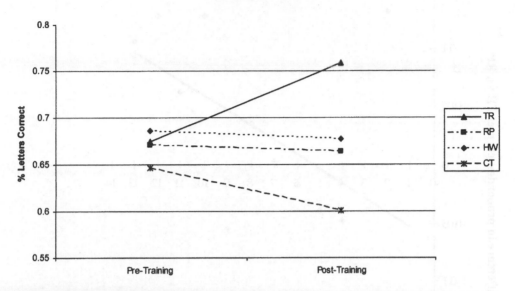

Figure 3. Percent letters correct at pre and post training (combined over two administrations of each list at each time point). TR = trained list, RP = repeated list, HW = homework list, and CT = control list (*n* = 228 letters for each word list at each time point).

Control words at post-treatment that is statistically significant with one-tailed testing, $\chi^2(1) = 2.91$, $p < .01$, 1-tailed. However, this benefit for Homework words cannot be distinguished from a benefit for repeated testing, as Homework

TABLE 7
CBD's written responses to Trained words at the first pre-treatment evaluation and at the final post-treatment evaluation

Target	PRE	POST
DIME	DINE	√
MAZE	MASE	MAC
BONE	√	√
BOMB	DOOM	BOME
PAPER	PAPAR	√
TWIST	TIST	√
GHOST	SO	GOST
FLAME	FASME	FALM
TOUGH	THOUT	TUS
PIANO	PION	PIPO
CANDLE	CANDLED	DANLL
SHIELD	SHERD	SHEID
PHRASE	CA	PRAC
TALENT	TALLANT	TALINT
SKETCH	SKECK	SKECK
JOURNAL	GO	JORNE
ANTIQUE	ANTIC	ANTQUE
QUESTION	√	√
BACTERIA	BATINC	BTERI
ORDINARY	ONR	√

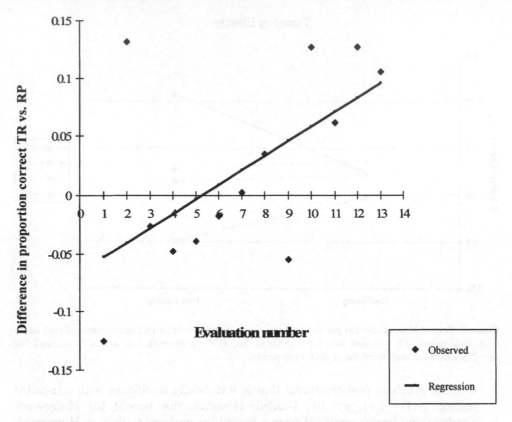

Figure 4. Differences in proportions correct on Trained (TR) minus Repeated (RP) word sets at each of 13 evaluations (from baseline to post-training) are represented with diamonds. Also included is the best linear fit to the data (slope = .012, F = 5.57; p < .04).

words were not produced significantly more accurately at Post-treatment than Repeated words, $\chi^2(1) = .04$, *ns*.

3. We could not discern any *generalisation effects* as performance with Control words declined from Pre to Post training, although this decline only trended towards being significant, T = 1914 (N = 97) p < .1. As indicated above, it is possible that performance with Control words declined less than it would have without treatment, but there is no experimental methodology that allows us to determine whether that was the case in the context of the neurodegenerative disease.

4. With regard to a *repetition effect,* we first note that accuracy on Repeated words did not significantly improve from Pre to Post treatment, T = 1675 (N = 86) p > .4. However, there was a suggestion of a benefit of repetition as Repeated words were spelled more accurately than Control words at post-treatment, although this difference was not significant, $\chi^2(1) = 1.98$, *ns*.

Analysis 2. The strongest finding from Analysis 1 is that of a treatment benefit for Trained words. The finding of a treatment benefit is indicated by a significant accuracy difference between Trained words at Pre and Post-treatment as well as by a significant difference between Trained and Repeated words at Post-treatment. The difference between Trained and Repeated words is critical for establishing the benefits of treatment and this second analysis provides a more stringent test of this difference between conditions. It does so by comparing the Trained and Repeated not only at the endpoints of the intervention period, but by including all of the intermediate evaluations as well.

The question addressed in this analysis is whether or not the differences between the Trained and Repeated words increase systematically with training. This is evaluated by means of a regression analysis that essentially determines the degree to which the accuracy differences between Trained and Repeated words are related to the evaluation number. Figure 4 reports the difference scores (difference in proportion correct) for Trained and Repeated word sets for each of the individual 13 evaluations (including two Pre-treatment evaluations). Also included in the figure is the best linear fit to these difference scores ($R^2 = .34$). The positive slope of this line indicates that the differences in accuracy between Trained and Repeated words are increasing with training session—indicating a training benefit. The critical statistical question is whether or not the positive slope of this line is significantly greater than 0. In fact, the regression analysis indicates a clearly significant positive slope ($F = 5.57$, $p < .04$), confirming the significant treatment effect established in Analysis 1. A number of variations on this analysis were carried out as well as evaluations of various characteristics of the data. These findings were incorporated into a more complex regression analysis (described in footnote 3). All additional analyses revealed significant findings, comparable to those reported just above.[3]

Maintenance of benefits and medium- to long-term treatment effects

Figure 5 reports the accuracy for each of the four stimulus conditions ut Pre and Post-treatment as well as Follow-up 1 (6 months post treatment) and Follow-up 2 (12 months post treatment). It provides an overview of the entire intervention and the trajectories of all stimulus conditions.

---

[3] The regression analysis can be carried out on the raw proportion differences depicted in Figure 5 or on statistically appropriate transformations of the data. For example, we also applied a logit transformation to the proportion scores obtained for each of the two kinds of word sets in each session. The logit transformation is the log-odds or logarithm of the odds ratio of the proportion of letters correctly identified. In this case, this provides us with transformed scores that are on the real line and, consequently, greater comfort with the assumptions in the linear model. We modeled the differences in the logit of the scores in terms of a simple linear regression set-up with time as the explanatory variable. The differences in log-odds ratios of the trained and repeated sets varied significantly with time (coefficient = 0.0567, $p = .0403$). (In the context of the original untransformed data, this implies that the relative proportions of the odds ratios of the scores for the repeated and trained word sets increases exponentially by 0.0567 for every unit change in time.) The model reported an R-squared of 0.3293 and an adjusted R-squared of 0.2684. Detailed diagnostics of the residuals indicates that the set of scores for the second observation was both outlying as well as influential. Otherwise, the homoscedasticity and normal assumption for the errors in the differences of logit-transformed scores was reasonable. Given this, the analysis was redone with the second set of observations omitted. The main finding of a significant relationship over time (slope = 0.0184, $p = .0003$) was strongly supported. The residuals have an autocorrelation coefficient of –0.329, so a model incorporating a first-order autocorrelation structure was also fitted, yielding significant results comparable to those of all previous analyses (slope = 0.08903; $p < .0001$). Finally, a chi-squared test statistic evaluating the goodness of fit of the model incorporating the autocorrelation ($\chi^2 = 2.49$) indicates that the first-order autoregressive structure for the model is not significant (p-value = .115). In other words, the previous model that did not include the autocorrelation was adequate.

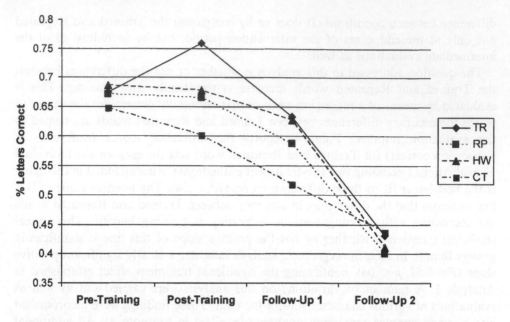

Figure 5. Accuracy for all word sets (TR = trained, RP = repeatedly tested, HW = homework, and CT = control (*n* = 228 letters for all sets at all time points, except Follow-up 2 where *n* = 58 letters for TR and RP and *n* = 56 for HW and CT).

Maintenance: From post-treatment to follow-ups. The degree to which treatment benefits were *maintained* over the 12-month period following the end of treatment can be evaluated by comparing post-treatment accuracy levels with those at Follow-ups 1 and 2.

Comparisons of Post-treatment accuracy levels with those at Follow-up 1 reveal a numerical decline in performance for all stimulus categories. These changes were statistically significant for all categories except for Homework words—Homework: T = 1365 (*N* = 82) *p* < .12, Trained: T = 1287 (*N* = 94) *p* < .0001, Control words: T = 2281 (*N* = 108) *p* < .04, Repeated words: T = 1560 (*N* = 93) *p* < .02. Despite this decline, 6 months after the end of treatment at Follow-up 1, Trained words still remained significantly more accurate than Control words, $\chi^2(1) = 6.18$, *p* < .05, although they were no longer statistically more accurate than either Repeated, $\chi^2(1) = 0.97$, *ns*, or Homework words, $\chi^2(1) = 0.01$, *ns*. Furthermore, at Follow-up 1 both Homework and Repeated words continued to be more accurate than Control Words, although this difference was statistically significant only for the Homework set—Homework: $\chi^2(1) = 5.60$, *p* < .05—with only a trend towards significance for the Repeated set—Repeated: $\chi^2(1) = 2.27$, *p* < .1.

From 6 to 12 months after the end of treatment there continued to be a decline for all stimulus categories. All of these decreases were statistically significant except for the Control words—Control words: T = 296.5 (*N* = 36) *p* < .6, Trained: T = 118.5 (*N* = 35) *p* < .002, Repeated words: T = 177 (*N* = 38) *p* < .006, and Homework: T = 841.5 (*N* = 70) *p* < .02. Finally, by 1 year after the end of treatment at Follow-up 2, there were no statistically significant differences among the four word categories. In sum, there was clear evidence of the benefit of treatment, although the magnitude of the post-treatment benefit to Trained words had reduced by 6 months after treatment. This is indicated by the fact that at 6 months after the end of treatment, Trained words were still spelled significantly more accurately than Control words. Furthermore, both Homework and Repeated words maintained their advantage over Control words from post-treatment to Follow-up 1, although this difference was only significant for Homework words. Finally, no benefits of treatment were discernible for any of the word sets 12 months after the end of the treatment.

Medium- and long-term treatment benefits: From pre-treatment to follow-ups. An evaluation of the medium- and long-term effectiveness of treatment was carried out by comparing *Pre*-treatment accuracy levels with levels at Follow-ups 1 and 2.

Compared to the pre-treatment accuracy levels, at 6 months after the end of treatment there were numerical declines in performance for all stimulus categories. These declines were statistically significant only for Control words, $T = 1849$ $(N = 110)$, $p < .0005$, while accuracy levels for Homework words, $T = 1708.5$ $(N = 93)$, $p < .07$, Repeated words, $T = 2248.5$ $(N = 103)$ $p < .2$, and Trained words, $T = 1883$ $(N = 94)$ $p < .2$, were statistically unchanged. This is evidence that, in the face of clear deterioration of untrained items, the training protocol helped to *maintain* the integrity of Trained, Homework, and Repeated items through the treatment period and out to 6 months beyond the end of treatment.

Compared to pre-treatment, at 12 months after the end of treatment there were significant declines in all four categories (all $ps < .01$). Therefore, despite the immediate (post-treatment) improvement for Trained words and medium-term maintenance of pre-treatment accuracy levels for Trained, Homework, and (to a lesser extent) Repeated words, there was no evidence of any treatment benefits by 1 year after the end of treatment.

Summary of results

The results can be summarised as follows:

1. The spell-study-spell treatment provided a modest (10% of letters), but statistically significant, advantage to words that are trained compared to words that were either untrained, practised in homework, or simply repeatedly tested.
2. The benefit for Trained words was fragile, such that by 6 months after the end of the study Trained words could not be statistically distinguished from Homework and Repeated items.
3. However, the intermediate range benefits of treatment manifested themselves at 6 months after the end of treatment in the maintenance of pre-treatment levels of accuracy for Trained words. This occurred in the face of clearly declining spelling abilities as indexed by deteriorating performance with Control words.
4. More modest benefits of homework practice or repeated testing were indicated by the greater stability in the accuracy levels of Homework and Repeated items relative to control items in comparisons of pre-treatment with post-treatment and with the 6-month follow-up.
5. No generalisation effects could be documented.
6. No benefits of treatment could be discerned by one year after the end of treatment.

GENERAL DISCUSSION

We find both immediate and short-term benefits of behavioural intervention for dysgraphia in a case of primary progressive aphasia. Immediately following treatment, accuracy on Trained words increased relative to pre-treatment baseline and relative to all other control word types. Six months after the end of treatment, Trained words were protected from the significant deterioration experienced by untrained Control words. Repeated testing or practice at home yielded modest benefits, resulting in accuracies intermediate to those of the Trained and untrained Control words. These findings are among the first to provide empirical support for the potential of behavioural therapy to prolong language abilities in primary progressive aphasia. This occurred in a context of non-intensive training (typically 2 sessions/week) with overall relatively modest input (11 sessions).

The relationship between treatment in progressive and non-progressive disorders

A fundamental question in the study of PPA is the extent to which the response to treatment is similar or different in progressive compared to non-progressive disorders resulting from stroke, surgery, or head injury. Of course, in non-progressive disorders there may be changes in symptomatology subsequent to the neurological insult, but given that the aetiology is not degenerative the changes tend to be quantitative rather than qualitative. In previous work, Rapp and Kane (2002) and Rapp (2005) reported three individuals with acquired dysgraphia subsequent to stroke who were tested with essentially the same treatment protocol (without the Homework condition) as was used in the case of CB. Although none of the individuals had both the orthographic lexicon and graphemic buffering deficits that CB demonstrated, one (MMD) had a clear lexicon deficit and the other two (JRE, RSB) suffered from graphemic buffer deficits. These differences notwithstanding, it may be informative to consider the similarities and differences between CB's response to treatment and the responses of these individuals with non-progressive deficits. Figure 6 presents the results from MMD, JRE,[4] and CB. For MMD and JRE we include results from follow-ups at 5 and 10 months post treatment as these are the closest to CB's 6 and 12 month follow-ups.

First of all, Rapp and Kane (2002) and Rapp (2005) found that all individuals (regardless of deficit type) exhibited a benefit for Trained words. That is, all three significantly improved their performance for Trained words pre to post treatment, and Trained words were spelled more accurately than Repeated words at the end of training. Furthermore, this treatment benefit persisted until 10 months after the end of treatment, such that although performance decreased on the Trained words during this time period, accuracy on these words was still significantly better at 10-month follow-up than it had been prior to the onset of treatment. In this regard, CB's response to treatment was very similar to the individuals with non-progressive deficits. She too showed significant improvement for Trained words and the effects of this treatment were still evident at 6 months after the end of treatment. However, for CB, the benefits at the 6-month follow-up were manifested not in continued

---

[4] Both JRE and RSB responded very similarly to treatment except that JRE's maintenance of benefits was more short-lived than RSB's; for the sake of brevity, we report only the results for JRE.

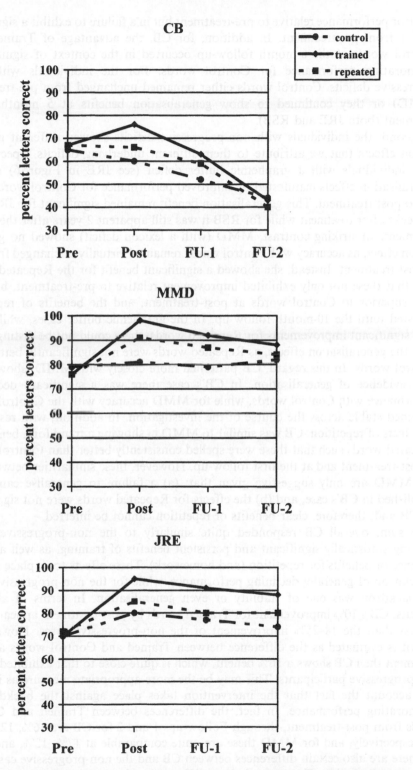

Figure 6. Letter accuracy at Pre-intervention, Post-intervention, Follow-up 1, and Follow-up 2 for CB, MMD, and JRE (details regarding MMD and JRE's data are available in Rapp, 2005, and Rapp & Kane, 2002).

superior performance relative to pre-treatment but in a failure to exhibit a significant decline from pre-treatment. In addition, for CB, the advantage of Trained over Control words at the 6-month follow-up occurred in the context of significantly deteriorating performance for Control words. For the individuals with non-progressive deficits, Control words either remained unchanged from pre-treatment (MMD) or they continued to show generalisation benefits at 5 months post-treatment (both JRE and RSB).

Second, the individuals with non-progressive deficits showed different general-isation effects that we attribute to their different underlying deficits. Specifically, both individuals with a graphemic buffer deficit (see JRE in Figure 6) showed generalisation effects manifested by improved performance for Control words from pre to post treatment. This generalisation benefit remained significant for JRE until 12 weeks after treatment while for RSB it was still apparent 2 years after the end of treatment. In striking contrast, MMD (with a lexicon deficit) showed no general-isation effect, as accuracy with control words remained virtually unchanged from pre to post treatment. Instead, she showed a significant benefit for the Repeated words such that these not only exhibited improvement relative to pre-treatment, but they were superior to Control words at post-treatment, and the benefits of repetition persisted until the 10-month follow-up. In the graphemic buffer cases, while there were significant improvements for Repeated words, these could not be distinguished from the generalisation effects, as Repeated words were not significantly better than Control words. In this regard, CB patterned more closely with MMD, showing no clear evidence of generalisation. In CB's case there was a significant decline in performance with Control words, while for MMD accuracy with the Control words remained stable across the course of the investigation. In addition, with respect to the effects of repetition, CB was similar to MMD in showing a trend for a benefit for Repeated words such that these were spelled consistently better than Control words at post-treatment and at the first follow-up. However, these similarities between CB and MMD are only suggestive given that: (a) a failure to generalise cannot be established in CB's case, and (b) the effects for Repeated words were not significant for CB and, therefore, clear benefits of repetition cannot be inferred.

In sum, overall CB responded quite similarly to the non-progressive cases, showing statistically significant and persistent benefits of training, as well as some evidence of benefits for repetition (and homework). These effects took place against a backdrop of generally declining performance, while for the non-progressive cases the backdrop was one of stability or even generalisation. In terms of absolute benefits, CB's 10% improvement for Trained words by post-treatment appears more modest than the 18–25% improvement of the non-progressive cases. However, if benefit is evaluated as the difference between Trained and Control words at post-treatment then CB shows a 16% benefit, which is quite close to that exhibited by the non-progressive participants. This may be the more appropriate measure as it takes into account the fact that the intervention takes place against the backdrop of deteriorating performance. In fact, the differences between Trained and Control words from post-treatment, through Follow-ups 1 and 2 for CB are 16%, 12%, and 0% respectively, and for MMD these are quite comparable at 17%, 13%, and 6%.

There are also certain differences between CB and the non-progressive cases that are worth discussing. The most obvious difference is the deteriorating performance of Control words across the entire intervention period. In addition there is the deterioration for all word classes from pre-treatment to 12 months post-treatment.

More subtle differences include the fact that during the treatment sessions, CB required a greater number of repetitions of each item. She averaged 1.8 repetitions, while the individuals with non-progressive deficits averaged only .22 to .45 repetitions. Furthermore, non-progressive participants received training until reaching the criterion of 95% accuracy or better for two consecutive sessions. CB was never able to achieve these accuracy levels; instead training was discontinued when accuracy for Trained words stabilised between 70% and 75% of letters correct. Nonetheless, for both groups, stable effects were achieved with roughly comparable numbers of training sessions (11 for CBD, 11–20 for the non-progressive cases). Overall, therefore, CB's ability to relearn the spellings of words or recover some of her ability to access these words seemed roughly comparable to that of individuals who did not suffer from neurodegenerative disease, yet there is clear evidence from the number of repetitions required, the level of accuracy at which asymptotic performance is reached, and the fragility of the training benefits, that CB's relearning was hampered by the neurodegenerative disease.

Costs, benefits, and other considerations

Therapy is costly in terms of time and financial resources, and therefore it is important to weigh the costs and benefits of any therapy approach. Unfortunately, it is of course difficult to evaluate cost/benefit ratios in the best of circumstances, and clearly not possible with the limited data from this study. Nonetheless, it may be worthwhile to consider some of the relevant issues.

This study serves as a type of "proof of concept" study demonstrating that it is possible to get improvement and "protection" from degeneration for specific words that are trained. It is clear that the degree of improvement or protection conferred on the Trained words is not sufficient to make an impact on CB's quality of life. This is not only because the benefits were quantitatively modest, but also because the words that were selected for treatment were not words that were important to CB's everyday life (words such as CANDLE, TOUGH, BACTERIA). However, the study does show that, even under these less than optimal functional circumstances, measurable and significant benefits can be obtained. Certainly it will be important to evaluate the degree to which effectiveness of training is affected by the personal relevance of the items, as well as by whether or not the training itself explicitly works to integrate the words into activities of daily living.

In the context of evaluating the benefits of this treatment, one might also question the wisdom of expending resources on written rather than spoken language rehabilitation. One thing that is relevant in this regard is that, in the context of non-progressive deficits, it has been sometimes reported that for certain individuals with both spoken and written language impairments, remediation of the written language deficits is sometimes more successful than remediation of the spoken deficits (Beeson, 1999; Robson et al., 2001). This is not entirely surprising given the fairly extensive evidence showing the independence of a number of the cognitive mechanisms involved in written and spoken language production. That is, there have been a number of cases of individuals who can write words they cannot say, and vice versa (for a review see Rapp et al., 1997). In the context of progressive aphasia we noted in the Introduction that it has been reported that, for some individuals, written language remains a relative strength and they therefore rely on this for communication (Cress & King, 1999; Holland et al., 1985; Kertesz et al., 1994;

Mesulam & Weintraub, 1992; Murray, 1998; Weintraub et al., 1990). Cress and King (1998) specifically remarked on relative preservation of reading in the course of PPA, at least in with regard to overlearned written materials. They state (p. 257):

> It is important to determine whether people with PPA can successfully overlearn critical written information during periods of better reading and language skills or whether this skill is restricted to highly familiar environmental writing.... if deliberate practice of specific written vocabulary can keep those vocabulary items in active use, *then overlearning of essential information may be an effective strategy in maintaining functional reading and recognition skills for persons with PPA* [italics added].

Given the findings we have reported here indicating that learning of written material is possible in cases of PPA, it will be important for future research to examine the role that the timing of the intervention plays in the development and strengthening of skills and representations that will be durable in the face of the degenerative process.

Conclusions

In sum, we have reported evidence that the relearning, strengthening, or improved accessibility of word spellings are possible in a case of primary progressive aphasia. This recovery, at least superficially, resembles what is observed in cases of non-progressive dysgraphia. Certainly, however, the underlying nature and mechanisms of the improvement are not understood in any of these cases and this represents yet another area that will require future investigation. However, what is most encouraging is that the benefits provided by the training allow the targeted words to remain available for use for a longer period of time. The study raises a number of questions regarding the best means of harnessing this learning capacity so as to best serve the needs of individuals with neurodegenerative language disorders.

REFERENCES

Aliminosa, D., McCloskey, M., Goodman-Schulman, R., & Sokol, S. M. (1993). Remediation of acquired dysgraphia as a technique for testing interpretations of deficits. *Aphasiology, 7*(1), 55–69.

Ardila, A., Matute, E., & Inozemtseva, O. V. (2003). Progressive agraphia, acalculia, and anomia: A single case report. *Applied Neuropsychology, 10*(4), 205–214.

Beeson, P. M. (1999). Treating acquired writing impairment: Strengthening graphemic representations. *Aphasiology, 13*(9), 767–785.

Beeson, P. M., & Hirsch, F. M. (1998, November). *Writing treatment of severe aphasia.* Paper presented at the Annual Convention of the American Speech-Language-Hearing Association, San Antonio, TX.

Beeson, P. M., Hirsch, F. M., & Rewega, M. A. (2002). Successful single-word writing treatment: Experimental analyses of four cases. *Aphasiology, 16*(4), 473–491.

Beeson, P. M., & Rapcsak, S. Z. (2002). Clinical diagnosis and treatment of spelling disorders. In A. E. Hillis (Ed.), *Handbook on adult language disorders: Integrating cognitive neuropsychology, neurology, and rehabilitation* (pp. 101–120). Philadelphia: Psychology Press.

Beeson, P. M., Rewega, M. A., Vail, S., & Rapcsak, S. Z. (2000). Problem solving approach to agraphia treatment: Interactive use of lexical and sublexical spelling routes. *Aphasiology, 14*(5), 551–565.

Beeson, P. M., Rising, K., & Volk, J. (2003). Writing treatment for severe aphasia: Who benefits? *Journal of Speech, Language, and Hearing Research, 46*(5), 1038–1060.

Behrmann, M. (1987). The rites of righting writing: Homophone remediation in acquired dysgraphia. *Cognitive Neuropsychology, 4*(3), 365–384.

Behrmann, M., & Byng, S. (1992). A cognitive approach to the neurorehabilitation of acquired language disorders. In D. I. Margolin (Ed.), *Cognitive neuropsychology in clinical practice* (pp. 327–350). Oxford, UK: Oxford University Press.

Benton, A. L., & Hamsher, K. (1976). *Multilingual aphasia examination* (2nd ed.). Iowa City: IA: AJA Associates.

Benton Sivan, A. (1991). *Benton Visual Retention Test – 5th edition.* San Antonio, TX: Harcourt Assessment.

Carlomagno, S., Iavarone, A., & Columbo, A. (1994). Cognitive approaches to writing rehabilitation: From single case to group studies. In M. J. Riddoch & G. W. Humphreys (Eds.), *Cognitive neuropsychology and cognitive rehabilitation* (pp. 485–502). Hillsdale, NJ: Lawrence Erlbaum Associates Inc.

Carlomagno, S., & Parlato, V. (1989). Writing rehabilitation in brain damaged adult patients: A cognitive approach. In X. Seron & G. Deloche (Eds.), *Cognitive approaches in neuropsychological rehabilitation* (pp. 175–209). Hillsdale, NJ: Lawrence Erlbaum Associates Inc.

Clausen, N. S., & Beeson, P. M. (2003). Conversational use of writing in severe aphasia: A group treatment approach. *Aphasiology, 17*(6), 625–644.

Cress, C. J., & King, J. M. (1999). AAC strategies for people with primary progressive aphasia without dementia: Two case studies. *AAC: Augmentative and Alternative Communication, 15*(4), 248–259.

Croisile, B., Carmoi, T., Adeleine, P., & Trillet, M. (1995). Spelling in Alzheimer's disease. *Behavioural Neurology, 8*(3), 135–143.

de Partz, M., Seron, X., & Van der Linden, M. (1992). Re-education of a surface dysgraphia with a visual imagery strategy. *Cognitive Neuropsychology, 9*(5), 369–401.

Dunn, L. M., & Dunn, L. M. (1981). *Peabody Picture Vocabulary Test – Revised.* Circle Pines, MN: American Guidance Service.

Folstein, M. F., Folstein, S. E., & McHugh, P. R. (1975). Mini-Mental State: A practical method for grading the state of patients for the clinician. *Journal of Psychiatric Research, 12*, 189–198.

Golden, C. J., & Freshwater, S. M. (2002). *Stroop Color and Word Test.* Wood Dale, IL: Stoelting Co.

Graham, N. L. (2000). Dysgraphia in dementia. *Neurocase, 6*(5), 365–376.

Graham, N. L., Patterson, K., & Hodges, J. R. (1997). Progressive dysgraphia: Co-occurrence of central and peripheral impairments. *Cognitive Neuropsychology, 14*(7), 975–1005.

Graham, N. L., Zeman, A., Young, A. W., Patterson, K., & Hodges, J. R. (1999). Dyspraxia in a patient with corticobasal degeneration: The role of visual and tactile inputs to action. *Journal of Neurology, Neurosurgery & Psychiatry, 67*(3), 334–344.

Hanna, P. P., Hanna, J. S., & Hodges, R. E. (1996). *Phoneme–grapheme correspondences as cues to spelling improvement.* Washington, DC: US Government Printing Office.

Hatfield, M. F. (1983). Aspects of acquired dysgraphia and implications for re-education. In C. Code & D. J. Mueller (Eds.), *Aphasia therapy.* London: Arnold.

Hatfield, M. F., & Weddel, R. (1976). Re-training in writing in severe aphasia. In R. Hoops & Y. Lebrun (Eds.), *Recovery in aphasics* (pp. 65–78). Amsterdam: Swets & Zeitlinger.

Hillis, A. E. (1992). Facilitating written production. *Clinics in Communication Disorders, 2*(1), 19–33.

Hillis, A. E. (1989). Efficacy and generalisation of treatment for aphasic naming errors. *Archives of Physical Medicine and Rehabilitation, 70*(8), 632–636.

Hillis, A. E. (1991). Effects of separate treatments for distinct impairments within the naming process. *Clinical Aphasiology, 19*, 255–265.

Hills, A. E., & Caramazza, A. (1987). Model-driven treatment of dysgraphia. In R. H. Brookshire (Ed.), *Clinical aphasiology* (pp. 84–105). Minneapolis, MN: BRK Publishers.

Hillis, A. E., Heidler-Gary, J., Newhart, M., Chang, S., Ken, L., & Bak, T. H. (2006). Naming and comprehension in primary progressive aphasia: The influence of grammatical word class. *Aphasiology, 20*, 246–256.

Hillis Trupe, A. E. (1986). Effectiveness of retraining phoneme to grapheme conversion. In R. H. Brookshire (Ed.), *Clinical aphasiology.* Minneapolis, MN: BRK Publishers.

Holland, A. L., McBurney, D. H., Moossy, J., & Reinmuth, O. M. (1985). The dissolution of language in Pick's disease with neurofibrillary tangles: A case study. *Brain and Language, 24*(1), 36–58.

Hughes, J. C., Graham, N., Patterson, K., & Hodges, J. R. (1997). Dysgraphia in mild dementia of Alzheimer's type. *Neuropsychologia, 35*, 533–545.

Kaplan, E., Goodglass, H., & Weintraub, S. (1983). *Boston Naming Test.* New York: Lee & Febiger.

Kay, J., Lesser, R., & Coltheart, M. (1992). *PALPA: Psycholinguistic Assessments of Language Processing in Aphasia.* Hove, UK: Lawrence Erlbaum Associates Ltd.

Kertesz, A., Hudson, L., Mackenzie, I. R. A., & Munoz, D. G. (1994). The pathology and nosology of primary progressive aphasia. *Neurology*, *44*(11), 2065–2072.

Luzzatti, C., Colombo, C., Frustaci, M., & Vitolo, F. (2000). Rehabilitation of spelling along the sub-word-level routine. *Neuropsychological Rehabilitation*, *10*(3), 249–278.

Luzzatti, C., Laiacona, M., & Agazzi, D. (2003). Multiple patterns of writing disorders in dementia of the alzheimer type and their evolution. *Neuropsychologia*, *41*(7), 759–772.

Luzzatti, C., Laiacona, M., & Agazzi, D. (2002). Dysgraphia in dementia of the Alzheimer's type. *Cortex*, *38*(5), 887–890.

Luzzi, S., & Piccirilli, M. (2003). Slowly progressive pure dysgraphia with late apraxia of speech: A further variant of the focal cerebral degeneration. *Brain and Language*, *87*(3), 355–360.

McNeil, M. R., Small, S. L., Masterson, R. J., & Fossett, T. R. D. (1995). Behavioural and pharmacological treatment of lexical-semantic deficits in a single patient with primary progressive aphasia. *American Journal of Speech-Language Pathology*, *4*(4), 76–87.

Mesulam, M. M. (1982). Slowly progressive aphasia without generalised dementia. *Annals of Neurology*, *11*(6), 592–598.

Mesulam, M. M., Grossman, M., Hillis, A., Kertesz, A., & Weintraub, S. (2003). The core and halo of primary progressive aphasia and semantic dementia. *Annals of Neurology*, *54*(Suppl 5), S11–14.

Mesulam, M. M., & Weintraub, S. (1992). Spectrum of primary progressive aphasia. *Bailliere's Clinical Neurology*, *1*(3), 583–609.

Mortley, J., Enderby, P., & Petheram, B. (2001). Using a computer to improve functional writing in a patient with severe dysgraphia. *Aphasiology*, *15*(5), 443–461.

Murray, L. L. (1998). Longitudinal treatment of primary progressive aphasia: A case study. *Aphasiology*, *12*(7), 651–672.

O'Dowd, B. S., & Zubicaray, G. I. D. (2003). Progressive dysgraphia in a case of posterior cortical atrophy. *Neurocase*, *9*(3), 251–260.

Osterreith, P. A. (1944). Le test de copie d'une figure complexe. *Archives de Psychologie*, *30*, 206–356.

Pattee, C., Von Berg, S., & Ghezzi, P. (2006). Effects of alternative communication on the communicative effectiveness of an individual with a progressive language disorder. *International Journal of Rehabilitation Research*, *29*(2), 151–153.

Platel, H., Lambert, J., Eustache, F., & Cadet, B. (1993). Characteristics and evolution of writing impairment in Alzheimer's disease. *Neuropsychologia*, *31*(11), 1147–1158.

Pound, C. (1996). Writing remediation using preserved oral spelling: A case for separate output buffers. *Aphasiology*, *10*(3), 283–296.

Rapcsak, S. Z., Arthur, S. A., Bliklen, D. A., & Rubens, A. B. (1989). Lexical agraphia in Alzheimer's disease. *Archives of Neurology*, *46*(1), 65–68.

Rapp, B. (2005). The relationship between treatment outcomes and the underlying cognitive deficit: Evidence from the remediation of acquired dysgraphia. *Aphasiology*, *19*(10), 994–1008.

Rapp, B., Benzing, L., & Caramazza, A. (1997). The autonomy of lexical orthography. *Cognitive Neuropsychology*, *14*, 71–104.

Rapp, B., & Caramazza, A. (2002). Selective difficulties with spoken nouns and written verbs: A single case study. *Journal of Neurolinguistics*, *15*, 373–402.

Rapp, B., & Kane, A. (2002). Remediation of deficits affecting different components of the spelling process. *Aphasiology*, *16*(4), 439–454.

Rey, A. (1942). L'examen psychologique dans les cas d'encephalopathie traumatique. *Archives de Psychologie*, *28*, 286–340.

Riddoch, M. J., & Humphreys, G. (1993). *Birmingham Object Recognition Battery*. New York: Psychology Press.

Raymer, A. M., Cudworth, C., & Haley, M. A. (2003). Spelling treatment for an individual with dysgraphia: Analysis of generalisation to untrained words. *Aphasiology*, *17*(6), 607–624.

Reitan, R. M. (1992). *Trail Making Test (Adult Version) (TMT)*. Tucson, AZ: Reitan Neuropsychology Laboratory.

Robson, J., Marshall, J., Chiat, S., & Pring, T. (2001). Enhancing communication in jargon aphasia: A small group study of writing therapy. *International Journal of Language & Communication Disorders*, *36*(4), 471–488.

Schmalzl, L., & Nickels, L. (2006). Treatment of irregular word spelling in acquired dysgraphia: Selective benefit from visual mnemonics. *Neuropsychological Rehabilitation*, *16*(1), 1–37.

Schmidt, M. (1996). *Rey Auditory Verbal Learning Test (RAVLT) – a Handbook*. Los Angeles: Western Psychological Services.

Schneider, S. L., Thompson, C. K., & Luring, B. (1996). Effects of verbal plus gestural matrix training on sentence production in a patient with primary progressive aphasia. *Aphasiology*, *10*(3), 297–317.

Seron, X., Deloche, G., Moulard, G., & Rousselle, M. (1980). A computer-based therapy for the treatment of aphasic subjects with writing disorders. *Journal of Speech & Hearing Disorders*, *45*(1), 45–58.

Trites, R. (1984). *Grooved Pegboard Test*. Lafayette, IN: Lafayette Instrument.

Warrington, E. K. (1984). *Recognition Memory Test*. London: NFER-Nelson Publishing Co., Ltd.

Weekes, B., & Coltheart, M. (1996). Surface dyslexia and surface dysgraphia: Treatment studies and their theoretical implications. *Cognitive Neuropsychology*, *13*(2), 277–315.

Weintraub, S., Rubin, N. P., & Mesulam, M. M. (1990). Primary progressive aphasia. longitudinal course, neuropsychological profile, and language features. *Archives of Neurology*, *47*(12), 1329–1335.

Wechsler, D., & Stone, C. P. (1973). *Manual: Wechsler Memory Scale*. New York: Psychological Corporation.

Westbury, C., & Bub, D. (1997). Primary progressive aphasia: A review of 112 cases. *Brain and Language*, *60*(3), 381–406.

APHASIOLOGY, 2009, 23 (2), 266–285

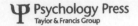

Promoting strategic television viewing in the context of progressive language impairment

Jade Cartwright and Kym A. E. Elliott

Neurosciences Unit, Perth, Western Australia

Background: Television viewing is one of the most common and readily accessible leisure pursuits in the developed world today. Unfortunately, access to this powerful form of mass communication is frequently diminished in individuals experiencing progressive language impairment, with deficits in both the comprehension and expression of television content reported from the very early stages of the illness. Considering the wide appeal of television viewing in today's culture, it seems reasonable to conclude that improving access to television content should be considered as an ecologically valid goal for intervention in clinical populations with progressive language impairment who have demonstrated difficulties comprehending and speaking about this powerful form of mass communication. This consideration becomes more pressing when we attend to recent research highlighting the potential neuroprotective effect of engagement in cognitively and intellectually stimulating social and leisure pursuits by individuals with dementing illness.

Aims: This pilot therapy programme aimed to explore the effectiveness of aphasia-friendly television viewing formats for improving discourse comprehension and production in people with progressive language impairment. It was predicted that following intervention, group participants would (1) recall significantly more story information units from the episode, (2) achieve higher transactional success, and (3) demonstrate improved comprehension when viewing aphasia-friendly television episodes than they did prior to group intervention.

Methods & Procedures: Four participants with progressive language impairment attended eight sessions of group-based intervention as part of their usual language therapy programme. Each session aimed to instantiate strategic television viewing capabilities in participants through the application of aphasia-friendly television viewing principles to novel episodes of a popular 30-minute documentary programme. Repeated measures ANOVA was used to analyse the differences between participants' pre-therapy viewing patterns and supported post-therapy measures of episode-related story information unit production, while paired *t*-tests were used for analysis of discourse comprehension measures.

Outcomes & Results: Participants demonstrated significant increases in story information unit reporting and comprehension indicated by performance on concrete and opinion based questions post-therapy. There was no significant difference in participants' post-therapy comprehension of inferential questions.

Address correspondence to: Jade Cartwright, Neurosciences Unit, cnr John XXIII Ave and Mooro Drive, Mt Claremont, WA 6010, Australia. E-mail: Jade.cartwright@health.wa.gov.au

Thanks to Jemma Selby and Stephanie Danker (final year Human Communication Science students, Curtin University), who helped facilitate the treatment group; to our colleagues at the Neurosciences Unit for their ongoing support; and to Lyndsey Nickels and Karen Croot for comments on an earlier version of this manuscript. Most importantly, we would like to thank our clients with progressive language impairment and their families who are the source of our inspiration and who have made this project so rewarding.

http://www.psypress.com/aphasiology   DOI: 10.1080/02687030801942932

Conclusions: This pilot therapy programme affirms the prediction that aphasia-friendly television viewing formats are successful in achieving significant improvements in episode related discourse production, communication effectiveness, comprehension of concrete question forms, and opinion generation in individuals with progressive language impairment. It supports the notion that novel, ecologically based intervention techniques can be beneficial in enhancing access to preferred leisure activities in individuals with progressive language impairment.

Keywords: Language; Therapy; Dementia; Aphasia friendly; Television.

We are currently experiencing a dramatic worldwide rise in dementia prevalence (Cummings & Jeste, 1999). Communication difficulties are one of the major obstacles faced by this client group, resulting in the gradual dissolution of a fundamental human skill that is so often taken for granted. The loss of language ability inevitably affects an individual's independence and participation in activities of daily living, sense of self, and overall quality of life (Lyon, 2000). Sufficient evidence is emerging to support the benefit of psychosocial and behavioural intervention programmes in dementia (Burns, 2004). It seems, however, that dementia care continues to receive low prioritisation in clinical service provision and there is an immense need for further applied research.

The Primary Progressive Aphasias described by Mesulam (1982) are the dementia syndromes directly characterised by a progressive and relentless deterioration of normal language function, with preservation of more global cognitive abilities for a period of at least 2 years (Mesulam, 2001; Nestor et al., 2003). The diagnosis and characterisation of progressive aphasia remains a contentious issue (Croot, 2009 this issue; Knibb, Xuereb, Patterson, & Hodges, 2006) with a number of classification systems proposed. Diagnostic debates aside, clinical speech pathology experience shows a clear need for focused behavioural and pharmacological intervention (Taylor, Miles-Kingma, Croot, & Nickels, 2009 this issue).

Duffy and Petersen (1992) predicted that individuals with primary progressive aphasia would appear in speech pathology clinics more frequently in the future, with obvious implications for diagnosis, assessment, and management. Empirical research investigating the efficacy of behavioural intervention programmes is still in its infancy. However, early findings are giving individuals with progressive aphasia a sense of hope in the possibility that language abilities can be prolonged and quality of life improved (McNeil, Small, Masterson, & Fossett, 1995; Rapp, Glucroft, & Urrutia, 2005).

BENEFITS OF COGNITIVELY STIMULATING ACTIVITIES

The concepts of cognitive reserve and neuroprotection have received much interest in recent dementia research. The cognitive reserve hypothesis accounts for the recognised link between little or no formal education and the risk of developing dementia (Liao et al., 2005). According to this hypothesis, individuals who engage in more cognitively stimulating education, work and leisure activities are believed to develop richer synaptic networks and greater ability to use alternative brain circuitry in the face of neurodegenerative decline (Liao et al., 2005). In clinical practice, these individuals may present with significantly better abilities than would be predicted by clinical investigations suggesting advanced pathology (Liao et al., 2005). Furthermore, the progression of dementia may be slowed by continued engagement in leisure and social activities that stimulate cognitive and communication processes (Coyle, 2003; Lindstrom et al., 2005).

A huge concern for individuals with neurodegenerative disease is that as symptomatology and disability increases, segregation and withdrawal from cognitively stimulating opportunities within the community often results. This may be due to disease-related consequences such as loss of driver's licence, difficulty navigating public transport systems, or feelings of inadequacy, embarrassment, and increased dependence. This can result in individuals adopting a more passive role during daily life, and can potentially hasten the rate of clinical decline, while reducing opportunities to develop effective compensatory strategies and/or alternative synaptic networks. As part of our role as clinical specialists in this field, our ethical responsibility should be extended to encouraging and supporting our clients to continue engaging in stimulating tasks, and setting new challenges to maximise benefit from their everyday environment. To do this we need to determine what situations and daily activities are accessible and motivating for our clients.

ACCESS TO EVERYDAY LEISURE PURSUITS: TELEVISION VIEWING

Premorbid leisure pursuits are often no longer accessible to individuals with aphasia. Huge shifts in free and obligated time activities have been reported (Lyon, 2000). Individuals with aphasia face a gamut of informational, structural, environmental, and attitudinal barriers (Parr, Byng, & Gilpin, with Ireland, 1997), which intensify withdrawal from and segregation within personal, family, vocational, and educational roles. There has been a worldwide push to foster aphasia-friendly environments and reduce the disability experienced by people with aphasia (Howe, Worrall, & Hickson, 2004).

Extensive research has focused on the accessibility of written information for individuals with aphasia. Brennan, Worrall, and McKenna (2005) highlighted the fact that written material is often inaccessible for people with aphasia, and proposed that aphasia-friendly formats be employed to enhance reading comprehension and ultimately improve access to this medium. Brennan's study concluded that applying such strategies to clinical practice might enable clients to have equal access to written information and to participation in society.

While the promotion of aphasia-friendly written material has begun to improve access to information provided through modified newspapers, newsletters, information brochures, and personal correspondence, research has yet to consider accessibility to information provided through the medium of television. Television viewing is one of the most common leisure pursuits in the developed world today (Lindstrom et al., 2005). The global average for hours of television viewed has been found to creep upward each year and TV is the most trusted source of information that Australians turn to (Free TV Australia, 2006).

Given the extent of language difficulties associated with progressive language impairment, it is almost inevitable that TV viewing would become a more challenging task for people with this disorder. Our clinical experience supports this claim. Clients with progressive language impairment have complained of, for example, difficulty in remembering episode plots from week to week and trouble engaging in social discussion about TV programmes. The primary barriers to TV viewing appear to be predominantly informational and environmental. Individuals may have trouble following complex informational content that may be presented too quickly or through non-literal language, with complex characters and hidden meanings. This is likely to influence the type of TV shows watched, with people with progressive language impairment choosing conceptually simpler programmes (like soap operas and sport) over more complex, cognitively stimulating shows (like documentaries or news programmes). This is a concern when we consider that over time our clients with progressive language impairment typically become more housebound, watch simpler programmes with less hypothesised neuroprotective value, and thus perhaps hasten the rate of neurodegenerative decline. This is all the more likely to occur once individuals with progressive language impairment lose the ability to be active decoders who select what they want to take from each television episode, critically appraise it, and share it in a social manner. Instead they may simply adopt TV viewing as a passive leisure activity to fill their free time.

With this in mind we sought to develop an ecologically valid intervention programme for our clients with progressive language impairment, acknowledging the very real power of television as a leisure activity in the lives of adults with neurodegenerative disease. At the same time we endeavoured to (a) enhance the hypothesised neuroprotective qualities of TV viewing through increased social and cognitive demands, and (b) harness episode content as the basis for promoting transactional success in conversational discourse. In a sense, the intervention programme aimed to capitalise on the inherent appeal of TV viewing, while morphing it into a cognitively stimulating social endeavour—ultimately removing the divide between "pleasurable" and "beneficial" leisure activities for our clients.

Based on Simmons-Mackie's (2000) "social model approach" to aphasia therapy, we created two overarching socially based principles to foster aphasia-friendly TV viewing. Our treatment model conceptualised TV viewing as a flexible and dynamic entity, encouraging the use of all available modes to enhance discourse comprehension and production during programme viewing, rather than insisting that individuals comprehend unmodified TV content. Target behaviours were viewed as collaborative achievements resulting from an interaction between the group facilitator and group members, rather than being the sole responsibility of the viewer. Considerable care was taken to select the TV series used within the therapy programme. The *Australian Story* TV series (Fleming, 2007) was chosen because of its consistently high ratings for Australian viewing audiences, its single story format (one story per episode), consistent documentary-based structure, and "real life" content about personal issues of salience to adults in contemporary Australian culture. Critical attention was also paid to identifying discourse comprehension and production measures that accurately captured the change our clients exhibited as they became active decoders over the course of the intervention programme.

PREDICTED OUTCOMES

The current pilot therapy programme aimed to investigate whether the act of television viewing could be transformed into an accessible and beneficial leisure activity for individuals with progressive language impairment. Predicted outcomes were:

1. Progressive language impairment participants would recall a higher number of story information units when speaking about aphasia-friendly TV episodes following intervention than they did prior to intervention.
2. Progressive language impairment participants would achieve higher transactional success in conversation when speaking about aphasia-friendly TV episodes than they did prior to intervention.
3. Progressive language impairment participants would demonstrate improved comprehension when answering concrete, opinion, and inferential-based questions about aphasia-friendly TV episodes than they did prior to intervention.

METHOD

Participants

Four people with progressive language impairment were selected from the Speech Pathology caseload for participation in this pilot therapy programme through the Neurosciences Assessment and Care Clinic (NACC) programme at the Neurosciences Unit, North Metropolitan Health Service, Western Australia. All participants had been diagnosed with a neurodegenerative disorder characterised by progressive language impairment on the basis of clinical assessment by a neurologist, neuropsychologist, and speech pathologist. Imaging confirmed the presence of neurodegenerative illness. Participants were aged between 59 and 66 years. All participants spoke English as their first language, had completed tertiary education, had visual acuity sufficient to view a TV monitor from 4 metres (with visual aids if required), along with auditory acuity sufficient to hear 60 dB television speaker volume. Participants had no other history of neurological disease or learning impairment.

Participants' language abilities were screened using the Language scale of the Cognitive Linguistic Quick Test (CLQT) (Helm-Estabrooks, 2001). The CLQT is a standardised screening tool designed to allow rapid evaluation of five cognitive domains (attention, memory, language, executive, and visuospatial skills) in adults between the ages of 18 and 89 with known or suspected neurological dysfunction. In this instance, only the language subtest was utilised in order to provide a brief, but unifying snapshot of participants' language capabilities (see Table 1). On the basis of scores achieved on the CLQT Language Severity Scale, it can be seen that participants presented with language impairment ranging from mild to severe (as indicated by scores ranging from 1 to 3).

Four gender-matched controls (aged between 38 and 52 years with normal language and no neurological history) provided normative samples of episode content.

Procedure

Participants with progressive language impairment viewed a total of 10 novel episodes of the *Australian Story* (Fleming, 2007) series over a total of 10 weeks (8 of these weeks being therapeutic and 2 being data collection). The control participants viewed the pre- and post-therapy episodes only. The number of story information units produced by controls provided a normative comparison for each episode.

TABLE 1
Participant demographics

Age Gender	Academic history	CLQT language severity score	Qualitative description of communicative competence
P1 65 F	Tertiary education.	Severe (1)	Marked non-fluency with overt breakdown at the levels of language conceptualisation and formulation. Heavy pantomime use as compensatory technique. Functional auditory comprehension despite susceptibility to information overload. Social disinhibition. Non-functional writing skills in the context of functional reading capabilities to paragraph level.
P2 59 F	Tertiary education.	Mild (3)	Overt non-fluency secondary to marked anomia (formulation phase breakdown). Relative preservation of auditory comprehension. Non-functional written language in the context of functional reading capabilities (to phrasal level).
P3 66 F	Tertiary education.	Moderate (2)	Severely non-fluent / agrammatic output (secondary to marked formulation and articulation phase deficits along with severe motor programming deficits). Relatively preserved auditory comprehension. Strong written language (used as primary compensatory strategy). Strong reading capabilities.
P4 62 M	Tertiary education.	Severe (1)	Dense semantic deficit across all modalities. Marked receptive language impairment. Fluent spoken output. Behavioural disinhibition and ideational perseveration. Relative preservation of reading capabilities and written language use (used as primary compensatory strategy).

Pre- and post-therapy measures

Weeks 1 and 10 of the programme were individual sessions used to obtain pre- and post-therapy measures of participants' discourse comprehension, production of story information units, and transactional success using two distinct episodes. Week 1's session aimed to capture each participants' level of episode recall and understanding prior to intervention. Following viewing of week 1's episode, each participant was required to produce a free recall of the storyline (which was recorded and transcribed verbatim) and answer 10 concrete, 5 inferential, and 5 opinion-based questions regarding the piece. In both pre- and post-therapy conditions, all participants were given access to a "feature analysis" guide (see Appendix A) and pen in order to take notes regarding the episode; however, it is important to note that no participant utilised this resource in the pre-therapy phase. Following both pre- and post-therapy sessions, individual recounts were read by volunteers (who were not communication experts and were naive to episode content) who then produced their own account of what they thought the episode was about. The number of story information units conveyed by the volunteers was then calculated, creating a measure of "transactional success" (Ramsberger & Rende, 2002).

Therapy session content and structure

Weeks 2 to 9 were group-based intervention sessions, which aimed to enhance participants' access to TV content through the provision of aphasia-friendly television support strategies. Specific therapeutic goals included improving each participant's comprehension of episode content and their transactional success during conversations about the episode. Each session occurred over a 90-minute period and consistently followed the outline described below:

1. Television glossary review. This involved formal review of a standard range of vocabulary items commonly used within the genre of television viewing. The word list was compiled into a "TV glossary" (see Appendix B). This was given to participants at the commencement of their first week of therapy, and was subsequently used in therapy and home television viewing, remaining in their possession throughout the course of the therapy programme. At the start of each therapy session, the clinician reviewed every vocabulary item within the TV glossary, defining and contextualising each word and related concept through the use of verbal explanation and pantomime (as in demonstrating the act of "pausing" or "fast forward" through an acted out sequence).

2. Priming episode content. Prior to viewing the episode, participants were led by the clinician in a period of ideational priming around the topic of the target episode for that session. In order to facilitate priming, the clinician read a synopsis of the episode, which was downloaded from the ABC *Australian Story* website (*Australian Story*, 2007). This helped participants to reflect on the topic in general terms, discussing any relevant personal experience or exposure to similar themes conveyed in the upcoming episode. Scaffolding techniques used by the clinician involved supportive questioning and collaborative discourse planning around the episode theme. Typical questions used to facilitate the priming period included; 'Can anyone tell us what they know about the topic of Alzheimer's disease?' (asked while priming story content about the episode in which the wife of a previous Australian prime minister talks about her journey with Alzheimer's disease; McRobert, 2003a). Participants were then encouraged to jointly brainstorm around the topic and seek clarification, draw associations from personal experience, or make predictions regarding the upcoming episode prior to commencement of the viewing period.

3. Orientation to modified viewing schedule. Participants were reminded of the modified viewing schedule for the upcoming episode, with the clinician describing (and drawing) the altered play/pause schedule being employed. This schedule involved pausing the episode one quarter, half-way, and three-quarters of the way along the course of the episode and it was explained that these "pause periods" would be used to allow group-based review and synthesis of individual story elements, plot detail, and character development. Participants were encouraged to make requests for clarification during these intervals to ensure incremental consolidation of episode content.

4. Paused intervals. Paused intervals were used by the clinician to facilitate group-based recall of key story information units and to describe plot development to date.

Relevant plot information was written (and drawn in iconic form for participants with limited reading skills) in chronological and thematic form on a whiteboard. The whiteboard remained in full view of group members throughout the session and provided permanent tangible support to participants during viewing periods, pause periods, and group discussion (see Appendix C).

5. Clinician summary. Following completion of the episode, the clinician used the whiteboard to guide the production of a verbal summary of the major content of the TV show.

6. Supported group discussion. Group members were supported to participate in debate and discussion about episode content, offering their perspectives on the storyline, characters, and conclusion. Participants were then engaged in a formal question period in which they were asked 10 concrete questions (such as, "Who was flying the plane that crashed?"), 5 inferential questions (such as, "What else could Victoria and Geoff have done to get rescued sooner?"), and 5 opinion-based questions (such as, "Do you think Geoff should have flown the plane even though there was thick cloud cover?"). All questions were directly related to the episode they had just viewed. The question examples provided above were from the episode "On the Mountain" (McRobert, 2003c) viewed during week 1 of the treatment group.

7. Feature analysis guide. The session concluded with clinician-supported completion of the feature analysis guide sheet. The guide was completed in a manner that provided each participant with an accessible summary of episode content. Prior to leaving the session, participants were given the opportunity to use their completed feature analysis guide as a conversational springboard for group-based discourse practice. Participants were encouraged to use the feature analysis guide when watching television programmes at home.

8. Carer training. Following session 1 of therapy, at least one carer of each participant was trained in the purpose of the group, typical session structure, the use of home based aphasia-friendly viewing principles, and accurate completion of the feature analysis guide. Carers were generally the participants' spouses, however one friend also participated in the training session. Carers were given individualised strategies to support comprehension and discussion of TV shows within the home context.

9. Home practice. As home practice, group participants were encouraged to view two novel TV episodes (of any preferred genre) with their trained carer in the week prior to the next session. It was explained that both the participant and their carer should use any advertisement break periods in the same way that clinicians used the paused schedules in therapy sessions (that is, for review of content and provision of clarification as required). The carer and participant were asked to jointly complete a feature analysis guide following each home practice episode. They were informed that the participant would be required to bring both feature analysis guides to the next session and use one of them as the basis for group discussion about the episode they had watched.

RESULTS

We took a range of measures, which allowed qualitative and quantitative analysis of our participants' TV viewing skills and progress made during the treatment period. Our pre- and post-therapy measures included (a) the number of episode story information units produced, (b) measures of transactional success, and (c) discourse comprehension questions.

Story information units

After the first and tenth episodes of *Australian Story* (pre- and post-treatment) our participants were asked to engage in discussion about the show providing a recount or summary to their conversational partner. The participants were informed that the recount would be given to a non-expert listener, to ensure they gave as much information as possible. No time limits were imposed on the conversations, with participants encouraged to continue until they felt that they had achieved maximal exchange of ideas. After transcribing the discourse sample, the number of story information units produced was calculated and compared to that provided by unimpaired control speakers.

All of the participants with progressive language impairment produced more story information units following the treatment period. Participant P4 demonstrated the greatest change in story information unit production with his pre- and post-discourse samples, provided in Table 2.

We conducted a two-way ANOVA with repeated measures on condition to compare the effect of group (control versus progressive language impairment) and condition (pre- versus post-treatment) on our participants' story information unit production. The performance of individual participants is shown in Figure 1, while Figure 2 compares the group performance of the progressive language impairment and control participants. Significant main effects were achieved for group, $F(1, 7) = 7.22$, $p = .031$, and condition, $F(1, 7) = 11.10$, $p = .013$, indicating that the control participants reported significantly more story information units than the participants with progressive language impairment and, overall, more story information units were reported in the post condition. A significant interaction effect was also obtained, $F(1, 7) = 24.36$, $p = .007$, which is due to the fact that the participants with progressive language impairment demonstrated a significantly greater increase in story information unit reporting in the post condition, after group therapy. While their performance was markedly worse than the control group at pre-test, after they had received therapy the number of story information units they produced was approaching that of the control group.

Transactional success

We also looked at our participants' increase in transactional success. This provides an indication of the number of story information units that were correctly interpreted by a non-expert listener (Ramsberger & Rende, 2002). The non-expert listeners were asked to read the transcribed retell samples that were produced by the participants with progressive language impairment and then to provide their own account or understanding of what the TV programme was about. The non-expert listeners reported no prior exposure to the *Australian Story* episodes. The number of

TABLE 2
Example of pre- and post-treatment discourse samples from P4

Pre-treatment discourse sample
Boots and All Episode (McRobert, 2003b)
The story of Peter Brocklehurst's amazing rise from the cobblers shop to the concert hall.

OK. There was one guy named Peter...Peter...his name began with 'H'.

Pete, Pe, Pe, I can't remember the word.

But he was singing initially and then he was talking. And singing several times.

Right to the end. Um...and there was another lady who was talking about it.

And...She was sitting there talking.

Occasionally. I can't remember her name. She was, she was talking quite a lot.

The guy was singing...they did some singing. Then she'd talk, then they'd sing, and sing and talk and sing and talk. The other guy who was singing was playing with his guitar. Is that the right word, guitar? Doing this [gestures playing guitar]

P: He was doing that sometimes. And other times he was just standing and singing initially.

And then several times in the middle of it he was talking.

Talking about things. Don't know what he was saying.

He did singing several times, probably about...he might have done singing about ten times.

Um the first one he was doing he was just singing by himself with a guy, with a guy with a, with a guy with a.... That was the first one. And then a bit later on I think he was singing some music from somewhere and later, towards the end there was a whole crowd of people all playing music and playing items and things. Right towards the end there was um...don't know how many, maybe twenty or more. Big group in, in the place doing a show for everyone to watch.

And quite lovely, all meeting each other and kissing their friends.

And then they all get dressed up as well. Originally he was, he wasn't dressed, he was just like this [gestures; tugs on his casual shirt]

But later on he got jackets on and stuff. Formal? What does that mean? Dressy. All the dressy...Clothes? Um...big black ones like that. And he went over it with a jack, with a jack, with a um...thing down here [gestures tie around neck]...he had one of those on towards the end.

Um...now the, the, the, a lot of the singing wasn't in English....it was, some, only a couple of times I heard some English stuff but a lot of times they were singing in different words that I didn't understand the words. So they must have been singing from somewhere else. I'd rather watch the English one. Um...I think there was only one...ahh...ten different songs he sang different words and I, I, he might have only sung one.

And bits of some were only briefly English words. Cos I'm sure that wasn't correct, no. But the same guy was doing it all the time. That, that guy Peter. And he was doing lots of talking all the time to, to somebody, some people...I don't know who he was talking to. You saw him standing around just speaking. Don't know who he was speaking to.

That lady he was speaking to, I'm not sure. Sorry, I don't understand all that stuff.

Post-treatment discourse sample
And Justice for All Episode (McRobert, 2000)
The episode concerns a man who has helped to revolutionise police practices around the world. He's been praised for his pioneering work in Restorative Justice where offenders are brought face to face with their victims.

It is a movie or a documentary...*Australian Story* Classics.

It was Terry O'Connell and the chief policeman...Pollard...the chief constable...

Terry O'Connell, Pollard, Kevin Wales...Walls and Ted Watchell...from the US.

Three important things that happened in the show is Terry made a new way to fix problems like stealing which is taking something that is not yours...shoplifting

And then he went to the UK to teach problems...and then he went to see children who steal and meet the people who they have hurt ...children who steal meet the people...sorry...children who steal meet the people who they have hurt. Terry was a police man for 28...no, 29 years.

Then it says what do you think will happen next, and I think Terry will retire.

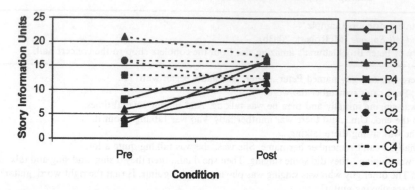

Figure 1. Number of story information units produced by participants with progressive language impairment and normal controls following pre- and post-treatment episodes.

story information units then produced by the non-expert listeners was calculated and divided by the mean number of story information units produced by the control group. This gave the number of story information units conveyed successfully by each speaker with progressive language impairment as a proportion of story information units conveyed by the controls (i.e., an index of their transactional success). It is important to note that this measure was based purely on the transcribed discourse samples, without access to the participants' use of gesture or alternative forms of communication and is therefore a conservative measure of communicative effectiveness. All of the participants with progressive language impairment demonstrated an increase in transactional success in the post condition, successfully conveying a greater number of episode story information units successfully to the non-expert listeners. That is, the non-expert listeners interpreted and produced more story information units from the participants' discourse samples about the post-treatment episode compared to the pre-treatment episode. This is shown in Figure 3, with P4 again showing the greatest improvement in performance.

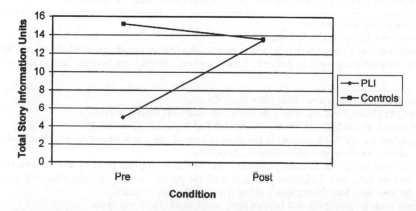

Figure 2. Number of story information units produced by the progressive language impairment (PLI) and control groups under the pre- and post-treatment conditions.

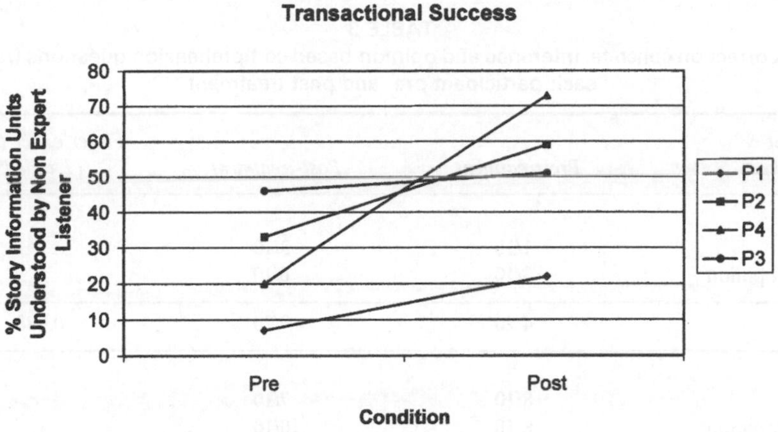

Transactional Success

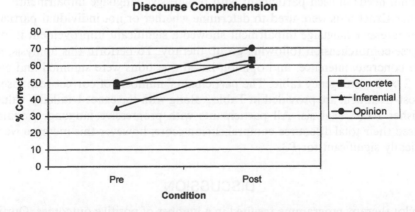

Figure 3. Transactional success achieved by participants with progressive language impairment across the pre- and post-treatment conditions.

Discourse comprehension

After watching the episodes of *Australian Story*, the participants with progressive language impairment were asked to answer 20 discourse comprehension questions, which tested their ability to retain and recall the key story elements, draw inferences, and state their opinions. These questions were based on the types of information that may be required during everyday social commentary about TV programmes. Figure 4 demonstrates that as a group the participants with progressive language impairment answered more questions successfully in the post condition. The inferential questions were on the whole more difficult to answer. Paired *t* tests were used to determine whether or not discourse comprehension scores differed significantly across the pre and post group therapy conditions. Statistical significance was reached for the concrete, $t(3) = 4.73$, $p = .002$, and opinion-based, $t(3) = 2.49$, $p = .048$, questions, but not inferential questions, $t(3) = 1.31$, $p = .231$.

Individual comprehension profiles provided insight into the heterogeneous nature of discourse comprehension ability in progressive language impairment. For example, on initial testing P1 experienced most difficulty answering concrete

Discourse Comprehension

Figure 4. Accuracy of discourse comprehension (concrete, inferential, and opinion based) by the progressive language impairment group pre- and post-treatment.

TABLE 3
Number correct on concrete, inference and opinion-based comprehension questions ($n = 20$) for each participant pre- and post-treatment

Participant & question type	Pre-treatment	Post-treatment	Fisher exact p-value (1 tailed*)
P1			
Concrete	1/10	3/10	
Inference/opinion	3/10	6/10	
Total	4/20	9/20	0.088
P2			
Concrete	8/10	7/10	
Inference/opinion	8/10	10/10	
Total	16/20	17/20	0.4999
P3			
Concrete	5/10	8/10	
Inference/opinion	6/10	9/10	
Total	11/20	17/20	0.004*
P4			
Concrete	5/10	7/10	
Inference/opinion	0/10	1/10	
Total	5/10	8/10	0.25

questions, while P4 found these easier to answer. P1 stated that she couldn't remember concrete facts. However P1 was able to state her opinions and inference a lot better than P4, suggesting that she was still able to form an overall gist and emotional appreciation of what the episode was about. P4 on the other hand found it particularly difficult to form the bigger picture. He could, for example, tell you the character's names but couldn't explain how the characters were related or what contribution they made to the overall story. These individual performance profiles were used to tailor support strategies and aphasia-friendly principles to the individual needs of each participant with progressive language impairment.

Fisher Exact tests were used to determine whether or not individual participants with progressive language impairment showed a significant improvement in overall discourse comprehension following group therapy. To perform this analysis, scores for the concrete, inference, and opinion-based questions were summed and entered into a 2 × 2 contingency table. The participants' numbers of correct responses pre- and post-treatment are provided in Table 3 along with the exact 1-tailed *p* values for the Fisher Exact analysis. All participants with progressive language impairment increased their total discourse comprehension score; however this increase was only statistically significant for P3.

DISCUSSION

This pilot therapy programme resulted in a number of positive outcomes. Our initial predictions were supported, with the aphasia-friendly TV viewing principles resulting in the participants with progressive language impairment:

1. Recalling a significantly higher number of episode story information units in spoken discourse in the post-treatment condition.
2. Achieving greater transactional success, by conveying more story information units to a naive non-expert listener in the post-treatment condition.
3. Demonstrating improved ability to answer discourse comprehension questions about aphasia-friendly TV episodes in the post-treatment condition.

These results add to emerging research demonstrating that individuals with progressive language impairment can benefit considerably from formal speech and language therapy services. It is clear they have the potential to learn new skills and benefit from individualised strategic support, at least in the early to mid stages of neurodegenerative disease. This capacity should be harnessed by speech-language pathologists in attempt to maximise communicative abilities, enhance life participation and ultimately foster quality of life for as long as possible.

One of the primary aims of this therapy programme was to determine whether it was possible to capitalise on the inherent appeal of TV viewing, while transforming it into a beneficial, cognitively stimulating social endeavour for our client's with progressive language impairment. TV viewing has the potential to be a passive leisure activity, which may indeed become more passive as an individual's neurodegenerative disease progresses. It is a concern that TV viewing may take the place of more intellectually stimulating pursuits (Lindstrom et al., 2005). The participants' performance on the pre-assessment highlighted that individuals with progressive language impairment have difficulty following TV content, extracting and recalling key story details, engaging in meaningful discussion, stating their opinions, and making inferences from story content. Such impairments could have real-life costs for individuals with progressive language impairment, limiting their potential to access information provided through this powerful medium and to participate in the full range of topical conversations that arise during daily interactions.

Through the provision of aphasia-friendly formats the group treatment successfully facilitated TV viewing performance. Group participants were receptive to structured support and strategic behaviours, resulting in a number of positive improvements. Based on the work of Simmons-Mackie (2000), TV viewing was seen as a flexible and dynamic exercise throughout the group process, encouraging use of all available modes of communication to enhance discourse comprehension and production. Target behaviours were achieved collaboratively, resulting from active interaction between the facilitators and viewers, rather than being the sole responsibility of the viewer. Group facilitators made every attempt to ensure that the TV programmes were presented in an aphasia-friendly format, providing group participants with greater access to the modified TV content. Aphasia-friendly modifications included priming episode content prior to viewing, pausing the programme at regular intervals to allow reflection, clarifying and consolidating main story details, providing written and picture support to enhance comprehension, and discourse production, as well as synthesising episode content for group discussion. These support strategies were effective in facilitating the progressive language impairment participants' appreciation (and recall) of the most important people, places, and story elements, while providing a supportive environment for engaging in meaningful social discussion about the programme with their peers.

Post-therapy measures revealed significant improvement in TV viewing ability. After watching the post-treatment episode of *Australian Story*, all of the progressive language impairment participants recalled a greater number of story information units in their recount discourse. As a group, this was a significant change, with the progressive language impairment speakers' performance approaching the range of the control participants. Improved transactional success was also achieved, with non-expert listeners drawing more meaningful information from the episode recounts following the intervention period. This indicated that not only did the speakers with progressive language impairment have greater access to the story content, but they also had enhanced potential to share this with a naive listener and engage in meaningful social interaction.

The improvement in discourse comprehension was also encouraging. Following the post-treatment episode of *Australian Story* the participants with progressive language impairment were able to answer more concrete, inferential, and opinion-based questions about episode content. However, this improvement was statistically significant only for one individual overall, and only for the concrete and opinion-based questions in the group analysis. This suggests that not all individuals with progressive language impairment will benefit equally from the aphasia-friendly formats, and they may require additional support, practice, and resources to be able to draw inferences about TV content effectively.

The participants with progressive language impairment presented with different profiles of TV viewing strengths and weaknesses, highlighting the need to tailor support strategies to individual language needs. For example, P4's TV viewing experience was frequently disrupted by word comprehension difficulties with the inability to comprehend single words or concepts having a devastating effect on his comprehension and use of TV content. For example, during an episode about drug traffickers in Bali (McRobert, 2006), P4 asked the group facilitators, "What are drugs?" Without support, P4 had been unable to ascertain the meaning of the word "drug", which was extremely disruptive to his general understanding of the episode's content. Such semantic difficulties occurred frequently and P4 required considerable one-to-one support to maximise his comprehension and fill in semantic gaps via picture, written, and gestural support. This helped to focus his attention on the most important details and ultimately reduce confusion. Given the improvement in P4's comprehension performance at post-assessment, it seems that these tailored strategies were effective in improving his access to the semantic content of the *Australian Story* episodes. It is important to recognise that the differences inherent in the participants' language profiles meant that each individual made gains in different areas; however all participants benefited from the group and clearly enjoyed the process.

It is important to acknowledge the limitations of this pilot therapy programme and make suggestions for future research or replication. First, the sample size was small, investigating the effect of the treatment programme on only four individuals with progressive language impairment. As a result, replication of the study on a larger cohort of participants is strongly recommended. Furthermore, the pilot therapy programme did not control for the age, sex, language symptomatology, or impairment severity of individual participants, which may have contributed to the variable performance profiles. Participants responded to the group treatment in different ways, making it difficult to capture statistically significant change when relying predominantly on group-based analyses. Future research could utilise multiple case study (case series) designs to look more closely at the treatment gains and performance profiles of individual participants. This should be explored to help quantify treatment gains with participants acting as their own experimental control.

The pilot therapy programme also had some methodological limitations, which make interpretation of the results less certain. In particular, the control group only watched two episodes of the television programme, rather than the ten watched by the participants with progressive language impairment. As a result, we cannot be confident that post-treatment gains were due to the intervention itself, or simply to the fact that the participants with progressive language impairment received greater exposure to the TV programme and story content.

In addition, this pilot therapy programme did not control for the informational content, complexity, and need for conceptual abstraction in the pre- and post-treatment episodes. As much as possible, future studies should attempt to ensure that pre- and post-therapy episodes are matched, in order that interpretation of differences in performance due to the intervention are not confounded by differences between the stimuli used in the two assessments. Finally, we would recommend that future aphasia-friendly TV viewing interventions establish whether the benefits in the clinical context transfer into the participants' home and community contexts through the use of, for example, measures of Quality of Life and TV viewing satisfaction.

SUMMARY AND FUTURE DIRECTIONS

The results of this pilot therapy programme have demonstrated that with innovative flair we can turn passive leisure activities into cognitively and socially stimulating tasks, which are of great benefit to our clients with neurodegenerative disease. This is extremely important, given the tendency for our clients with progressive language impairment to withdraw from social and intellectually stimulating activities and spend more time within their home environments engaged in less stimulating tasks.

In conclusion, speech pathologists should not be afraid to take up the challenge to explore new and innovative ways to "dig around the communication roadblocks" faced by individuals with progressive language impairment. By not accepting our mandate to reduce these barriers (McNeil & Duffy, 2001), we run the risk not only of contributing to the social isolation of our clients, but also of missing out on some of the most rewarding and enjoyable clinical interactions of our career.

REFERENCES

Australian Story. (2007).[Programme synopses] retrieved 8 August 2007 from http://abc.net.au/austory/.

Brennan, A., Worrall, L., & McKenna, K. (2005). The relationship between specific features of aphasia-friendly written material and comprehension of written material for people with aphasia: An exploratory study. *Aphasiology, 19,* 693–711.

Burns, A. (2004). Psychosocial and behavioural interventions in dementia. *Current Opinion in Psychiatry, 17,* 433–437.

Coyle, J. T. (2003). Use it or lose it: Do effortful mental activities protect against dementia. *The New England Journal of Medicine, 348,* 2489–2490.

Croot, K. (2009). Progressive aphasia: Definitions, diagnoses, and prognoses. *Aphasiology, 22,* 302–326.

Cummings, J. L., & Jeste, D. V. (1999). Alzheimer's disease and its management in the year 2010. *Psychiatric Services, 50,* 1173–1177.

Duffy, J. R., & Petersen, R. C. (1992). Primary progressive aphasia. *Aphasiology, 6,* 1–15.

Fleming, D. (Executive Producer). (2007). *Australian story* [television series]. Brisbane: ABC.

Free TV Australia. (2006, 13 September). *50 years of television – a lot to celebrate.* Retrieved 11 July 2006, from http://www.freetv.com.au/SiteMedia/w3svc087/Uploads/) Documents/7f5781 e6-2da3-4875-9434-531f524da1fd.pdf.

Helm-Estabrooks, N. (2001). *Cognitive Linguistic Quick Test*. San Antonio, TX: The Psychological Corporation.

Howe, T. J., Worrall, L. E., & Hickson, L. M. H. (2004). What is an aphasia-friendly environment? *Aphasiology, 18*, 1015–1037.

Knibb, J. A., Xuereb, J. H., Patterson, K., & Hodges, J. R. (2006). Clinical and pathological characterization of progressive aphasia. *Annals of Neurology, 59*, 156–165.

Liao, Y. C., Liu, R. S., Teng, E. L., Lee, Y. C., Wang, P. N., & Lin, K. N. et al. (2005). Cognitive reserve: A SPECT study of 132 Alzheimer's disease patients with an education range of 0–19 years. *Dementia and Geriatric Cognitive Disorders, 20*, 8–14.

Lindstrom, H. A., Fritsch, T., Petot, G., Smyth, K. A., Chen, C. H., & Debanne, S. M. et al. (2005). The relationships between television viewing in midlife and the development of Alzheimer's disease in a case-control study. *Brain and Cognition, 58*, 157–165.

Lyon, J. (2000). Finding, defining and refining functionality in real life for people confronting aphasia. In L. Worrall & C. Frattali (Eds.), *Neurogenic communication disorders: A functional approach* (pp. 137–161). New York: Thieme.

McNeil, M. R., & Duffy, J. R. (2001). Primary progressive aphasia. In R. Chapey (Ed.), *Language intervention strategies in aphasia and related neurogenic communication disorders* (5th ed., pp. 472–486). Philadelphia: Lippincott Williams & Wilkins.

McNeil, M. R., Small, S. L., Masterson, R. J., & Fossett, T. R. D. (1995). Behavioural and pharmacological treatment of a lexical-semantic deficits in a single patient with primary progressive aphasia. *American Journal of Speech-Language Pathology, 4*, 76–87.

McRobert, T. (Director). (2000). And justice for all [Television series episode]. In D. Fleming (Executive Producer), *Australian Story*. Brisbane: Australian Broadcasting Commission.

McRobert, T. (Director). (2003a). The big A [Television series episode]. In D. Fleming (Executive Producer), *Australian Story*. Brisbane: Australian Broadcasting Commission.

McRobert, T. (Director). (2003b). Boots and all [Television series episode]. In D. Fleming (Executive Producer), *Australian Story*. Brisbane: Australian Broadcasting Commission.

McRobert, T. (Director). (2003c). On the mountain [Television series episode]. In D. Fleming (Executive Producer), *Australian Story*. Brisbane: Australian Broadcasting Commission.

McRobert, T. (Director). (2006). Road to Keroboken [Television series episode]. In D. Fleming (Executive Producer), *Australian Story*. Brisbane: Australian Broadcasting Commission.

Mesulam, M. M. (1982). Slowly progressive aphasia without generalized dementia. *Annals of Neurology, 11*, 592–598.

Mesulam, M. M. (2001). Primary progressive aphasia. *Annals of Neurology, 49*(4), 425–431.

Nestor, P. J., Graham, N. L., Fryer, T. D., Williams, G. B., Patterson, K., & Hodges, J. R. (2003). Progressive non-fluent aphasia is associated with hypometabolism centred on the left anterior insula. *Brain, 126*, 2406–2418.

Parr, S., Byng, S., & Gilpin, S., with Ireland, C. (1997). *Talking about aphasia: Living with loss of language after stroke*. Buckingham, UK: Open University Press.

Ramsberger, G., & Rende, B. (2002). Measuring transactional success in the conversation of people with aphasia. *Aphasiology, 16*, 337–353.

Rapp, B., Glucroft, B., & Urrutia, J. (2005). The protective effects of behavioural intervention in a case of primary progressive aphasia. *Brain and Language, 95*, 18–19.

Simmons-Mackie, N. N. (2000). Social approaches to the management of aphasia. In L. Worrall & C. Frattali (Eds.), *Neurogenic communication disorders: A functional approach* (pp. 162–188). New York: Thieme.

Taylor, C., Miles-Kingma, R., Croot, K., & Nickels, L. (2009). Speech pathology services for primary progressive aphasia: Exploring an emerging area of practice. *Aphasiology, 22*, 161–174.

APPENDIX A

Feature analysis guide

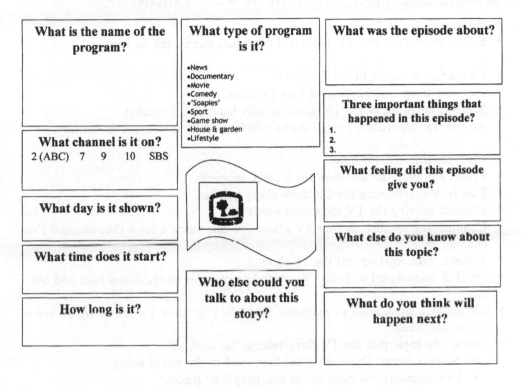

What is the name of the program?	**What type of program is it?** •News •Documentary •Movie •Comedy •'Soapies' •Sport •Game show •House & garden •Lifestyle	**What was the episode about?**
What channel is it on? 2 (ABC) 7 9 10 SBS		**Three important things that happened in this episode?** 1. 2. 3.
What day is it shown?		**What feeling did this episode give you?**
What time does it start?		**What else do you know about this topic?**
How long is it?	**Who else could you talk to about this story?**	**What do you think will happen next?**

APPENDIX B

Sample TV glossary

TV GLOSSARY: WHAT DO ALL THOSE WORDS MEAN?

- Episode: a single TV show.
- Series: more than one TV show that continues from week to week.

- Character: a person in the TV show.
- Plot: the story that happens in that TV show.
- Scene: a small bit of the TV show (usually between ad breaks).
- Ad breaks: advertising / small shows which talk about things you can buy.

- Play: starting the TV show.
- Pause: stopping the TV show for a quick moment.
- Fast forward: moving the TV show along quicker.
- Rewind: moving the TV show backwards.
- Channel: the number on your TV where you can watch a show (like channel 7 or channel 9).
- Volume: how loud or soft the TV show is.
- DVD: a special part of your TV, which lets you play programmes over and over again.
- TV guide: a small book or magazine that tells you when TV shows are on every day of the week.
- Genre: the topic that the TV show belongs to, such as:
  - News – stories about what has happened in the world today.
  - Documentary – a story about real people or places.
  - Comedy – a story that makes us laugh.
  - Suspense – a story that makes us a bit worried or scared about what's going to happen next.
  - Horror – a story that can make us very frightened.
  - Soapie – a story that tells us about the lives of a group of people (not real).
  - Sport – a show where you watch people play a game (like football or cricket or tennis).
  - Game show – a show where people win money or prizes.
  - Lifestyle show – shows us how to fix our house or garden or where to go on holidays.

APPENDIX C

Sample whiteboard summary: "On the Mountain" (*Australian Story*, 12 May 2003)

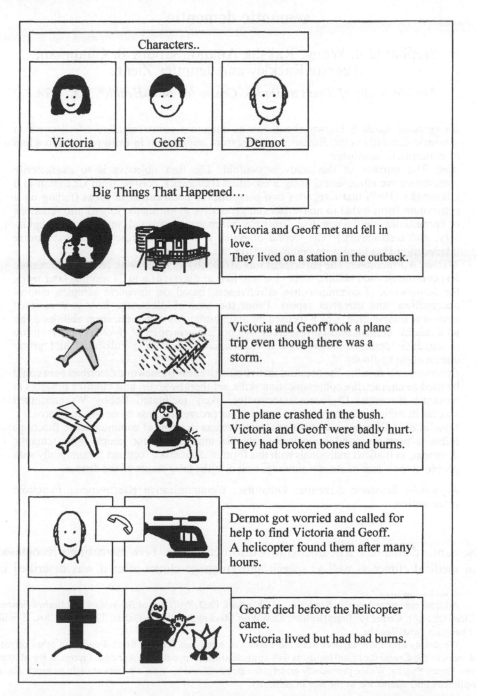

Characters..

Victoria   Geoff   Dermot

Big Things That Happened...

Victoria and Geoff met and fell in love.
They lived on a station in the outback.

Victoria and Geoff took a plane trip even though there was a storm.

The plane crashed in the bush.
Victoria and Geoff were badly hurt.
They had broken bones and burns.

Dermot got worried and called for help to find Victoria and Geoff.
A helicopter found them after many hours.

Geoff died before the helicopter came.
Victoria lived but had bad burns.

APHASIOLOGY, 2009, 23 (2), 286–301

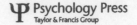

When nouns and verbs degrade: Facilitating communication in semantic dementia

Stephanie B. Wong, Raksha Anand, Sandra B. Chapman, Audette Rackley and Jennifer Zientz

The University of Texas at Dallas, Center for BrainHealth®, TX, USA

Background: Little is known about how to maintain communicative effectiveness in semantic dementia as the disease progresses from impairment in word retrieval to a loss of conceptual knowledge.

Aim: The purpose of this study is twofold. The first objective is to characterise communicative effectiveness using a modified framework derived from Chapman and Ulatowska (1997) that integrates two components: codification of ideas (falling on a continuum from verbal to nonverbal and generative to automatic forms) and functions of communication (imaginative, heuristic, informative, personal, interactional, regulatory, and instrumental). The second objective is to outline principles of a discourse intervention that focuses on communicative effectiveness.

Method & Procedures: The participant was Mr Bobby V, a man with semantic dementia. His communication abilities were characterised at diagnosis and 24 months later using the framework of communicative effectiveness, based on discourse samples, clinical observation, and caregiver report. From the time of diagnosis, Bobby V received discourse intervention, which focused on maintaining his communication abilities using all available communication resources. We outline principles of discourse intervention in semantic dementia based on our experience of delivering individual and group intervention to Bobby V.

Outcomes and Results: The communicative effectiveness framework described here could be used to characterise communication skills, set therapy goals, and monitor progress in semantic dementia. Discourse intervention likely facilitated Bobby V's continued success in maintaining communication despite progressive loss of nouns and verbs.

Conclusions: Targeting conversational effectiveness in terms of communicative functions offers a promising and ecologically valuable intervention for people with semantic dementia, as it allows individuals with this form of dementia to connect meaningfully with people in their immediate surroundings well into the later stages of the disease.

Keywords: Semantic dementia; Discourse; Communicative effectiveness; Function; Intervention.

Semantic dementia is a neurocognitive disorder that has been increasingly recognised in medical clinics as well as speech and language clinics after it was described in

Address correspondence to: Sandra Bond Chapman, PhD, Professor of Behavioral and Brain Sciences, Chief Director, Center for BrainHealth®, 2200 West Mockingbird Lane, Dallas, TX 75235 USA. E-mail: schapman@utdallas.edu

We deeply appreciate support from the Frank Garrott Fund, Temple Stark Fund, and other private donors to the Center for BrainHealth, as well as professional support from Anne M. Lipton, Katy Milton, and Garen Sparks. We are profoundly grateful for Bobby V and his wife, who have taught us much about optimism and adaptation in the face of difficulty.

http://www.psypress.com/aphasiology   DOI: 10.1080/02687030801943112

detail in the 1990s (Hodges, Patterson, Oxbury, & Funnell 1992; Neary et al., 1998). This degenerative dementia, also known as fluent primary progressive aphasia or temporal variant frontotemporal dementia, is characterised by loss of vocabulary (Grossman, 2005; Hodges et al., 1992). Individuals with this form of dementia present with a semantic deficit which progresses from word retrieval problems in the mild stages to a greater loss of conceptual meaning in the moderate to late stages. Their repertoire of nouns and verbs in discourse production narrows, and the specificity of the stored representation of meaning diminishes as the disease progresses.

Individuals with semantic dementia experience communication difficulties in day-to-day interactions even in the early stages of the disease (Hodges et al., 1992). Inability to retrieve words causes frustration, leading to distressing breakdowns in communication with both familiar and unfamiliar partners. The research character-ising the impact of semantic dementia on communication is scant. A few studies have found that individuals with early semantic dementia are able to stay on topic and expand the topic when narrating a story and during conversation (Ash et al., 2006; Chapman et al., 2005). Unfortunately, the conceptual skills underlying topic maintenance and elaboration appear to degrade with disease progression as meaning loss becomes more pervasive (Chiu & Chapman, 2003). Jarrar, Orange, Kertesz, and Peacock (1998) found press of speech as reflected in the increased number of words per utterance, stereotyped phrases, and problems with idea sequencing and idea completion in individuals with semantic dementia.

To our knowledge, no study to date has examined the effects of discourse-based intervention on communication abilities in semantic dementia. The majority of intervention research in individuals with semantic dementia has focused on word retrieval in isolation (Cress & King, 1999; Graham, 2001; Jokel, Rochon, & Leonard, 2002; Reilly, Nadin, & Murray, 2005). These intervention strategies can be broadly categorised into two types. The first type of intervention involves repetition drills of isolated words. To facilitate word retrieval, words are presented alongside pictures or word definitions. Word drills typically result in transient learning because successful naming is supported by rote recognition rather than stable long-term conceptual knowledge (Graham, 2001; Reilly et al., 2005). Although this form of intervention may have some validity, it has limited application in terms of maintaining functional communication. Perhaps, as Reilly and team (2005) suggest, drills may be more effective and functional with a finite set of personally relevant words.

A second type of intervention approach involves use of communication boards to augment the communicative repertoire (Cress & King, 1999). A visual assembly of printed personally salient objects and comments (e.g., calendar with events, sketch and name of daughter, question mark) are used for joint reference between the individual with semantic dementia and his or her listener. This form of intervention may be beneficial when verbal output is significantly reduced. However impaired recognition of words and pictures at later stages may impede the effectiveness of communication boards.

The purpose of this paper is twofold. The first objective is to characterise communicative effectiveness in semantic dementia using a modified framework derived from Chapman and Ulatowska (1997), illustrated with examples from a case study. The second objective is to outline, using illustrations from the case study, principles of discourse-focused intervention that aim to maintain communicative effectiveness.

FRAMEWORK OF COMMUNICATIVE EFFECTIVENESS

Chapman and Ulatowska (1997) described communicative effectiveness in individuals with Alzheimer's disease (AD) using a framework that integrates two components. The first component is the *codification of ideas and desires*, and the second component comprises the *functions of communication* (see Table 1).

The codification of ideas refers to the ability to convey a message with available linguistic and non-linguistic cognitive resources. Codification processes can be characterised as falling on a continuum from generative (novel) to automatic (rote) expressions, as well as verbal (e.g., words) to nonverbal (e.g., gestures) forms of communication (Van Lancker, 1990). Generative expression represents an ability to initiate and respond to a communication context using creative and meaningful messages. On the other hand, automatic expression represents the ability to use overlearned stereotypic responses. This distinction between generative and automatic expression has already been shown to be useful in documenting selective patterns of preservation and impairment in communication in Alzheimer's disease (Chapman & Ulatowska, 1997).

The second component of communicative effectiveness incorporates functions of communication defined by Halliday (1977). These functions of communication include: the *instrumental function* (satisfying material needs, e.g., I want ...); the *regulatory function* (affecting the behaviour of others); the *interaction function* (for social exchange); the *personal function* (expressing personal feelings); the *informative function* (sharing information); the *heuristic function* (gathering knowledge and information); and the *imaginative function* (creative function in generating output) (see Table 1).

TABLE 1
Components of communicative effectiveness

Components	Definition	Examples
Codification of ideas		
• Generative	Spontaneously created responses generated to initiate or reply to a particular communicative context	Conversational interactions
• Automatic	Non-creative and fixed over-learned responses	Routine social exchanges Recurrent stereotyped utterances
Functions of communication		
• Imaginative	Serves a creative function in generating stories	What would you do if
• Heuristic	Operates to gather knowledge and information	Tell me why
• Informative	Serves to share information	Explanations and instructions
• Personal	Represents statements of personal feelings	I think
• Interactional	Reflects the use of language for social exchange	Greetings
• Regulatory	Serves to control the behaviour of others	Could you please

According to Chapman and Ulatowska (1997), functions of communication can be achieved in individuals with AD through use of generative or automatic expression. However, the range of communication functions achieved by these individuals may vary depending on their ability to codify ideas. For instance, individuals with AD experience a decline in generative language use and an increase in automatic utterances with disease progression (Chapman & Ulatowska, 1992; Hamilton, 1994). Although these automatic utterances are useful in maintaining the interaction function and the personal function, a marked deficit is observed in the informative function (Blanken, Dittmann, Haas, & Wallesch, 1987; Bohling 1991; Chapman & Ulatowska, 1997; Obler & Albert, 1981; Ripich & Terrell, 1988). Integrating information about an individual's ability to both codify ideas and fulfil communicative functions enables a clinician to characterise communication and to measure treatment effectiveness.

We believe that this framework of communicative effectiveness can also be applied in the assessment and monitoring of semantic dementia. We hypothesise that in early stages of semantic dementia the codification of ideas will be similar to that described in mild stages of AD. In particular, codification of ideas in semantic dementia will be predominantly verbal and generative in nature yet somewhat vague and empty. However, we anticipate that the individual in early stages of semantic dementia will achieve a wider range of communication functions than that observed in individuals with mild AD because of relative strengths in cognitive functions of episodic memory, reasoning, and problem solving (Hodges & Patterson, 1996; Kramer et al., 2003). In later stages of semantic dementia we anticipate more automatic and nonverbal communication. Unlike marked loss of initiation in individuals with AD, individuals with semantic dementia may continue to initiate interaction with progression of the disease (Schwartz & Chawluk, 1990).

DISCOURSE-FOCUSED INTERVENTION IN DEMENTIA

Discourse-focused intervention approaches communication by focusing on the client's intended message in connected language. The purpose of discourse-focused intervention in dementia is to maintain an optimum level of communication and social connectedness. In most forms of dementia we see that the desire to communicate and stay connected remains relatively preserved well into the later stages of the disease (Chapman & Ulatowska, 1992; Hamilton, 1994). Since communication using discourse requires joint construction of the message by the listener(s) and speaker(s), all participants jointly share the responsibility of communication (Ferguson, 2000). Thus, discourse-focused intervention involves both the client as well as their communication partner.

Discourse-focused intervention has been investigated in individuals with Alzheimer's disease. These studies demonstrated significant improvements in the richness of language and discourse interactions as well as reduction in anxiety, relative to controls who did not undergo intervention (Arkin & Mahendra, 2001; Chapman, Weiner, Rackley, Hynan, & Zientz, 2004; Moss, Polignano, White, Minichiello, & Sunderland, 2002). To our knowledge, no study has yet addressed discourse-focused intervention in the semantic dementia population. We anticipate that this intervention will have potential benefits in maintaining functional communication abilities in semantic dementia into the later stages of the disease.

In the following section we will characterise communicative effectiveness in a case of semantic dementia using the modified framework of Chapman and Ulatowska (1997). We discuss principles of discourse-focused intervention, which aims to utilise residual ability to convey a message rather than to improve word retrieval in isolation.

CASE ILLUSTRATION

Initial diagnostic evaluation

Bobby V, a right-handed Caucasian male, was 61 years old at the time of diagnosis of semantic dementia. He was a retired broadcast engineer with 14 years of formal education. At the time of diagnosis, he independently maintained a busy recreational schedule and organised his time using a personal digital assistant. Despite his independence, his wife was concerned about the change in his language and behaviour. She reported difficulty in making sense of his vague and nonspecific communication. She was growing tired of his long monologues, inflexibility, and his apparent lack of interest in her concerns. She reported that previously "he so wanted to discuss things" and that he had always encouraged her to express her views. She interpreted his recent antagonism as purposeful rather than the result of internal frustration and degenerative brain disease. Neither of them understood what was happening, and they each blamed the other. After months of tension and conflict in their marriage, Bobby V's wife began to seek help.

Initially, Bobby V was prescribed an antidepressant medication that did not alleviate his difficulties. While several diagnoses were being considered (AD, a vascular aetiology and frontal lobe degeneration), he was referred to the Alzheimer's Disease Center (ADC) at The University of Texas Southwestern Medical Center for further medical investigation. At the ADC, Bobby V was diagnosed with semantic dementia based on a neurological evaluation along with input from a neuropsychologist and our discourse team at the University of Texas at Dallas, Center for BrainHealth. Functional brain-imaging results using single photon emission computed tomography (SPECT) showed significant hypoperfusion restricted to Bobby V's left temporal lobe. These findings concur with previous brain-imaging studies wherein localised disruption in the left temporal lobe was associated with semantic dementia (Chapman et al., 2005; Mummery et al., 1999).

Overall, the results of Bobby V's cognitive assessment (see Table 2) suggested impairment in verbal skills with relative preservation of nonverbal skills and memory. His Mini Mental State Examination score (23/30) may not be reflective of his general cognitive ability since this screening tool is heavily dependent on verbal language. His performance on verbal fluency and naming tasks indicated word retrieval deficits. For instance, his performance on 15 items from the Boston Naming Test was significantly below average (Kaplan & Weintraub, 1983). On the Peabody Picture Vocabulary Test (Dunn & Dunn, 1997), in which the client matches an auditorily presented word with one of four line drawings, Bobby V performed at the 16th percentile. On a subset of items from the Pyramids and Palm Trees test (Howard & Patterson, 1992), he matched 15/15 picture pairs and 14/15 word pairs based on semantic relatedness. Although these scores suggest intact semantic concepts, further probing revealed marked deficits in his ability to explain the relationship in these semantic pairs. For example, he could not explain how a bat

TABLE 2
General cognitive assessment at time of diagnosis

Test	Score
The Mini Mental State Examination	23/30
Wechsler Adult Intelligence Scale	
Verbal IQ	81
Performance IQ	100
Peabody Picture Vocabulary Test	16th percentile
Boston Naming test	10/15
Category Fluency	10
Letter Fluency	
F; A; S	2; 2; 2
Pyramids and Palm Trees	
Picture–picture	14/15
Word–word	15/15
Word–picture	13/22
Boston Diagnostic Aphasia Examination	
Naming	7/10
Complex Ideational	
Sentences	4/4
Complex Ideational Paragraphs	7/8
Repetition of phrases	
Repetition of high probability phrases	8/8
Repetition of low probability phrases	7/8
Rey Auditory Verbal Learning Test	
Repetitive list learning	7/15
Recall	2/15
Delayed Recall	3/15
Recognition	14/15

and an owl are more related than a bat and a woodpecker, despite accurately matching the bat and owl.

Bobby V's performance on the recognition task of the Rey Auditory Verbal Learning Test (RAVLT) (14/15) suggests relatively preserved memory function. Recall on RAVLT (2/15) is likely to be impaired due to verbal retrieval deficits. He presented no obvious impairment in phonology, syntax, or phrase repetition, suggesting that he did not have prominent language difficulties outside of semantic knowledge and lexical retrieval. Also he exhibited relatively preserved ability to draw common animate and inanimate objects. His ability to draw distinct semantic features of less familiar objects was impaired.

Discourse-based evaluation

Bobby V's narrative discourse, procedural discourse, and proverb interpretation ability were examined by our team at the Center for BrainHealth as part of the diagnostic investigation (see Table 3). Discourse samples were elicited by a clinician experienced in discourse assessment. Bobby V's responses were tape recorded, transcribed, and later analysed by the examiner and a second discourse rater. On the narrative task his verbal responses of gist were vague, as reflected by scores of 2/5 and 2/10 for main idea and lesson generation respectively. However, he gave some indication of having comprehended the gist. Similar to his performance on Rey

TABLE 3
General discourse assessment at time of diagnosis

Measure	Task	Ability assessed	Scoring	Bobby V
Narrative discourse	Provide a summary statement about a long biographical narrative in a sentence (main idea)	Generating abstract inferences	Total possible points: 5 (points range from 0 (incorrect) to 5 (correct and transformed)	2/5
	Formulate a lesson learned from the narrative (lesson)	Generating abstract inferences	Total possible points: 10 (points range from 0 (incorrect) to 10 (correct and transformed)	2/10
	Recall the careers that the character had and the outcome of each career	Recall memory for details	Total possible points: 24	5/24
	Recognise specific information from the story	Recognition memory for details	Total possible points: 8	6/8
Procedural discourse	Provide a detailed description of steps involved in making scrambled eggs. The steps were evaluated in terms of :	Generating, organising, and sequencing steps and producing specific language appropriate to the task		
	Gist steps: Crack the eggs Stir the eggs Add ingredients Cook the eggs		Total possible points: 4	2/4
	Core steps: Get the eggs Mention of pan Turn on heat Put butter in skillet Pour in milk Stir while cooking Put eggs on plate		Total possible points: 7	6/7
	Specificity of nouns and verbs		Total possible score: 100%	43%
Proverb interpretation	Interpret familiar and unfamiliar proverbs	Generating abstract inferences	Total possible points: 40 (10 points for each of 4 proverbs, ranging from 0 (incorrect) to 10 (correct)	4/40
	Choose appropriate meaning when presented with choice	Choosing appropriate abstract inferences	Total possible points: 8 (2 points for each of 4 proverbs, ranging from 0 (incorrect) to 2 (correct)	6/8

Auditory Verbal Learning Test (RAVLT), his ability to recognise details from the narrative on a recognition task was relatively preserved (6/8) in comparison to his ability to provide these details verbally (5/24) in a spoken recall task.

On the procedural discourse task he included 2/4 essential gist steps and 6/7 additional core steps. His discourse was characterised by vague and empty output.

The language sample below, taken from his description of how to make scrambled eggs, illustrates his confusion with object labels and meanings.

> ... You stir it up with a, you know a brush or a handle or something. (Examiner: What additional ingredients could you use?) You could use, I know they're green in color, we have lots, but it's just hard for me to realize. They're not mustard, they're uh, I'm sorry ...You stir that up, whatever with the something and then you put a little milk in it and stir that up and then you put it in, uh, whatever you want to put it in, some sort of dish uh or fry pan or something ... then you put it on a stove and you set it at some rating I don't know what uh 480.

In the above sample, Bobby V's semantic errors (e.g., he called a mixing tool a "brush or a handle" and spoke of setting the stovetop to 480 degrees) and nonspecific vocabulary and pronoun references (e.g., "You stir that up, whatever with the something") suggest semantic impairment. Nonetheless, Bobby V was able to stay on topic, maintain the goal of the discourse task, and complete his description. An individual with AD, on the other hand, would likely get confused, lose the goal, and produce a disorganised sequence of steps (Chapman, Chiu, Zientz, Lipton, & Rosenberg, 2002).

On a task involving interpretation of proverbs, Bobby V demonstrated difficulty expressing the meaning of the given proverbs, and his output was "empty" of informational content. For the familiar proverbs he gave partially correct but concrete responses (e.g., responded to the proverb "Rome wasn't built in a day" with "...that was a normal thing. I think probably there were beaucoup years involved in building Rome. If that's what they were talking about ... something along those lines that it does move on there are things that seem just you know come into being you know."). For the unfamiliar proverbs his responses were incorrect (e.g., he responded to "Anyone can hold the helm when the sea is calm" with "... if someone says to me this is how, or the helm, hold the helm, the sea is calm that's what I think about is only this is a boat this is its job in life. When I look at it in an overview, it does have a different way of looking at it a little different. I don't see it that way, generally because to me, it's if this is a boat this is what I think about, if this is somebody else this is something else I think about. ...). When asked to apply the proverbs to more generalised ideas, his responses became tangential. In contrast to this generative difficulty (4/40), he was able to choose the correct interpretation on multiple choice (6/8). In contrast, individuals with AD show marked impairment in generating as well as selecting meaning for the proverbs (Chapman et al., 1997).

Overall, Bobby V presented core features of semantic dementia in that he had severe anomia, continuous but empty spontaneous language, preserved single word repetition, and preserved drawing in conjunction with relatively preserved every day memory (Neary et al., 1998).

Communicative effectiveness

Bobby V's communicative effectiveness was evaluated twice. The first assessment was done after the initial diagnosis before we began discourse intervention. During this period Bobby V was in the early stages of the disease. The second assessment followed the discourse intervention, 2 years after initial diagnosis. The aim of the first assessment was to establish Bobby V's baseline communicative effectiveness.

The second assessment examined change in communicative effectiveness associated both with disease progression and with the discourse intervention. The assessments focused on two broad areas: (1) Bobby V's ability to codify his thoughts, and (2) his ability to achieve various functions of communication.

One of the clinicians who led the intervention programme carried out both of these assessments using activities such as topic-centred conversation (topics: work, family, vacation, and hobbies), social exchange, and caregiver interviews. Sample probes that were used by the clinician to elicit certain communicative functions are listed in Table 4 along with Bobby V's responses. The clinician qualitatively rated Bobby V's ability to codify ideas and to meet various functions of communication based on the discourse samples and the caregiver report. We acknowledge that lack of documentation in terms of the frequency of response could be a limitation. However, we believe that since various factors such as context, client's need, and listener's response determined the functions of communication achieved by the client and the manner in which the message was codified, obtaining a frequency count was less important than knowing that the client was capable of achieving these functions as needed. Despite the limitations of our approach with regard to quantitative data, considerable insight was gleaned from this case to foster future clinical approaches for assessing and treating communication skills in semantic dementia.

On the first assessment Bobby V predominantly codified his thoughts using generative verbal language despite problems with lexical specificity. In the early stage of semantic dementia, Bobby V was able to independently achieve all the functions of communication except imaginative and heuristic functions. His message was often clear, despite manifesting a loss of linguistic specificity and a loss of detailed ideas. He primarily enjoyed interactions on personally relevant emotional topics and appeared emotionally disengaged when discussing other topics such as the 9/11 anniversary.

The clinician was concerned about Bobby V's lack of awareness of the impact of his language on the listeners. For example, his regulatory utterances often seemed aggressive, and he did not effectively make polite requests. When he was ready to leave the house and wanted to tell his wife to get her purse, he said, "You need to get your act together." In addition, he often spoke at length without relinquishing his conversational turn.

During the second assessment the clinician observed that Bobby V's ability to use generative verbal language had reduced. At this later stage of the disease he primarily used automatic utterances or nonverbal modalities to communicate. Nonetheless, he could still convey a message and achieve personal, interactional, instrumental, and at times informative functions of communication when gestures, facial expressions, and props were considered part of his communicative repertoire. At this stage of the disease he needed more assistance from his communication partners compared to the early stage. Table 5 provides examples that illustrate Bobby V's communicative effectiveness (best performance) based on the dimensions of codification of ideas and communication functions at early and later stages of the disease.

DISCOURSE INTERVENTION WITH BOBBY V

Our discourse intervention with Bobby V focused on both the client and the caregiver, based on the premise that both jointly share the responsibility of communication exchange. Based on 4 years of experience working with Bobby V, we

TABLE 4
Samples from the assessment of communicative functions in Bobby V

Communicative function	Activity	Clinician probe	Early stage	Late stage
Imaginative	Topic-centred conversation (topic: work)	If you could have changed anything about your job, what would you change?	I was there. I did it all.	Yeah yeah, that's right.
Heuristic	Topic-centred conversation (topic: work)	Can you ask me questions to see if I have the skills to do your job?	You can't do that job. You can't.....	uh ah
Informative	Topic-centred conversation (topic: work)	Tell me something about your job.	I know when I used to explain to the engineers in the group how to get something put together in proper way I can remember we would talk about that, that this is how I see how to put this together.	That's right
Personal	Topic-centred conversation (topic: work)	What was it like doing your job?	It was amazing. We got along very well. They were all there. Time of life.	Only in America!
Interactional	Socialisation	Let me introduce you to someone. This is RS.	Hi. What's your gig?	Yeah yeah (with varied intonation)
Regulatory	Caregiver interview	Does Bobby V enlist your assistance when he needs something?	Get me a brush or a handle. (Interpretation: Get me a spoon)	Snaps fingers and points to capture clinician/caregiver's attention to enlist help
Instrumental	Caregiver interview/clinician observation	Does Bobby V take the initiative to meet some of his own needs?	Come on. Let's go.	Collects nametags at end of group, indicating he's ready to go

TABLE 5
Codification of ideas and functions of communication

Functions of communication	Early stage	Late stage
Imaginative	*Generative/Nonverbal* Example: To thank people he gave away music CDs that he created	*Automatic/Nonverbal* Example: Brought pictures from his trips to share
Heuristic	*Generative/Nonverbal* Example: Using gestures towards his personal digital assistant, he requested that clinicians insert their names and contact information	*Automatic/Verbal* Example: "Yeah?" to ask his wife about the day's agenda
Informative	*Generative/Verbal* Example: "Yeah, Chris. Chris works in the store. You give him something and he puts it on paper. But he really just doesn't, yeah" when asked about his son, where he works (a print shop), and if he enjoys his work	*Automatic/Verbal* Example: "You got that right" in response to a clinician reading aloud excerpts from his Life Stories Collection
Personal	*Generative/Verbal* Example: "Oh no, not that rap stuff" when asked if he liked rap music	*Generative/Nonverbal* Example: He expressed his distaste for a video through facial expression
Interactional	*Generative/Verbal* Example: "And you? and the other one?" to ask about two clinicians who worked with him	*Automatic/Verbal* Example: "Only in America!" was used in a variety of communicative situations, including greetings and conversational turns
Regulatory	*Generative/Verbal* Example: "These wires go over there, these wires go to that place" to give direction to others while at work	*Automatic/Nonverbal* Example: Snapped his finger to gain the attention of others
Instrumental	*Generative/Verbal* Example: "Let's get a break" to request a break during testing	*Automatic/Nonverbal* Example: Using a prewritten card, he was able to order lunch at Wendy's, which was the same thing every time

outline here two principles of discourse intervention. The first principle was to maintain communicative effectiveness by drawing on the whole repertoire of possible responses (client-focused). The second principle was to facilitate communicative effectiveness with education and training (caregiver-focused).

Maintaining communicative effectiveness

Discourse intervention with Bobby V was carried out in both individual and group sessions by experienced clinicians. The group included individuals diagnosed with Alzheimer's disease and frontotemporal lobar degeneration. Based on the baseline assessment of communicative effectiveness, the goal of both individual and group sessions was to maintain informative, personal, and interactional skills using all available communication resources. In addition, attempts were made to improve his listening skills during individual treatment sessions.

In both individual and group sessions, five specific activities were carried out to facilitate maintenance of communicative effectiveness. These activities were adapted from a previous intervention study (Chapman et al., 2004). These included social

TABLE 6
Examples of activities carried out during intervention

Activity	Description
Social exchange	Informal interaction at beginning of session consisting of social greetings, conversation about family or outings since the previous session. Bobby V was encouraged to bring pictures, flyers, or other items to share with the clinician and the group
Current events (sports event; politics, world news; local news; personal activities)	Participant-initiated discussions based on individual interest. Bobby V was encouraged to bring newspaper articles from previous week to share
Informational topic (vaccine; what is dementia?; genetics of dementia; current research; drug approval process)	Interactive discussion about dementia designed to stimulate questions, and promote interaction
Book club	Interactive discussion about a chapter from the book *The Greatest Generation* by Tom Brokaw. Clinician helped expand topic as necessary and involved Bobby V by asking questions, making comments, and drawing members in based on their individual world knowledge
Life story collection (parents/siblings; early childhood; education; marriage and children; work; hobbies)	Eight or more personal photographs paired with rich narratives capturing individual life experiences, salient memories, wisdom, and wit derived from Bobby V's retelling of the life events

exchange, current events, information topics, book club, and life stories. Table 6 provides a description of each of these activities. All of the activities targeted each of the three communicative functions, i.e., informative, personal, and interactional functions. Probes similar to those used during assessment of communicative function (illustrated in Table 4) were utilised to elicit the best possible response from Bobby V. We emphasised that he use residual verbal abilities along with props, gestures, and facial expressions to codify his message, thereby expanding his communicative repertoire.

During individual sessions the clinician worked on developing Bobby V's awareness of turn-taking in addition to working on informative, personal, and interactional functions of communication. The importance of turn-taking behaviour in conversation and its relevance in maintaining social functions of communication was described and practised. He was asked to monitor the clinician for nonverbal cues such as a head nod to relinquish his turn during interactions. Bobby V was interrupted if he did not demonstrate sensitivity to the cues that exhibited a desire to take a turn. He was then reminded that it was time to relinquish his turn. Interrupting and redirecting him did not disrupt his flow of thought. He successfully responded to explicit cues (e.g., raised hand) suggesting time to relinquish a turn in both individual and group situations, however he was unable to self-regulate turn taking.

Overall, in both individual and group sessions, Bobby V practised the ability to combine all modes of expression (verbal and nonverbal) to interact with others and share information, as well as express his personal opinions despite deteriorating word-finding ability. For instance, he read descriptions from his life story book (a collection of completely developed episodes of events that are emotionally salient) and pointed to the pictures in the book to supplement his verbal output while interacting with others. He brought in music CDs that he created to share information about music with the clinician and as well as group members.

In the later stages of semantic dementia, as Bobby V's verbal skills continued to decline, he was encouraged to continue using a combination of automatic utterances, facial expressions, and props to maintain personal, interactional, and informative functions of communication. For example, with his life story book in hand, Bobby V did not have to struggle to introduce a topic. He just opened the book and pointed to a picture paired with a few automatic utterances, establishing a topic understood by the listener.

FACILITATING COMMUNICATIVE EFFECTIVENESS WITH CAREGIVER TRAINING

Since discourse exchange requires joint construction of the message by the listener(s) and speaker(s), educating and training communication partners is crucial for maintaining communicative effectiveness. As described previously, Bobby V's wife was extremely frustrated with his communication skills at the time of diagnosis. Thus, our intervention plan with her (the primary communication partner) was to educate her about the changes in his communication and provide her with strategies to facilitate communication, as described below.

We counselled his wife about the profound effects of word retrieval deficits on Bobby V's communication abilities. We explained how his difficulty in lexical specificity could lead to lengthy conversational turns, limited topics, limited depth, and apparent egotism. She realised that he was not intentionally uncooperative, thus mitigating her frustration. We counselled her about his residual abilities such as relatively good memory for past events, retention of learned information over time, relatively good auditory comprehension for small amounts of information, and the ability to initiate and maintain interactions on topics of emotional relevance. We also informed her of the changes that she could anticipate with progression of his condition.

To help Bobby V's wife facilitate communicative effectiveness we provided strategies for her as a listener. First, we trained her to focus on the global message her husband was trying to convey rather than on lexical specificity. She was told that insisting on specific word retrieval might perpetuate frustrating guessing games. As a partner, she was asked to encourage him to use all modalities of communication (e.g., verbal output, written output, gestures, pictures etc.) during interactions.

Second, we trained her to use verbal and nonverbal contextual information to interpret his message. We pointed out that Bobby V utilised stereotypic responses to compensate for a loss of generative language. However, his limited repertoire of words and fixed phrases was used to convey a variety of messages. As Chapman and Ulatowska (1997, p. 183) stated, a "preserved ability to use automatic (stereotypic) responses for communicative purposes serves as a caution to look beyond the mere words to understand" the message of an individual with dementia. Often an individual with semantic dementia has an underlying idea to express and the cognitive ability to maintain it, whereas an individual with Alzheimer's disease may not (Chiu & Chapman, 2003). Thus, other cues (e.g., awareness of previous topic of conversation, immediate physical environment, personal history, or nonverbal cues) may help a listener decipher the message.

For example, in early stages, Bobby V would frequently say in conversation "That's kind of flaky" without further explanation. The clinician recognised this statement as compensation for his degraded ability to express his thoughts using language (Duchan, 1994). Depending on the context of the previous conversation topic, the fixed phrase "That's kind of flaky" was sometimes interpreted as acknowledging a poor description of an object (e.g., a cooking grill), and other times a description of poor behaviour (e.g., his reaction to a stressful situation). The caregiver was shown how she could discern his intended message by asking questions, requesting clarifications, and providing an explanation, and asking him if that is what he meant rather than dismissing the utterance as an insult or as vague and meaningless.

A third strategy given to Bobby V's wife was the instruction to serve as a liaison between Bobby V and other communication partners. As a liaison she was instructed to provide words, clarify his message as needed, accept his conversational turns, and expand his conversational turns. She was also trained to utilise the life story book as a tool to facilitate his interactions with others, especially in the later stages of the disease. This strategy expanded his circle of conversation partners and addressed a primary concern of Bobby V's wife. She had noted that Bobby V was withdrawing during social occasions and commented that "People tend to talk around him. It's like he is becoming an object in the room." Her support as a liaison for communication thus helped Bobby V maintain social connections.

CONCLUSION

One of the most important contributions of this case report is the description of a promising approach of communicative effectiveness that could be used to characterise communication skills, set therapy goals, and monitor progress in semantic dementia. As anticipated, Bobby V used verbal language to communicate in the early stages of semantic dementia. His language was generative in nature. He was able to achieve informative, personal, interactional, regulatory, and instrumental functions of communication despite word-finding difficulty. With disease progression his spoken output reduced drastically. Despite this he was able to achieve various functions of communication by combining automatic verbal and nonverbal language with support from the communication partner. We believe that our discourse intervention likely facilitated Bobby V's continued success in participating in conversation rather than withdrawing in frustration. To date he continues to attend group sessions and maintain social interactions despite the progression of semantic dementia. Helping his wife focus on residual abilities has enabled Bobby V to maintain meaningful interactions with immediate family members and others.

We are cautious in drawing conclusions about the general application of this framework due to the exploratory nature of this single-case intervention. In the future, carefully controlled studies are needed to further characterise communicative effectiveness in various stages of semantic dementia. Future studies should also determine the results of discourse therapy that focuses on communicative effectiveness across individual and group settings. Studies that specifically examine the effect of discourse therapy on functional communication, social interaction, quality of life, engagement, and affect are crucial. The outcome of discourse intervention on communicative effectiveness should be explored with listeners who are trained versus untrained in discourse strategies. Dose of intervention that produces optimal treatment outcomes should be determined, in addition to the maintenance of positive treatment effects. Also, the outcome of discourse therapy in individuals who differ in severity of semantic dementia, as well as severity of the behavioural and personality changes that often accompany it, needs examination.

We believe that interventions that aim to improve linguistic specificity in people with semantic dementia have limited functional value, considering the fact that semantic dementia is characterised by progressive disintegration in precisely this aspect of language. Contrastively, targeting conversational effectiveness in terms of communicative functions and means of expression offers a promising and an ecologically valuable intervention method as it allows individuals with semantic dementia to connect meaningfully with people in their immediate surroundings well into the later stages of the disease. Training Bobby V to supplement his verbal language with other modes of expression (e.g., gestures, props, facial expressions) has helped him to meet the basic need for human communication despite deterioration in semantic knowledge. At the present state of knowledge, such intervention in progressive brain disease may prove to be beneficial to quality of life and level of functionality alongside developing pharmacological treatments (Chapman et al., 2004).

REFERENCES

Arkin, S., & Mahendra, N. (2001). Discourse analysis of Alzheimer's patients before and after intervention: Methodology and outcomes. *Aphasiology, 15*, 533–569.

Ash, S., Moore, P., Antani, S., McCawley, G., Work, M., & Grossman, M. (2006). Trying to tell a tale: Discourse impairments in progressive aphasia and frontotemporal dementia. *Neurology, 66*, 1405–1413.

Blanken, G., Dittmann, J., Haas, J. C., & Wallesch, W. W. (1987). Spontaneous speech in senile dementia and aphasia: Implications for a neurolinguistic model of language production. *Cognition, 27*, 247–274.

Bohling, H. R. (1991). Communication with Alzheimer's patients: An analysis of caregiver listening patterns. *International Journal of Aging and Human Development, 33*, 249–267.

Chapman, S. B., Bonte, F. J., Wong, S. B. C., Zientz, J. N., Hynan, L. S., & Harris, T. S. et al. (2005). Convergence of connected language and SPECT in variants of frontotemporal lobar degeneration. *Alzheimer Disease and Associated Disorders, 19*, 202–213.

Chapman, S. B., Chiu, S. B., Zientz, J., Lipton, A. M., & Rosenberg, R. (2002). *Discourse fluency distinctions in frontotemporal dementia vs. Alzheimer's.* Poster session presented at Frontotemporal Dementia and Pick's Disease Conference, London, Canada.

Chapman, S. B., & Ulatowska, H. K. (1992). The nature of language disruption in dementia: Is it aphasia? *Texas Journal of Audiology and Speech Pathology, 17*, 3–9.

Chapman, S. B., & Ulatowska, H. K. (1997). Discourse in dementia: Consideration of consciousness. In M. I. Stamenov (Ed.), *Language structure, discourse and the access to consciousness* (pp. 155–188). Philadelphia: John Benjamin Publishing Company.

Chapman, S. B., Ulatowska, H. K., Franklin, L. R., Shobe, A. E., Thompson, J. L., & McIntire, D. D. (1997). Proverb interpretation in fluent aphasia and Alzheimer's disease: Implications beyond abstract thinking. *Aphasiology, 11*, 337–350.

Chapman, S. B., Weiner, M., Rackley, A., Hynan, L., & Zientz, J. (2004). Effects of cognitive-communication stimulation for Alzheimer's disease patients treated with Donepezil. *Journal of Speech, Language, and Hearing Research, 47*, 1149–1163.

Chiu, S. B., & Chapman, S. B. (2003). *Dissolution of script knowledge in semantic dementia.* Poster session presented at the Clinical Aphasiology Conference, Orcas Island, WA, USA.

Cress, C., & King, J. (1999). AAC strategies for people with primary progressive aphasia without dementia: Two case studies. *Augmentative and Alternative Communication, 14*, 248–259.

Duchan, J. (1994). Approaches to the study of discourse in the social sciences. In R. Bloom, L. Obler, S. DeSanti, & J. Erlich (Eds.), *Discourse studies in adult clinical populations* (pp. 1–14). Hillsdale, NJ: Lawrence Erlbaum Associates Inc.

Dunn, L. M., & Dunn, L. M. (1997). *Peabody Picture Vocabulary Test-III*. Circle Pines, MN: American Guidance Service.

Ferguson, A. (2000). Maximizing communication effectiveness. In N. Muller (Ed.), *Pragmatics in speech language pathology* (pp. 53–88). Philadelphia: John Benjamins Pub. Co.

Graham, K. S. (2001). Can repeated exposure to "forgotten" vocabulary help alleviate word-finding difficulties in semantic dementia? An illustrative case study. *Neuropsychological Rehabilitation, 11*, 429–454.

Grossman, M. (2005). Dawning hope for "the other dementia". *Cerebrum, 7*, 27–38.

Halliday, M. A. K. (1977). *Learning how to mean: Explorations in the development of language*. New York: Elsevier.

Hamilton, H. E. (1994). *Conversations with an Alzheimer's patient*. Cambridge, UK: Cambridge University Press.

Hodges, J. R., & Patterson, K. E. (1996). Nonfluent progressive aphasia and semantic dementia. A comparative neuropsychological study. *Journal of International Neurospychological Society, 2*, 511–524.

Hodges, J. R., Patterson, K. E., Oxbury, S., & Funnell, E. (1992). Semantic dementia: Progressive fluent aphasia with temporal lobe atrophy. *Brain, 115*, 1783–1806.

Howard, D., & Patterson, K. E. (1992). *The Pyramids and Palm Trees Test*. Windsor, UK: Thames Valley Test Co.

Jarrar, G., Orange, J. B., Kertesz, A., & Peacock, J. (1998). Pragmatics in frontal lobe dementias and primary progressive aphasia. *Journal of Neurolinguistics, 11*, 153–177.

Jokel, R., Rochon, E., & Leonard, C. (2002). Therapy for anomia in semantic dementia. *Brain and Cognition, 49*, 241–244.

Kaplan, E., & Weintraub, S. (1983). *Boston Naming Test*. Philadelphia: Lea & Febiger.

Kramer, J. H., Jurik, J., Sha, S. J., Rankin, K. P., Rosen, H. K., & Johnson, K. et al. (2003). Distinctive neuropsychological patterns in frontal-temporal dementia, semantic dementia, and Alzheimer's disease. *Cognitive Behavioral Neurology, 16*, 211–218.

Moss, S. E., Polignano, E., White, C. L., Minichiello, M. D., & Sunderland, T. (2002). Reminiscence group activities and discourse interaction in Alzheimer's disease. *Journal of Gerontological Nursing, 28*, 36–44.

Mummery, C. J., Patterson, K. E., Wise, R. J. S., Vandenbergh, R., Price, C. J., & Hodges, J. R. (1999). Disrupted temporal lobe connections in semantic dementia. *Brain, 122*, 61–73.

Neary, D., Gustafson, L., Passant, U., Stuss, D., Black, S. E., & Freedman, M. et al. (1998). Frontotemporal lobar degeneration: A consensus on clinical diagnostic criteria. *Neurology, 51*, 1546–1554.

Obler, L. K., & Albert, M. L. (1981). Language in the elderly aphasic and in the dementing patient. In M. T. Sarno (Ed.), *Acquired aphasia* (pp. 385–398). Orlando, FL: Academic Press.

Reilly, J. R., Nadin, M., & Murray, G. (2005). Verbal learning in semantic dementia: Is repetition priming a useful strategy? *Aphasiology, 19*, 329–339.

Ripich, D. N., & Terrell, B. Y. (1988). Patterns of discourse cohesion and coherence in Alzheimer's disease. *Journal of Speech and Hearing Disorders, 53*, 8–15.

Schwartz, M. F., & Chawluk, J. B. (1990). Deterioration of language in progressive aphasia: A case study. In M. F. Schwartz (Ed.), *Modular deficits in Alzheimer-type dementia. Issues in the biology of language and cognition* (pp. 245–296). Cambridge, MA: MIT Press.

Van Lancker, D. (1990). The neurology of proverbs. *Behavioral Neurology, 3*, 169–187.

APHASIOLOGY, 2009, 23 (2), 302–326

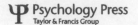

Progressive language impairments: Definitions, diagnoses, and prognoses

Karen Croot

University of Sydney, NSW, Australia

Background: Speech pathologists have much to contribute to diagnosis of, intervention in, and education about the clinical syndromes that present with selective and progressive impairments in spoken or receptive language processing, reading, writing, and semantic knowledge. However, there is no single agreed classification system for these disorders, with the result that different research and clinical groups may use the same terms with subtly or substantially different meanings, or use different terms for similar phenomena. Understanding of the neuropathology and prognosis of these disorders is increasing rapidly.

Aims: This paper reviews (i) the major approaches to classifying the clinical presentations of these disorders, (ii) progress in relating the clinical syndromes to neuropathology, and (iii) currently available information about prognoses.

Main Contribution: Two main classification approaches based on clinical syndromes have emerged for these disorders. The first uses the label *primary progressive aphasia* to describe gradual and selective deterioration in word finding, object naming, or word comprehension without identifying subtypes, following criteria published by Mesulam and colleagues during and subsequent to 2001. The second approach, initially associated with the Lund consensus meetings in the 1990s, identifies the clinical syndromes of nonfluent progressive aphasia (with and without apraxia of speech) and semantic dementia as subtypes of frontotemporal dementia. There are two main neuropathologies responsible for progressive language impairments: a spectrum of diseases classed under the term frontotemporal lobar degeneration, and Alzheimer's disease. Semantic dementia is most often associated with frontotemporal lobar degeneration with motor neuron disease-type inclusions. Apraxia of speech in neurodegenerative disease is most often associated with the tau-positive subtypes of frontotemporal lobar degeneration. Alzheimer-type neuropathology has been found in both semantic dementia and nonfluent progressive aphasia. Information about survival and autonomy in these disorders, and about incidence of behaviour and personality change and motor impairment, is just beginning to emerge.

Conclusions: The range of classification systems in use emphasise the importance of specifying the criteria used to reach a particular diagnosis, and the clinical symptoms on which the diagnosis is based. As pharmacological or other treatments become available to target the neuropathological mechanisms in these diseases, a primary diagnostic goal will be to identify the likely neuropathology in order to match clients to appropriate therapies at the earliest opportunity.

Keywords: Primary progressive aphasia; Frontotemporal dementia; Semantic dementia; Diagnosis; Prognosis.

Address correspondence to: Karen Croot, School of Psychology A18, University of Sydney, NSW, Australia 2006, E-mail: karenc@psych.usyd.edu.au

Thank you to Lyndsey Nickels and two anonymous reviewers for helpful feedback on an earlier version of this manuscript.

---

http://www.psypress.com/aphasiology   DOI: 10.1080/02687030801942981

PROGRESSIVE APHASIA: AN EMERGING FIELD OF SPEECH PATHOLOGY PRACTICE

As recently as 20 years ago, speech pathology training made little or no mention of the management of speech, language, and communication changes associated with dementia. The speech pathologist's role was limited to differential diagnosis between language impairments associated with dementia and language impairments subsequent to stroke. Since then there has been growing recognition that progressive brain pathology can result in selective language impairments where the expertise of the speech pathologist is invaluable.

This shift has come about for four main reasons. First, knowledge of the diseases that cause dementia has increased exponentially as the ageing population in both the developed and developing worlds provides an increasing number of people at risk for dementia (di Carlo, Baldereschi, Inzitari, & Amaducci, 1999). Second, progress in cognitive theory and neuropsychological assessment has allowed a more precise understanding of the cognitive and behavioural changes that occur in these diseases. Third, advances in imaging technologies reveal the integrity of brain structure and function in vivo. Finally, rapid developments in molecular pathology made possible by large-scale brain tissue donation (McLean, Beyreuther, & Masters, 2001) are beginning to identify the causes of the degenerative changes in brain tissue. Alongside these groundbreaking shifts, earlier views of speech pathology practice that largely excluded people with dementia from a typical adult caseload are undergoing major change (Ripich & Horner, 2004).

A speech pathologist can now argue for a number of important roles on a dementia health and social care team. These include assessment, education of people with dementia and their families and communities, delivery of impairment- and activity- and participation-based speech, language, communication and swallowing interventions, and advocacy and policy development roles (Royal College of Speech and Language Therapists, 2005). There is a burgeoning literature on language, communication, and other neuropsychological interventions in dementia that considers the client within a holistic framework embracing physical health, cognitive strengths and limitations, and social and physical environment. Leading examples of these include Attix and Welsh-Bohmer (2006), Bayles and Tomoeda (1997), Bourgeois (1991), Bryan and Maxim (2006), Clare (2001), Killick and Allan (2001), Lubinski (1995), Lubinski and Orange (2000), and Ripich (1994).

In this context of growing interest in dementia, the subset of disorders in which there are selective and progressive impairments of language have received particular attention from the speech pathology community. The most well known of these is primary progressive aphasia (PPA, Mesulam, 1982, 2001; Mesulam & Weintraub, 1992). However, there is a broad constellation of clinical syndromes in which the most prominent, initial, and ongoing symptom is deterioration in spoken or receptive language processing, reading, writing, or some combination of these. There may or may not be other accompanying cognitive impairments. When a collective term is required in the current paper, such symptoms will be described as "progressive language impairments".

Speech pathologists have much to contribute to diagnosis and intervention in these disorders because of the focal speech and language symptoms. Published work on appropriate interventions is only just beginning to appear, however, and lags behind the resources available on speech pathology interventions in dementia in general. There is nonetheless a small emerging literature on this client group that includes expert opinion on therapy approaches (McNeil & Duffy, 2001; Robinson, 2001; Rogers, King, & Alarcon, 2000; Snowden & Griffiths, 2000; Thompson & Johnson, 2006), and two-to-three dozen or so published therapy reports ranging from descriptions of therapy activities included as part of a case report (Hart, Beach, & Taylor, 1997; Holland, McBurney, Moossy, & Reinmuth, 1985) to controlled studies (K. S. Graham, Patterson, Pratt, & Hodges, 1999; McNeil, Small, Masterson, & Tepanta, 1995; Schneider, Thompson, & Luhring, 1996), including the reports in this special issue of *Aphasiology*. We pick up some of the key themes emerging from this literature in the final paper of this special issue (Croot, Nickels, Laurence, & Manning, 2009 this issue).

At this point in time we have much to learn about optimal interventions for progressive language impairments. Many crucial questions, such as "Which intervention for which client?", "Which intervention at which stage in disease progression?", "How long should therapy be continued?", "What will the benefits be?", and "How well can treatment effects be maintained?" are still a long way from evidence-based answers. Further, there are indications that people with these disorders are under-referred for speech pathology services (Taylor, Kingma, Croot, & Nickels, 2009 this issue), a situation that can be improved with increased awareness of available therapy options. This paper will address some commonly-asked questions about progressive language impairments which are relevant background for those considering providing intervention: questions about the range of clinical presentations, the disease processes involved, and the likely prognosis for various clinical presentations.

MANY DIAGNOSTIC CATEGORIES: CLINICAL SYNDROMES AND NEUROPATHOLOGY

One does not have to read far in the literature on progressive language impairments before encountering a range of diagnostic labels, such as fluent progressive aphasia, semantic dementia, progressive non-fluent aphasia, primary progressive anomia, progressive apraxia of speech, dementia of the frontal type, primary progressive dysgraphia, and (many) others in similar vein. References to frontotemporal lobar degeneration (FTLD), Pick's disease, and dementia lacking distinct histology (DLDH) are likely to be close behind. There are two main reasons for this "bewildering array of diagnostic terms" (Hodges & Miller, 2001, p. 31): (i) the distinction between labels for clinical syndromes and neuropathological classifications, and (ii) the independent development of several classification systems towards the end of the twentieth century.

Clinical syndromes

Some classification labels (for example, fluent progressive aphasia, semantic dementia, progressive non-fluent aphasia, progressive apraxia of speech, dementia of the frontal type, primary progressive dysgraphia) primarily describe the *clinical syndrome*, i.e., the particular set of symptoms with which the client presents at the clinic. Others (for example, frontotemporal lobar degeneration, Pick's disease, and dementia lacking distinct histology) primarily imply the *neuropathology* (neurodegenerative disease process) presumed or proven to be present in the brain (Hodges & Miller, 2001).

The range of signs and symptoms that make up the clinical syndrome presented by a person with neurodegenerative disease reflect the location of damaged tissue in the brain (Mesulam, Grossman, Hillis, Kertesz, & Weintraub, 2003; Neary, 1999), just as they do in acquired language disorders caused by stroke, traumatic brain injury, or tumour. In the case of progressive language impairments, the neuropathologies involved may target any one or more of a number of frontal, temporal, parietal, and/or subcortical regions involved in a range of speech and language functions. Speech, language, communication, and other abilities that were previously reliant on these brain regions will be compromised, and the person, their family, and colleagues will begin to notice a decline in those abilities. Because any or many parts of the brain networks supporting speech and language may be affected by the disease process involved, there are diverse patterns of speech and language symptoms that may develop. Further, the functioning of a particular brain region may be affected either directly when tissue in that region is diseased, or indirectly when it is connected in a brain network to another structure that is diseased, resulting in distal or "diaschesis" effects (Hillis et al., 2002; Price, Warburton, Moore, Frackowiak, & Friston, 2001). For example, the anomia in semantic dementia is attributed to hypoperfusion (reduced blood flow) in posterior temporal regions thought to be caused by the neuropathology located in the anterior temporal lobe (Lambon Ralph, McClelland, Patterson, Galton, & Hodges, 2001; Mummery et al., 1999).

Frontotemporal dementia

One of the most important syndrome labels found in the literature on progressive language impairments is *frontotemporal dementia* (FTD), which refers to a range of non-Alzheimer-type dementia syndromes caused by focal atrophy of the frontal and anterior temporal brain regions (Hodges, Davies, Xuereb, Kril, & Halliday, 2003; Hodges et al., 2004). The earliest and dominant symptom in frontotemporal dementia is often a gradual and progressive speech and/or language impairment (the *language variant of frontotemporal dementia*; McKhann et al., 2001), yielding clinical syndromes characterised by progressive language impairments. An earlier term for the language variant was *temporal (lobe) variant of frontotemporal dementia* (e.g., Edwards-Lee et al., 1997), so-named because of the brain region most affected in these cases.

A second major category of frontotemporal dementia primarily involves progressive changes in behaviour, including personality change and socially inappropriate behaviour (McKhann et al., 2001). This *behavioural variant of frontotemporal dementia* (also called *frontal variant frontotemporal dementia*; Hodges & Miller, 2001) will not be addressed in detail in this paper. However, behaviour changes do often emerge with progression in cases of progressive aphasia, (as neuropathology spreads to brain regions responsible for these functions), so these will be discussed in relation to disease progression and prognosis.

Neuropathology

The neuropathological findings in frontotemporal dementia include a spectrum of disease processes described under the umbrella term of *frontotemporal lobar degeneration* (FTLD; McKhann et al., 2001). There are a range of alternative names and classifications for these neuropathologies, described in more detail below. Sometimes, however, a person can present with clinical symptoms unlike classical Alzheimer-type dementia and consistent with those described for frontotemporal dementia, but be found to have Alzheimer-type neuropathology at autopsy. Thus the other major disease associated with progressive language impairments is Alzheimer's disease (Hodges et al., 2003; Knibb, Xuereb, Patterson, & Hodges, 2006). Neuropathological diagnosis is almost always made at autopsy following donation of brain tissue, although in rare cases biopsy may be used to rule out infection and cancer. Standard diagnostic criteria for Alzheimer's disease do not allow entirely reliable differentiation between Alzheimer's disease and frontotemporal lobar degeneration during life (Varma et al., 1999), and many studies in recent years have sought to refine the diagnostic criteria for these two diseases (Mendez & Perryman, 2002; Rascovsky et al., 2002; Rosen et al., 2002).

Classification systems developed by different research teams

Investigations of progressive language disorders took off in a number of centres in Europe and North America from the 1980s onwards. It was apparent from early on that there was considerable similarity between clinical presentations that were later shown to be associated with different neuropathologies and, conversely, that there were similar neuropathology findings post-mortem for syndromes that had been clinically dissimilar in life. To some extent, various research centres found different coherent ways of carving the clinical presentations and neuropathologies into diagnostic categories; sometimes creating new labels and new categories, and sometimes defining existing categories in slightly different ways.

The following section describes some of the major clinical classification systems currently in use. The range of classification systems, and the fact that different research groups may use somewhat different criteria in applying the same diagnostic label, emphasise the need for speech pathologists to be specific about which criteria they are using in reaching a particular diagnosis.

CLASSIFICATION SYSTEMS BASED ON CLINICAL SYNDROME

There is no single agreed classification system for progressive language impairments (Josephs et al., 2006a), with Knibb et al. (2006), for example, identifying five prominent approaches in current use. However, two main classification approaches based on clinical syndromes have emerged: one that summarises a range of progressive language impairments under the label *primary progressive aphasia*, and one that makes a core distinction between the syndromes of semantic dementia and non-fluent progressive aphasia (Hodges & Patterson, 1996; Neary, 1999) within the broader diagnostic category of frontotemporal dementia. Below are outlined the development of the current criteria for diagnosing primary progressive aphasia, then summarise the alternative approach taken by the Lund group of researchers and recent developments within this approach.

Primary progressive aphasia: Early reports and subtypes

The diagnosis of *primary* progressive aphasia (italics added) as described by Mesulam and colleagues (Mesulam, 1982, 1987, 1990, 2001; Mesulam et al., 2003;

Mesulam & Weintraub, 1992) is reserved for people with gradual language decline over a period of at least 2 years, with language difficulties being the only factor compromising activities of daily living (Mesulam & Weintraub, 1992; Weintraub, Rubin, & Mesulam, 1990). The early reports (Mesulam, 1982, 1987) described individuals for whom the deficits were predominantly language-based over a long period (up to 10 years) without generalised dementia, thus the neuropathological process was presumed to differ from Alzheimer's disease. Today a diagnosis of primary progressive aphasia is still assumed to indicate a non-Alzheimer pathology for some research and clinical groups—however, as described below, a person may meet current clinical criteria for primary progressive aphasia (Mesulam, 2001), yet prove to have Alzheimer-type pathology at post-mortem investigation.

The earliest explicit classification of progressive language impairments distinguished three subtypes of primary progressive aphasia along a fluency dimension, with a broad division into *fluent, non-fluent and mixed* subtypes (Grossman & Ash, 2004; Mesulam & Weintraub, 1992; Snowden, Neary, & Mann, 1996). The fluent subtype was defined by phrase length greater than four words and grammatically intact language, with language resembling anomic, conduction, Wernicke's, and transcortical sensory aphasia as defined by the "classical" aphasia batteries (Mesulam & Weintraub, 1992). Some of the (otherwise) fluent cases were noted to have word-finding difficulties that introduced long pauses into their spoken language, a subtype of fluent primary progressive aphasia that Mesulam and Weintraub described as logopenic. The non-fluent subtype was characterised by agrammatic speech with reduced phrase length, resembling Broca's and transcortical motor aphasias. An earlier report by the same authors had emphasised the prominence of errors in the production of speech sounds in four non-fluent cases (Weintraub et al., 1990), thus for some researchers and clinicians the presence of phonological or articulatory errors came to be viewed as the hallmark of the non-fluent subtype. Mixed primary progressive aphasia was proposed as the classification for people who met criteria for the non-fluent subtype but also had comprehension difficulties, a presentation resembling a global aphasia.

Snowden et al. (1996) described three very similar profiles, but noted that a number of the fluent cases (with fluent spoken language, anomia, and word comprehension deficits) also had difficulties recognising and knowing about objects and people, and developed personality and behaviour change with disease progression. They called this presentation *semantic dementia* (Snowden, Goulding, & Neary, 1989). However, Mesulam and colleagues (Mesulam, 2001; Mesulam et al., 2003) exclude people with semantic dementia defined this way (progressive loss of knowledge about objects and people occurring alongside a fluent progressive aphasia) from a diagnosis of primary progressive aphasia, and consider this a "primary progressive aphasia-plus syndrome" (see below). Confusingly, the term "semantic dementia" is sometimes used to label fluent progressive aphasia with impaired word comprehension *without* loss of object and face knowledge. For some groups this is on the basis that such deficits are expected to develop with disease progression, but for others the terms fluent progressive aphasia and semantic dementia are taken to be interchangeable. It is essential, therefore, to specify what deficits are present when using the label "semantic dementia" (Mesulam et al., 2003).

One of the clinical difficulties that has been faced by speech pathologists trying to apply the fluent/non-fluent categorisation is that the progressive language impairments encountered in the clinic and described in the published literature do not neatly correspond to the fluent versus non-fluent aphasia profiles associated with CVA (Josephs et al., 2006a; Mesulam, 2001). The problem is compounded by the fact that the fluency distinction is not straightforward in the CVA population (Gordon, 1998), and by clinical data showing that a high proportion of people with primary progressive aphasia may be fluent early in the disease course but progress to a non-fluent profile of language production over time (Kertesz, Davidson, McCabe, Takagi, & Munoz, 2003). Further, for clinicians who viewed the presence of phonological errors as diagnostic of the non-fluent subtype, clients who presented with phonological errors and fluent speech, or effortful, non-fluent speech without phonological errors, were particularly difficult to categorise. Mesulam and colleagues now acknowledge that basing a diagnosis of primary progressive aphasia subtype on the person's fluency is far from straightforward (Mesulam et al., 2003).

Current criteria for primary progressive aphasia: De-emphasis of subtypes

For the above reasons, Mesulam and colleagues (Mesulam, 2001, 2003; Mesulam et al., 2003; Sonty et al., 2002) have more recently taken a different approach that has been widely adopted in the USA, describing what is essentially a single category of primary progressive aphasia using the diagnostic criteria reproduced in Table 1. The central requirement is "insidious onset and gradual progressive impairment of word-finding, object naming, syntax or word comprehension" evident in conversation or formal assessment over a 2-year period (Mesulam, 2003, p. 1536). The aphasia may be fluent or non-fluent (Mesulam et al., 2003).

Structural brain imaging—i.e., using computerised tomography (CT) or structural magnetic resonance imaging (MRI)—in primary progressive aphasia shows tissue loss (atrophy) in frontal, temporal, and parietal regions associated with the left hemisphere language network (Mesulam, 2001). In the study of Josephs et al. (2006a), a group of participants with primary progressive aphasia without agrammatism, apraxia of speech, or semantic dementia had predominantly left-sided posterior temporal

TABLE 1
Diagnostic criteria for primary progressive aphasia

1. Insidious onset and gradual progression of word-finding, object-naming, or word-comprehension impairments as manifested during spontaneous conversation or as assessed through formal neuropsychological tests of language.
2. All limitation of daily living activities attributable to the language impairment, for at least 2 years after onset.
3. Intact premorbid language function (except for developmental dyslexia).
4. Absence of significant apathy, disinhibition, forgetfulness for recent events, visuospatial impairment, visual recognition deficits or sensory-motor dysfunction within the initial 2 years of the illness. (This criterion can be fulfilled by history, survey of daily living activities, or formal neuropsychological testing.)
5. Acalculia and ideomotor apraxia may be present even in the first 2 years (mild constructional deficits and perseveration—as assessed in the go-no-go task—are also acceptable as long as neither visuospatial deficits nor disinhibition influences daily living activities).
6. Other domains possibly affected after the first 2 years but with language remaining the most impaired function throughout the course of the illness and deteriorating faster than other affected domains.
7. Absence of specific causes such as stroke or tumour as ascertained by neuroimaging.

atrophy. Although structural imaging is typically one of the earliest investigations performed, functional brain imaging is likely to be more sensitive at the early stages in identifying regional changes associated with progressive language impairments, showing abnormalities earlier than structural imaging (Mesulam, 2001; Sinnatamby, Antoun, Freer, Miles, & Hodges, 1996). Such techniques include single positron emission tomography (SPECT) imaging, positron emission tomography (PET) imaging, perfusion-weighted MRI, and electroencephalography (EEG). Functional imaging of people with primary progressive aphasia shows that activation of classical language areas may be normal, although additional brain regions may participate in compensatory and/or increased inhibitory activity (Sonty et al., 2002).

Under the current approach of Mesulam and colleagues, people who initially receive a diagnosis of primary progressive aphasia but subsequently develop non-language symptoms (personality or behaviour or extrapyramidal motor symptoms, or neurological signs consistent with motor neuron disease)[1] are said to have a *primary progressive aphasia-plus syndrome* (Mesulam, 2001; Mesulam et al., 2003).

Semantic dementia and non-fluent subtypes of FTD

An alternative approach more common in Europe was strongly influenced by meetings on frontotemporal dementia held in Lund, Sweden, (Neary, 1999; The Lund and Manchester Groups, 1994) describing two main clinical presentations in which there is progressive language decline: *semantic dementia* and *non-fluent progressive aphasia* (identical to *progressive non-fluent aphasia*).

Semantic dementia, according to the early definitions (Hodges, Patterson, Oxbury, & Funnell, 1992; Snowden et al., 1989), is characterised by striking anomia and impaired word comprehension attributed to loss of semantic memory (e.g., concepts, facts, semantic features) (Hodges & Miller, 2001; Knibb et al., 2006). As noted by Snowden et al. (1989), these semantic memory deficits also impair recognition of visually presented objects, a symptom known as visual agnosia (Neary, 1999). This is the predominant usage of the term "semantic dementia", and in this sense the term is not interchangeable with a diagnosis of fluent primary progressive aphasia as defined by Mesulam and colleagues (Mesulam, 2001; Mesulam et al., 2003), as discussed above.

The early reports of imaging in semantic dementia were based on visual inspection of structural CT and MR images (Hodges et al., 1992; Snowden et al., 1996). These noted the consistently striking and focal atrophy of anterior temporal regions, especially the infero-lateral regions of the temporal pole visible on coronal MRI. All individuals showed left temporal atrophy, with involvement of anterior right temporal regions apparently associated with more severe object recognition deficits (Snowden et al., 1996). More recent studies that have sought to quantify the degree of atrophy have revealed that changes may be bilateral or involve the left hemisphere more than the right, and involve medial temporal structures, including the hippocampus and amygdala as well as infero-lateral regions (Chan et al., 2001; Galton et al., 2001; Gorno-Tempini et al., 2004).

Nonfluent progressive aphasia is defined by non-fluent spontaneous speech, and at least one of the following: anomia, errors in production of speech sounds, or

---

[1] For example, muscle weakness and atrophy, fasciculations, hyperactive reflexes, and spasticity (Borasio, Appel, & Buettner, 1996).

grammatical errors (Knibb et al., 2006; Neary, 1999). More recently, Gorno-Tempini et al. (2004) suggested that two non-fluent categories of primary progressive aphasia should be distinguished. One category they continued to call *non-fluent progressive aphasia*, characterised by apraxia of speech and agrammatism/syntactic comprehension deficits with spared single word comprehension. The other they called *logopenic progressive aphasia*, describing a clinical presentation with slow speech, impaired syntax comprehension, and anomia. Knibb et al. (2006) carried out a cluster analysis using 38 cases presenting with various progressive aphasia syndromes and also found that the non-fluent cases could be distinguished into two groups along the lines suggested by Gorno-Tempini et al. (2004).

In Gorno-Tempini et al.'s (2004) study, the subgroup of people with non-fluent progressive aphasia showed atrophy in Broca's area (Brodmann areas 44 and 45), a small region of Brodmann area 47, and the left precentral gyrus of the insula. The people with logopenic progressive aphasia showed a completely different distribution of atrophy, with angular gyrus and the posterior third of the middle temporal gyrus most affected (Brodmann areas 39, 40, and 21), with additional atrophy in left anterior hippocampus, right angular gyrus and precuneus (Brodmann area 31).

In another recent approach, Kertesz, McMonagle, Blair, Davidson, and Munoz (2005) described six subtypes, including *semantic dementia* and three subtypes of primary progressive aphasia meeting Mesulam's 2-year criterion: *anomic, logopenic*, and *non-fluent primary progressive aphasia*. Semantic dementia was defined by comprehension deficit, naming difficulty, and asking the meaning of nouns and objects (e.g., "What is parade?...shoe-polish?...steak?"; Kertesz et al., 2005, p. 2003). Anomic primary progressive aphasia described minimal impairment to fluency and speech rate but pronounced word-finding difficulty. Logopenic primary progressive aphasia described more severe word-finding difficulty combined with severely reduced output, but relatively preserved syntax, phonology, and articulation. Nonfluent primary progressive aphasia was characterised by agrammatism, errors in the production of speech sounds, and anomia. Kertesz et al. also noted two further subtypes: one they called *aphemic*, with difficulty in the production of speech approximately corresponding to apraxia of speech, and a *mute* subtype in which people were mute at presentation, but ambulant, cooperative and able to demonstrate relatively preserved comprehension.

In the newest development, Josephs et al. (2006a) advocated the need to distinguish when apraxia of speech is present, with or without aphasia. They noted that the non-fluent cases are frequently reported with "'laboured speech', 'laboured articulation', or 'distortion of speech'" (Josephs et al., 2006a, p. 1386), and suggested that the so-called "phonemic paraphasias" in these cases probably arise at an articulatory rather than a phonological level of processing. The perceptual features leading to a diagnosis of apraxia of speech by Josephs and colleagues (2006a, p. 1388) were consonant and vowel distortions; distorted sound substitutions; distorted sound additions; sound prolongations; trial and error attempts to correct articulation; slow overall rate; prolonged and often variable vowel duration and interword intervals; segregation of syllables; errors of stress assignment; and decreased phonetic accuracy with increased rate.

In this study, imaging of people with a selective progressive apraxia of speech showed atrophy to grey matter in superior premotor and supplementary motor areas, middle and inferior frontal gyri especially on the right, and basal ganglia (bilateral caudate and right globus pallidus). These individuals would not qualify for a diagnosis of primary progressive aphasia according to the criteria of Mesulam and colleagues (Mesulam, 2001; Mesulam et al., 2003) because no *language* disorder is present. People with progressive non-fluent aphasia (primarily denoted by agrammatic or telegraphic speech) and apraxia of speech showed similar premotor atrophy but more posterior inferior frontal atrophy (Josephs et al., 2006a) than the people with apraxia of speech only.

HOW USEFUL ARE SYNDROME-BASED CLASSIFICATIONS?

Purpose and limitations of syndrome labels

A syndrome label that captures the primary symptoms can be clinically beneficial for communicating the nature of the symptoms among clinicians, and for relating a particular case to similar previous cases, including communicating to the person with one of these syndromes and their family that their condition is a recognised disorder. For example, in the most literal sense, the label "primary progressive aphasia" communicates that the person's main (*primary*) symptom is an acquired language disorder (*aphasia*) that has a *progressive* course. Similarly, progressive pure *anomia* (K. S. Graham, Patterson, & Hodges, 1995) indicates that the progressive language disorder is primarily characterised by word-finding difficulties; primary progressive *conduction aphasia* (Hillis, Selnes, & Gordon, 1999) indicates there is similarity between the person's language symptoms and one of the existing conceptualisations of conduction aphasia, and primary progressive *apraxia of speech* (Josephs et al., 2006a) suggests that speech, more than language, is the domain affected ... and so on. Thus the proliferation of syndrome labels associated with these disorders provides a somewhat informative (if abbreviated) overview of the diversity of clinical presentations.

A problem arises, however, when different uses of a particular term by different researchers leads to misunderstanding about the clinical presentation being described. A syndrome label does *not* necessarily facilitate communication when there is no single agreed operational definition of the syndrome (Coltheart, 1984; Neary, 1999). For example, there are cases reported as semantic dementia with more or less comprehension impairment relative to anomia, or more or less behaviour and personality change. There are also people diagnosed with non-fluent progressive aphasia according to a range of definitions of "non-fluent", with or without apraxia of speech, and even with or without aphasia (when apraxia of speech is the only symptom) (Josephs et al., 2006a). It is unfortunately but unavoidably the case at present that different groups of clinicians and researchers hold subtly or substantially different understandings as to what symptoms, features, or neuro-pathology are implied by a number of these syndrome labels. It is *essential*, therefore, to explicitly identify the classification system used to reach a diagnosis (e.g., Mesulam, 2001, or the Lund criteria described by Neary, 1999 etc.), *and* to describe in detail the presenting symptoms, rather than simply assigning a syndrome label.

Change in syndrome with progression

Another difficulty in the application of syndrome labels to these disorders occurs because of the degenerative disease course. Impairments increase in severity over time and new impairments may become prominent that were not evident before. The clinical picture is far from static, and patterns of progression (as well as patterns of initial presentation) can be diverse.

It is not yet known to what extent the different neuropathologies responsible for progressive language impairments spread within language-specific networks of the brain versus spreading to brain regions involved in quite different cognitive functions. There are, however, three potential patterns of progression: (i) selective decline in language and/or speech abilities, (ii) initial language and/or speech decline, with additional impairments arising later in progression, and (iii) decline in language and/or speech alongside other deficits from onset.

To the extent that a person's impairments remain selective to language over a long period (as in the rare cases where there are isolated language symptoms over a 10- to 20-year period; Mesulam, 1982; Schwartz, De Bleser, Poeck, & Weis, 1998), it can be assumed that language-specific networks alone are compromised. These would clearly meet criteria for primary progressive aphasia as defined by Mesulam and colleagues (Mesulam, 2001; Mesulam et al., 2003). For many years, Mesulam and colleagues have taken the position that a selective language disorder for the first 2 years is predictive of a more language-specific clinical course, and a non-Alzheimer-type neuropathology, and this is why the 2-year criterion is central to their diagnosis of primary progressive aphasia.

Other authors, however, prefer to drop the designation "primary" and use the shorter term, *progressive aphasia* (Knibb et al., 2006). These authors argue that the 2-year limit is arbitrary, that the presence or absence of non-language symptoms is only ever a matter of degree, and that people who satisfy the 2-year criterion happen to fall within one region of a broad continuum of possible symptoms associated with various neuropathologies, but do not otherwise represent a useful clinical category. Which of these views will prove to be correct remains an open question, as the research to support a distinctive prognosis for people meeting the 2-year claim has not yet been reported (Knibb et al., 2006; McNeil & Duffy, 2001). Nonetheless, McNeil and Duffy point out that the diagnostic label "primary progressive aphasia" is clinically helpful in highlighting the need for aphasia management as the central component of client care for as long as the deficits remain specific to language. They note, however, that the diagnosis of primary progressive aphasia may need to be altered if or when the person's profile of impairments changes with disease progression (McNeil & Duffy, 2000).

In some cases, other deficits such as behavioural or personality change, impairments in additional cognitive domains (e.g., memory, visuo-spatial abilities, praxis, or attention), and non-speech motor impairments (gait rigidity, falls, vertical gaze palsy) can emerge during the disease course even when language impairments were the presenting symptom (profiles that Mesulam, 2001, would call primary progressive aphasia-plus syndromes). Diagnostic labels based on clinical symptoms alone clearly raise a problem in these disorders because a particular label may be appropriate at one point in time but not later. Kertesz et al. (2005) address this problem by describing the sets of clinical symptoms that emerge with disease progression in terms of the first syndrome, the second syndrome etc. For example, a person may have primary progressive aphasia (as per Mesulam's 2001 definition) as their first syndrome, but later develop a second syndrome of behavioural problems typical of a frontal dementia in addition to the language syndrome, and perhaps later still a third syndrome, characterised by motor symptoms including rigidity, limb apraxia, and alien hand (Kertesz et al., 2005). Conversely, one or more aspects of language decline can emerge later in a case for which other cognitive, behavioural, or motor deficits were the initial concern. In such cases, the language symptoms would constitute the second or third syndrome. Kertesz et al. (2005) use the term *primary progressive aphasia* when the language symptoms form the first syndrome for a period of 2 years or more, and call the disorder *progressive aphasia* when language decline is the second or third syndrome to appear.

The need for clinicopathologically based diagnostic categories

As pharmaceutical or other treatments become available to target the neuropathological mechanisms in these diseases, a primary diagnostic goal will be to identify the likely neuropathology in vivo, in order to match clients to appropriate therapies at the earliest opportunity. Even the development of such therapies requires "early and accurate prediction of pathology" (Davies et al., 2005, p. 1994; Whitwell et al., 2005). The most recent progress towards this goal comes from longitudinal studies analysing the clinical course and neuropathological findings in comparatively large case series of people who presented with or developed progressive language impairments (Davies et al., 2005; Hodges et al., 2003, 2004; Josephs et al., 2006a, 2006b; Kertesz et al., 2005; Knibb et al., 2006). These studies are beginning to clarify the relationship between the clinical course and the underlying disease process. The following section provides a brief introduction to the neuropathologies associated with progressive language impairments, then summarises current progress in relating clinical syndromes to the probable neuropathology. Finally, genetic mutations have been discovered in association with familial cases of frontotemporal lobal degeneration, and these will also be briefly reviewed.

NEUROPATHOLOGICAL DIAGNOSIS

Post-mortem examination of brain tissue classifies both the macroscopic and microscopic appearance of brain tissue. Macroscopic investigation notes regions of atrophy visible to the eye. Microscopic investigation (histology) involves treating slices of brain tissue with a range of chemical stains and agents that are sensitive to the molecular chemistry of a range of proteins that build up in the tissue in association with neurodegenerative disease. Treating the tissue with such techniques allows these atypical protein deposits (known as "inclusions") to be seen under a microscope. The type, frequency, and location of these inclusions form the main basis for classifying different neurodegenerative diseases. The two neuropathologies associated with progressive language impairments are Alzheimer's disease (Knibb et al., 2006), and the disease processes classed under the term frontotemporal lobar degeneration (or FTLD, McKhann et al., 2001).

Alzheimer's disease

The hallmark neuropathological inclusions in Alzheimer's disease are neurofibrillary tangles and neuritic plaques (The National Institute on Aging and Reagan Institute Working Group on Diagnostic Criteria for the Neuropathological Assessment of Alzheimer's Disease, 1997), characterised by the proteins *tau* and *beta amyloid*, respectively. Although the atrophy in Alzheimer's disease is usually widespread and symmetrical (Lantos & Cairns, 2001), it can be strikingly focal (localised to a small region of the brain) in people with progressive language impairments (Galton, Patterson, Xuereb, & Hodges, 2000; Knibb et al., 2006). Differential diagnosis of Alzheimer's disease versus frontotemporal lobar degeneration becomes more difficult in older individuals because of the increasing likelihood of neurofibrillary tangles and neuritic plaques with age (Johnson et al., 2005).

Frontotemporal lobar degeneration

Frontotemporal lobar degeneration is the current consensus term for a clinically and neuropathologically heterogeneous spectrum of diseases associated with the clinical syndrome of frontotemporal dementia. Diseases in the frontotemporal lobar degeneration spectrum were first reported by the German neurologist Pick (1892, 1904, cited in Kertesz, 2004), and are also described under the broad labels of *Pick's Disease*, *frontal lobe degeneration of non-Alzheimer-type* (Brun, 1987) and *Pick complex* (Josephs et al., 2006b; Kertesz, Hudson, Mackenzie, & Munoz, 1994). There is ongoing discussion as to whether the neuropathological subtypes should be considered as separate disorders (e.g., Dickson, 1999) or as different points on a single disease spectrum (Josephs et al., 2006b). In this paper we treat them as related because the clinical symptoms co-occur in many cases, the diverse syndromes are associated with the same set of histological findings, and, in an inherited subtype known as *frontotemporal dementia and parkinsonism linked to chromosome 17* (FTDP-17), any of the clinical syndromes associated with frontotemporal dementia may occur (Josephs et al., 2006b; Kertesz, 2004; Neary, 1999).

In frontotemporal lobar degeneration there is focal atrophy of frontal and/or temporal regions (McKhann et al., 2001; Neary, 1999). There are a number of approaches to classifying the neuropathological entities involved, based on the type of inclusions present and their distribution in the brain. The inclusions can be categorised according to whether they test positive for tau (collectively called *tauopathies*), or for another protein called *ubiquitin* (Lantos & Cairns, 2001; McKhann et al., 2001). The presence or absence of tau or ubiquitin may prove to be important given current debate about whether prognosis is better for the tauopathies (Hodges et al., 2003; Josephs et al., 2006b; Kertesz et al., 2005), attempts to develop biochemical therapies that modify tau metabolism (Josephs et al., 2006b), and genetic advances (see below).

Table 2 contains a simplified summary of five neuropathological subtypes of frontotemporal lobar degeneration described by Lantos and Cairns (2001) that have been found in association with progressive language impairments. It should be noted that additional subtypes are differentiated by other authors (Josephs et al., 2006b). Some of the additional subtypes discussed by Dickson (1999) and Josephs et al. (2006b) are discussed in the footnotes to Table 2.

PROGRESS IN RELATING CLINICAL SYNDROME TO NEUROPATHOLOGY

As recently as 2001, researchers were cautious about proposing links between clinical presentations and likely neuropathological subtype (Hodges & Miller, 2001; McKhann et al., 2001) because there was no clear pattern to the range of clinical presentations and the neuropathology results post-mortem. More recently still, however, a small number of studies have begun to suggest that some clinical

TABLE 2

Pathological subtypes of frontotemporal lobar degeneration described by Lantos and Cairns (2001), with notes on additional subtypes described by other researchers

Lantos & Cairns (2001) pathological subtype	Description and comments
Profile 1: Pick bodies	Spherical inclusions called *Pick bodies*, positive for both tau and ubiquitin.
Profile 2: Corticobasal degeneration (CBD)-type inclusions	Tau-positive inclusions as well as ballooned neurons (neurons that are colourless and swollen, also called Pick cells; Dickson, 2001) primarily in the cortex (Dickson, 1999), and other tau-positive inclusions in the glia (the cells that support and protect the neurons) (Hodges et al., 2003; Lantos & Cairns, 2001; McKhann et al., 2001).[a]
Profile 3: motor neuron disease (MND)[b]-type inclusions	Inclusions are tau-negative but ubiquitin-positive. This pathology may or may not be associated with clinical motor signs.[c]
Profile 4: Dementia lacking distinct histology (DLDH)[d]	Tests negative for the inclusions described above, and shows no ballooned Pick cells. There is focal atrophy of frontal and/or temporal regions and, typically, spongiform change (brain tissue takes on appearance of a sponge).[e]
Profile 5: frontotemporal dementia and parkinsonism linked to chromosome 17 (FTDP-17)	Inclusions similar to Pick bodies, CBD-type and PSP-type inclusions. Genetic testing shows mutation in the tau gene or progranulin gene on chromosome 17 (see text).

[a]Although corticobasal degeneration neuropathology has been found in people with progressive language impairments, it is more commonly associated with a clinical motor syndrome, the symptoms of which include limb apraxia, rigidity, and dystonia (Dickson, 1999). Both the clinical syndrome and neuropathology are typically referred to as corticobasal degeneration, although recently some authors have made the distinction by referring to corticobasal degeneration (or CBD-like) syndrome (Josephs et al., 2006b; Kertesz et al., 2005). Corticobasal degeneration inclusions have a similar protein structure but a different shape and location to the inclusions found in another motor syndrome known as *progressive supranuclear palsy* (PSP) (Dickson, 1999). Progressive supranuclear palsy is a syndrome usually characterised by falls, gait disturbance, and difficulty with vertical eye movements (Dickson, 1999), however on some occasions pseudosupranuclear palsy-type neuropathology has been found in people with progressive language impairments (Josephs et al., 2006a, 2006b; Knibb et al., 2006).

[b]A class of diseases, the most common of which is known as amyotrophic lateral sclerosis (ALS) in North America and continental Europe (Bak, O'Donovan, Xuereb, Boniface, & Hodges, 2001).

[c]When the person shows neurological signs characteristic of upper or lower MND at presentation or with disease progression, along with other language or behaviour symptoms associated with frontotemporal dementia, these inclusions are almost always found at autopsy (Josephs et al., 2006b). However, when these inclusions are found in people who showed *no* clinical features of MND at any time during disease progression (e.g., as in many cases of semantic dementia; Davies et al., 2005), the inclusions are found in frontal and temporal cortex and the dentate gyrus of the hippocampus (Whitwell et al., 2005), rather than the lower motor neurons of the brain stem and spinal cord as typical in classic MND. NB: The spinal cord may not be examined post-mortem in the absence of motor symptoms (Mackenzie & Feldman, 2005), so these inclusions may be present in lower motor neurons but not detected. Josephs et al. (2006b) make a helpful distinction between the neuropathology associated with positive MND signs (which they call *frontotemporal lobar degeneration with motor neuron disease*, or FTLD-MND) and the neuropathology with no MND signs but MND-type inclusions (which they call *frontotemporal lobar degeneration with ubiquitin-only immunoreactive neuronal changes*, or FTLD-U). Other terms also identifying the relationship of this frontotemporal lobar degeneration neuropathological profile to the pathology found in MND include *frontotemporal dementia-motor neuron disease* (FTD-MND; Knibb et al., 2006) and *motor neuron disease inclusion dementia* (Davies et al., 2005; Jackson, Lennox, & Lowe, 1996).

[d]Also reported as *frontal-lobe degeneration-type* (FLD) neuropathology (Neary, 1999), *dementia lacking distinct histopathological features*, or simply *frontotemporal lobar degeneration* (McKhann et al., 2001).

[e]Probably some cases reported as DLDH had MND-type inclusions (Profile 3) that were not detected because the test for ubiquitin was not carried out (Josephs et al., 2006a; Kertesz et al., 2005), and/or because the spinal cord was not examined (Mackenzie & Feldman, 2005).

presentations *are* more reliably associated with some neuropathologies than others (Davies et al., 2005; Hodges et al., 2004; Josephs et al., 2006a, 2006b; Kertesz et al., 2005; Knibb et al., 2006). Progress in this area is made possible by cases that are followed longitudinally with detailed clinical testing together with brain donation for post-mortem analysis of neuropathology. The rapid progress in this area over the past decade is likely to continue in the medium term at least.

Primary progressive aphasia

Using the Mesulam (1987) criteria for primary progressive aphasia, Kertesz et al. (2005) reported neuropathology for 22 people diagnosed with anomic, logopenic, or non-fluent primary progressive aphasia as described above, or "possible primary progressive aphasia" (so-named because memory difficulties were noted in the history over and above the aphasia that was prominent by the time of initial clinical examination). All but 1 of the 10 "possible primary progressive aphasia" cases had Alzheimer-type neuropathology, and most (90%) did not develop second or third syndromes. Of the 12 other primary progressive aphasia cases, the majority (92%) did develop behavioural or motor second syndromes, and the neuropathologies were corticobasal degeneration inclusions (5/12), frontotemporal lobar degeneration with motor neuron disease-type inclusions (4/12), and Pick body neuropathology (3/12).

Semantic dementia

A study combining cases from Sydney and Cambridge (Davies et al., 2005) over a 10-year period found that 13/18 cases (72%) with the clinical syndrome of semantic dementia following the Lund criteria (Neary, 1999) had frontotemporal lobar degeneration with motor neuron disease-type inclusions at autopsy. Only 1 of these 13 showed symptoms of motor neuron disease during life. Of the remaining five semantic dementia cases, three had Pick body neuropathology and two had Alzheimer's disease. Neuropathological results for people with semantic dementia in the Kertesz et al. (2005) cohort are not yet available.

Progressive non-fluent aphasia and apraxia of speech

In another Sydney/Cambridge study, 6/8 (75%) people with non-fluent progressive aphasia diagnosed by "disrupted speech output with phonological and/or syntactic errors" had Pick body neuropathology (Hodges et al., 2004). A report of 13 people with non-fluent progressive aphasia diagnosed on the basis of a prominent non-fluent aphasia "with hesitancy and phonetic errors" (Josephs et al., 2006b, p. 42) found that one had Pick body neuropathology, three had frontotemporal lobar degeneration with ubiquitin-only immunoreactive neuronal changes (FTLD-U), five had pseudo-supranuclear palsy-type neuropathology, and four had corticobasal degeneration-type neuropathology. Both these papers have been followed up by studies described below that pay more stringent attention to participants' clinical symptoms, and the results are promising for identifying neuropathology on the basis of clinical syndrome. Taken together, 16 of the 21 (76%) nonfluent cases reported by Hodges et al. (2004) and Josephs et al. (2006b) had tau-positive neuropathology.

Knibb et al. (2006) carried out a cluster analysis of measures of language deficits in 38 people with progressive language impairments. They identified 23 broadly non-fluent cases that could be further subdivided into two groups along lines similar to those proposed by Gorno-Tempini et al. (2004): a non-fluent progressive aphasia group (*n* = 14) and a logopenic progressive aphasia group (*n* = 7). Of the non-fluent progressive aphasia group, seven had Alzheimer's disease neuropathology and seven had one of the tauopathies (which ones and how many of each are not specified). Of the seven logopenic cases, three had progressive supranuclear palsy-type neuropathology, three had frontotemporal lobar degeneration with motor neuron disease-type inclusions, and the pathology for the final case was not given.

Josephs et al. (2006a) considered whether or not participants had apraxia of speech: 17 individuals with progressive apraxia of speech (diagnosed as described above) and/or aphasia could be further classified according to (i) whether apraxia of speech was the sole or dominant feature in the early years after presentation (the AOS group), (ii) whether they had agrammatic or telegraphic speech as well as apraxia of speech (a group Josephs and colleagues called progressive non-fluent aphasia – apraxia of speech, PNFA-AOS), or (iii) whether they had aphasic symptoms without agrammatic or telegraphic speech (a group called primary progressive aphasia not otherwise specified). Of the apraxia of speech group, five out of seven had progressive supranuclear palsy-type neuropathology, one had corticobasal degeneration-type neuropathology, and one Pick body neuropathology. Of the PNFA-AOS group, all three had corticobasal degeneration-type neuropathology. In the primary progressive aphasia not otherwise specified group, five of seven had frontotemporal lobar degeneration with motor neuron disease-type inclusions, one had corticobasal degeneration-type neuropathology, and one progressive supranuclear palsy-type neuropathology. In this latter case, indications of mild apraxia of speech had been present at onset. Thus the major contribution of this study was to show that 11 out of 11 participants with any hint of apraxia of speech showed tau-positive neuropathology. However, a report of of apraxia of speech is unlikely to predict tauopathy with 100% reliability in clinical practice, given the inconsistent criteria used across clinical and research groups to diagnose apraxia of speech (Croot, 2002), and the finding of Alzheimer-type neuropathology in a proportion of individuals who made articulatory/phonological errors in other studies (Croot, Hodges, Xuereb & Patterson., 2000; Knibb et al., 2006).

Summary of current findings on neuropathology

People who had a clinical syndrome of semantic dementia, or who were anomic without agrammatism or phonological errors, have most often been reported with frontotemporal lobar degeneration with ubiquitin-positive inclusions (FTLD-U Davies et al., 2005; Josephs et al., 2006a; Knibb et al., 2006). This neuropathology is rarely found when phonological errors and/or apraxia of speech are prominent. Where apraxia of speech *is* present, the neuropathology is most often one of the tauopathies (i.e., Pick bodies, corticobasal degeneration, or progressive-supranuclear palsy neuropathology). Kertesz et al. (2005) suggested that a tauopathy is the likely neuropathy when a movement disorder emerges as a second or third syndrome after the onset of primary progressive aphasia. Hodges et al. (2003) suggest that a tauopathy is more likely in people who are older, with a slower onset and a non-fluent profile.

Finally, Alzheimer's disease cannot be ruled out as a potential neuropathological diagnosis in either fluent or non-fluent progressive language impairments, including semantic dementia (Davies et al., 2005; Knibb et al., 2006). In the Knibb et al. (2006) study of 38 individuals, approximately one third of those with fluent progressive aphasia and one third of those with non-fluent progressive aphasia proved to have Alzheimer-type neuropathology. Alzheimer's disease *may* be identifiable by early memory difficulties (as suggested by Kertesz et al., 2005). Caution is required here, however, as memory difficulties at presentation do not reliably indicate Alzheimer's disease neuropathology (A. J. Graham et al., 2005; Hodges et al., 2004). At least some people with progressive aphasia caused by non-Alzheimer neuropathology exhibit mild memory difficulties (Knibb et al., 2006), and some people with autopsy-confirmed Alzheimer's disease do not show prominent episodic memory deficits at presentation (Galton et al., 2000). At this point in time, the above conclusions about the neuropathological process associated with the various subtypes of progressive aphasia are preliminary, as they are based on a small number of studies (Kertesz et al., 2005). Consequently, the use of diagnostic labels that presume a particular neuropathology would still be premature.

GENETIC DISCOVERIES

In some families the frontotemporal dementia is strongly heritable, with an autosomal dominant pattern of inheritance (50% likelihood of inheritance by male and female offspring). This subtype is known as frontotemporal dementia and parkinsonism linked to chromosome 17 (FTDP-17) because of the Parkinsonian symptoms that are frequently part of the syndrome[2] and because of the abnormalities found in a region of Chromosome 17 in individuals with this subtype (Lantos & Cairns, 2001). Families with FTDP-17 with tau-positive pathology have been found to have a mutation on the gene for tau that is located on this chromosome (Hutton et al., 1998). Families with ubiquitin-positive pathology have recently been shown to have a different mutation at a nearby location on Chromosome 17, a mutation affecting the gene that controls expression of progranulin, a growth factor associated with neuronal health (Baker et al. et al., 2006). Rowland (2006) notes this as a major genetic advance, opening the way for the development of genetic therapies.

PROGNOSIS FOR PEOPLE WITH PROGRESSIVE LANGUAGE IMPAIRMENTS

As the above review would suggest, many subtle (and not-so-subtle) differences are possible between individuals with progressive language impairments. Individuals differ in the initial speech or language symptoms present, the speech or language symptoms that appear with disease progression, and the non-speech/non-language symptoms that appear over time. More than 100 single cases or small case series have been published, typically with the aim of bringing to the attention of the clinical research community a previously unreported clinical syndrome (Kertesz et al., 2003), and such reports demonstrate that these disorders are clinically heterogeneous. However, how much information is available about the specific longitudinal course(s) likely to be associated with various clinical presentations? The best

---

[2] The symptoms typically seen in Parkinson's disease, including tremor, slow movements, decreased facial expression, rigidity, and postural instability (Oertel & Quinn, 1996).

information can be drawn from comparatively large group studies that used (fairly) consistent evaluations to follow participants over time (Davies et al., 2005; Hodges et al., 2003; Josephs et al., 2006a; Kertesz et al., 2003, 2005; Knibb et al., 2006; Le Rhun, Richard, & Pasquier, 2005).

Survival and autonomy

Age at onset (time when symptoms were first noticed) and duration of illness (calculated from onset until death) reported in a number of large longitudinal studies of individuals with progressive language impairments are summarised in Table 3. The typical cause of death in Alzheimer's disease and frontotemporal dementia is aspiration pneumonia (Lantos & Cairns, 2001; Le Rhun et al., 2005). One study (Hodges et al., 2003) found longer survival in progressive non-fluent aphasia than semantic dementia. Gender, presence of family history and age at diagnosis did not further influence survival.

Consistent with this, people with non-fluent progressive aphasia were likely to enter a care institution later than people with semantic dementia (on average 7–8 years after onset in non-fluent progressive aphasia versus 3–4 years after onset in semantic dementia; Hodges et al., 2003). In an apparent contrast, Le Rhun and colleagues reported a more benign course for people with fluent primary progressive aphasia than non-fluent primary progressive aphasia (with fluency determined by their profile on a French version of the Boston Diagnostic Aphasia Examination). However, Le Rhun and colleagues excluded people with semantic dementia from their fluent sample and only included those fluent individuals who met the Mesulam et al. criteria for primary progressive aphasia. Kertesz and colleagues have argued that people with fluent aphasia meeting the Mesulam et al. criteria are likely to be earlier in the course of the disease than people with a non-fluent language profile (Kertesz et al., 2003), which would explain the better prognosis for the fluent group in the Le Rhun et al. study.

Le Rhun et al. (2005) evaluated the possibility (Mesulam, 1987) that the course of primary progressive aphasia is more benign than Alzheimer-type dementia. Their study found that survival was actually shorter for people with primary progressive aphasia than people with Alzheimer-type dementia (consistent with the findings of Hodges et al., 2003), but that autonomy in activities of daily living was preserved longer in PPA. Loss of autonomy occurred at a median of 6–7 years post-onset and 1–2 years before death in people with primary progressive aphasia. Half the participants with primary progressive aphasia were autonomous with regard to toileting, personal hygiene, and dressing at 5 years post-onset, while half required assistance. By 7 to 8 years after onset, half were mute and half required assistance in eating and walking. Age at onset, gender, educational level, and vascular risk factors did not influence participants' likelihood of maintaining autonomy. In a comparison between semantic dementia and Alzheimer-type dementia, survival was found to be similar in both syndromes (Roberson et al., 2005), and gender, education, family history, and neuropsychiatric profile did not influence survival in semantic dementia.

Behaviour and personality change

Although speech and/or language impairments are most prominent in these disorders by definition, a high proportion of people also develop changes in

TABLE 3
Summary of age at onset and disease duration data

Study	Clinical syndrome(s)	Number of participants	Number of Males: Females	Age at onset (years)			Disease duration from onset to death (years)		
				Mean (SD)	Median	Range	Mean (SD)	Median	Range
Kertesz et al. (2003)	PPA	67	27:40	66.7 (7.9)	–	–	7.1 (3.2)*	–	2–15*
Kertesz et al. (2005)	PPA (FTLD neuropathology)	12	6:6	63.8 (8.3)	–	–	7.8 (4.0)	–	–
	PPA (AD neuropathology)	10	5:5	63.1 (10.3)	–	–	8.8 (2.3)	–	–
	PPA (Total)	22	11:11	63.8 (8.3)	–	–	7.8 (4.0)	–	–
Le Rhun et al. (2005)	PPA	49	21:28	63.8 (8.3)	62	49–73	–	7†	3–17†
Davies et al. (2005)	Semantic dementia	18	10:8	58.3 (7.0)		40–67	9.3 (4.5)		2.3–19.5
Hodges et al. (2003)	Semantic dementia	9	6:3	59.4 (8.6)		–		6–8	–
	PNFA	8	2:6	63.3 (5.1)		–		6–8	–
Knibb et al. (2006)	PNFA and semantic dementia	38	23:15	61.9		48–78	4:7		0:10–13:2
Josephs et al. (2006a)	AOS, AOS-PNFA, and PPA-NOS	17	8:9	63.8 (8.0)		53–79	7.8 (3.1)		3–16

PPA = primary progressive aphasia (Mesulam group criteria); AOS = apraxia of speech; AOS-PNFA = apraxia of speech with progressive non-fluent aphasia; PNFA = progressive non-fluent aphasia; PPA-NOS = primary progressive aphasia not otherwise specified; FTLD = frontotemporal lobar degeneration; * = for the 25 participants who died; † = for the 36 participants who died.

behaviour, personality, and social cognition. Chow, Miller, Boone, Mishkin and Cummings (2002) reported that for 30 people with the language presentations associated with frontotemporal dementia following the Lund and consensus criteria (McKhann et al., 2001; Neary, 1999; The Lund and Manchester Groups, 1994), three out of four showed neuropsychiatric symptoms or behavioural change. Participants were at various stages of disease progression in this study. Depression, apathy, and disinhibition were the most common symptoms. One third of participants showed depressed symptoms at onset, and just over 50% showed apathy and/or disinhibition at time of study. Participants who went on to demonstrate severe behaviour disturbance tended to already show behaviour changes early in progression. A similar proportion was reported by Kertesz et al. (2005), with 10/22 (46%) individuals with primary progressive aphasia (Mesulam 2001 criteria) developing behavioural difficulties as a second or third syndrome. Garrard and Hodges (1999) also observed that behaviour, personality, and social cognition changes commonly emerged during the progression of semantic dementia for a series of 20 cases. Especially common were fixations with particular types of food and time, and the hyperorality and sexual disinhibition frequently described as Klüver Bucy syndrome.

Motor disorders

Kertesz et al. (2005) found that 9 of 22 participants initially diagnosed with primary progressive aphasia developed clinical symptoms of corticobasal degeneration or pseudosupranuclear palsy as a second or third syndrome. Joseph et al.'s (2006a) study that subdivided participants according to whether they had apraxia of speech indicated that early apraxia of speech is predictive of a subsequent movement disorder. One individual in each of their subgroups (progressive apraxia of speech, primary progressive aphasia with apraxia of speech, and primary progressive aphasia without apraxia of speech) had motor features on initial clinical examination. In both groups with apraxia of speech, however, most individuals (six out of eight) with no initial movement disorder developed one or more of supranuclear gaze palsy, limb apraxia, rigidity, or bradykinesia when followed longitudinally. By contrast, in the primary progressive aphasia group without apraxia of speech, only one of the five who had no movement features at onset went on to develop a movement disorder. Motor neuron signs are less common with progression if not present initially. Johnson et al. (2005) found that approximately 3% of 153 people diagnosed with semantic dementia or non-fluent progressive aphasia at various stages of severity according to the Neary et al. (1998) criteria had developed symptoms of motor neuron disease at the time their study was carried out.

Factors associated with good or poor prognosis

One factor hypothesised to be associated with better prognosis in these studies included higher MMSE score at first visit (Le Rhun et al., 2005) potentially associated with milder language impairment and thus earlier stage of disease. Tau-positive neuropathology (Hodges et al., 2003; Roberson et al., 2005) is another, with tauopathies suggested to cause a slower rate of progression than the other neuropathologies in frontotemporal lobar degeneration (i.e., frontotemporal lobar degeneration with ubiquitin-positive inclusions or dementia lacking distinct histological features). However, this claim requires further research, as Kertesz et al. (2005) and Knibb et al. (2006) did not find longer survival for the tau-positive cases in their studies. Josephs et al. (2006b) found longer survival for people with tau-positive neuropathology, but noted that this was due to the very short disease duration for people with frontotemporal lobar degeneration and motor neuron disease in the tau-negative group. Josephs et al. (2006b) also found longer survival for the people with Pick body neuropathology than for people with pseudosupranuclear palsy-type and corticobasal-type neuropathology, attributing this to the higher level of brainstem neuropathology and thus aspiration risk in the latter two groups.

Factors associated with poor prognosis included the development of motor neuron disease features (Kertesz et al., 2005; Roberson et al., 2005), swallowing difficulty (Kertesz et al., 2003, 2005) and immobility (Kertesz et al., 2005), as well as relatively poor performance on a letter fluency task (Roberson et al., 2005).

CONCLUDING COMMENTS

As the above review shows, knowledge about the clinical presentations and neuropathologies associated with progressive language impairments, and information about prognosis, has increased substantially since Mesulam (1982) introduced the term "primary progressive aphasia" a quarter of a century ago. The range of classification systems that have developed since then emphasise how important it is to specify the criteria used to reach a particular diagnosis, and the clinical symptoms on which this diagnosis is based.

Frontier areas of research into progressive language impairments include pharmacological therapies (Burns & O'Brien, 2006; Huey, Putnam, & Grafman, 2006; McNeil et al., 1995; Reed, Johnson, Thompson, Weintraub, & Mesulam, 2004), early diagnostic indicators (Grossman et al., 2005) and genetics (Bertram & Tanzi, 2005; Blacker & Lovestone, 2006), ensuring that our knowledge of these disorders will continue to increase for many years to come. Given the emerging role of speech pathologists, psychologists, and other health professionals in assessment, education, intervention, advocacy, and policy development related to progressive language impairments (Croot et al., 2009 this issue; Taylor et al., 2009 this issue), it will be essential to follow the ongoing and rapid developments in clinicopathological diagnosis and treatment of these disorders. As pharmacological or other treatments become available to target the neuropathological mechanisms in these diseases, a primary diagnostic goal will be to identify the likely neuropathology to match clients to appropriate therapies at the earliest opportunity.

REFERENCES

Attix, D. K., & Welsh-Bohmer, K. A. (Eds.). (2006). *Geriatric neuropsychology: Assessment and intervention*. New York: Guilford Press.

Bak, T. H., O'Donovan, D. G., Xuereb, J. H., Boniface, S., & Hodges, J. R. (2001). Selective impairment of verb processing associated with pathological changes in Brodmann areas 44 and 45 in the motor neurone disease-dementia-aphasia syndrome. *Brain, 124*, 103–120.

Baker, M., Mackenzie, I. R., Pickering-Brown, S. M., Gass, J., Rademakers, R., Lindholm, C., et al. (2006). Mutations in progranulin cause tau-negative frontotemporal dementia linked to chromosome 17. *Nature, 442*, 916–919.

Bayles, K. A., & Tomoeda, C. K. (1997). *Improving function in dementia and other cognitive-linguistic disorders: Guide and resource book.* Tucson, AZ: Canyonlands.

Bertram, L., & Tanzi, R. E. (2005). The genetic epidemiology of neurodegenerative disease. *The Journal of Clinical Investigation, 115*(6), 1449–1457.

Blacker, D., & Lovestone, S. (2006). Genetics and dementia nosology. *Journal of Geriatric Psychiatry and Neurology, 19*(3), 186–191.

Borasio, G. D., Appel, S. H., & Buettner, U. (1996). Upper and lower motor neuron disorders. In T. Brandt, L. R. Caplan, J. Dichgans, H. C. Diener, & C. Kennard (Eds.), *Neurological disorders: Course and treatment.* San Diego, CA: Academic Press.

Bourgeois, M. S. (1991). Communication treatment for adults with dementia. *Journal of Speech and Hearing Research, 34,* 831–844.

Brun, A. (1987). Frontal lobe degeneration of non-Alzheimer type. I. Neuropathology. *Archives of Gerontology and Geriatrics, 6*(3), 193–208.

Bryan, K., & Maxim, J. (Eds.). (2006). *Communication disability in the dementias.* Chichester, UK: John Wiley.

Burns, A., & O'Brien, J. (2006). Clinical practice with anti-dementia drugs: A consensus statement from British Association for Psychopharmacology. *Journal of Psychopharmacology, 20*(6), 732–755.

Chan, D., Fox, N. C., Scahill, R. I., Crum, W. R., Whitwell, J. L., Leschziner, G., et al. (2001). Patterns of temporal lobe atrophy in semantic dementia and Alzheimer's disease. *Annals of Neurology, 49*(4), 433–442.

Chow, T. W., Miller, B. L., Boone, K., Mishkin, F., & Cummings, J. L. (2002). Frontotemporal dementia classification and neuropsychiatry. *The Neurologist, 8,* 263–269.

Clare, L. (Ed.). (2001). *Cognitive rehabilitation in dementia.* Hove, UK: Psychology Press.

Coltheart, M. (1984). Editorial. *Cognitive Neuropsychology, 1*(1), 1–8.

Croot, K. (2002). Diagnosis of AOS: Definition and criteria. *Seminars in Speech and Language, 23*(4), 267–279.

Croot, K., Hodges, J. R., Xuereb, J., & Patterson, K. (2000). Phonological and articulatory impairment in Alzheimer's disease: A case series. *Brain and Language, 75,* 277–309.

Croot, K., Nickels, L., Laurence, F., & Manning, M. (2009). Impairment- and activity/participation-directed interventions in progressive language impairment: Clinical and theoretical issues. *Aphasiology, 22,* 125–160.

Davies, R. R., Hodges, J. R., Kril, J. J., Patterson, K., Halliday, G. M., & Xuereb, J. H. (2005). The pathological basis of semantic dementia. *Brain, 128,* 1984–1995.

di Carlo, A., Baldereschi, M., Inzitari, D., & Amaducci, L. (1999). Dementias, the dimension of the problem: Epidemiology notes. In S. Govoni, C. L. Bolis, & M. Trabucchi (Eds.), *Dementias: Biological bases and clinical approach to treatment* (pp. 1–18). Milano: Springer-Verlag Italia.

Dickson, D. W. (1999). Neuropathologic differentiation of progressive supranuclear palsy and corticobasal degeneration. *Journal of Neurology, 246*(Suppl 2), II/6–II/15.

Dickson, D. W. (2001). Neuropathology of Pick's disease. *Neurology, 56*(Suppl. 4), S16–S20.

Edwards-Lee, T., Miller, B. L., Benson, D. F., Cummings, J. L., Russell, G. L., & Boone, K., et al. (1997). The temporal variant of frontotemporal dementia. *Brain, 120,* 1027–1040.

Galton, C. J., Patterson, K., Graham, K., Lambon Ralph, M. A., Williams, G., Antoun, N., et al. (2001). Differing patterns of temporal atrophy in Alzheimer's disease and semantic dementia. *Neurology, 57,* 216–225.

Galton, C. J., Patterson, K., Xuereb, J. H., & Hodges, J. R. (2000). Atypical and typical presentations of Alzheimer's disease: A clinical, neuropsychological, neuroimaging and pathological study of 13 cases. *Brain, 123*(3), 484–498.

Garrard, P., & Hodges, J. R. (1999). Semantic dementia: Implications for the neural basis of language and meaning. *Aphasiology, 13*(8), 609–623.

Gordon, J. K. (1998). The fluency dimension in aphasia. *Aphasiaology, 12*(7/8), 673–688.

Gorno-Tempini, M. L., Dronkers, N. F., Rankin, K. P., Ogar, J. M., Phrengrasamy, L., Rosen, H. J., et al. (2004). Cognition and anatomy in three variants of primary progressive aphasia. *Annals of Neurology, 55,* 335–346.

Graham, A. J., Davies, R., Xuereb, J., Halliday, G., Kril, J., Creasey, H., et al. (2005). Pathologically proven frontotemporal dementia presenting with severe amnesia. *Brain, 128,* 597–605.

Graham, K. S., Patterson, K., & Hodges, J. R. (1995). Progressive pure anomia: Insufficient activation of phonology by meaning. *Neurocase, 1,* 25–38.

Graham, K. S., Patterson, K., Pratt, K. H., & Hodges, J. R. (1999). Relearning and subsequent forgetting of semantic category exemplars in a case of semantic dementia. *Neuropsychology, 13*(3), 359–380.

Grossman, M., & Ash, S. (2004). Primary progressive aphasia: A review. *Neurocase, 10*(1), 3–18.

Grossman, M., Farmer, J., Leight, S., Work, M., Moore, P., Van Deerlin, V., et al. (2005). Cerebrospinal fluid profile in frontotemporal dementia and Alzheimer's disease. *Annals of Neurology, 57*, 721–729.

Hart, R. P., Beach, W. A., & Taylor, J. R. (1997). A case of progressive apraxia of speech and non-fluent aphasia. *Aphasiology, 11*(1), 73–82.

Hillis, A. E., Selnes, O., & Gordon, B. (1999). Primary progressive "conduction aphasia": A cognitive analysis of two cases. *Brain and Language, 69*(3), 478–481.

Hillis, A. E., Wityk, R. J., Barker, P. B., Beauchamp, N. J., Gailoud, P., Murphy, K., et al. (2002). Subcortical aphasia and neglect in acute stroke: The role of cortical hypoperfusion. *Brain, 125*, 1094–1104.

Hodges, J. R., Davies, R., Xuereb, J., Kril, J., & Halliday, G. (2003). Survival in frontotemporal dementia. *Neurology, 61*, 349–354.

Hodges, J. R., Davies, R. R., Xuereb, J. X., Casey, B., Broe, M., Bak, T. H., et al. (2004). Clinicopathological correlates in frontotemporal dementia. *Annals of Neurology, 56*, 399–406.

Hodges, J. R., & Miller, B. (2001). The classification, genetics and neuropathology of frontotemporal dementia: Introduction to the special topic papers: Part I. *Neurocase, 7*, 31–35.

Hodges, J. R., & Patterson, K. (1996). Non-fluent progressive aphasia and semantic dementia: A comparative neuropsychological study. *Journal of the International Neuropsychological Society, 2*, 511–524.

Hodges, J. R., Patterson, K., Oxbury, S., & Funnell, E. (1992). Semantic dementia: Progressive fluent aphasia with temporal lobe atrophy. *Brain, 115*, 1783–1806.

Holland, A. L., McBurney, D. H., Moossy, J., & Reinmuth, O. M. (1985). The dissolution of language in Pick's disease with neurofibrillary tangles: A case study. *Brain and Language, 24*, 36–58.

Huey, E. D., Putnam, K. T., & Grafman, J. (2006). A systematic review of neurotransmitter deficits and treatments in frontotemporal dementia. *Neurology, 66*, 12–77.

Hutton, M., Lendon, L., Rizzu, P., Baker, M., Froelich, S., Houlden, H., et al. (1998). Association of missense and 5'-splice-site mutations in *tau* with the inherited dementia FTDP-17. *Nature, 393*, 702–705.

Jackson, M., Lennox, G., & Lowe, J. (1996). Motor neurone disease-inclusion dementia. *Neurodegeneration, 5*, 339–350.

Johnson, J. K., Diehl, J., Mendez, M. F., Neuhaus, J., Shapira, J. S., Forman, M., et al. (2005). Frontotemporal lobal degeneration: Demographic characteristics of 353 patients. *Archives of Neurology, 62*, 925–930.

Josephs, K. A., Duffy, J. R., Strand, E. A., Whitwell, J. L., Layton, K. F., Parisi, J. E., et al. (2006a). Clinicopathological and imaging correlates of progressive aphasia and apraxia of speech. *Brain, 129*, 1385–1398.

Josephs, K. A., Petersen, R. C., Knopman, D. S., Boeve, B. F., Whitwell, J. L., Duffy, J. R., et al. (2006b). Clinicopathological analysis of frontotemporal and corticobasal degenerations and PSP. *Neurology, 66*, 41–48.

Kertesz, A. (2004). Frontotemporal dementia/Pick's disease. *Archives of Neurology, 61*, 969–971.

Kertesz, A., Davidson, W., McCabe, P., Takagi, K., & Munoz, D. (2003). Primary progressive aphasia: Diagnosis, varieties, evolution. *Journal of the International Neuropsychological Society, 9*, 710–719.

Kertesz, A., Hudson, L., Mackenzie, I. R. A., & Munoz, D. G. (1994). The pathology and nosology of primary progressive aphasia. *Neurology, 44*(Nov.), 2065–2072.

Kertesz, A., McMonagle, P., Blair, M., Davidson, W., & Munoz, D. (2005). The evolution and pathology of frontotemporal dementia. *Brain, 128*, 1996–2005.

Killick, J., & Allan, K. (2001). *Communication and the care of people with dementia.* Buckingham, UK: Open University Press.

Knibb, J. A., Xuereb, J. H., Patterson, K., & Hodges, J. R. (2006). Clinical and pathological charnoterisation of progressive aphasia. *Annals of Neurology, 59*, 156–165.

Knopman, D. S. (1993). Overview of dementia lacking distinctive histology: Pathological designation of a progressive dementia. *Dementia, 4*, 132–136.

Lambon Ralph, M. A., McClelland, J. L., Patterson, K., Galton, C. J., & Hodges, J. R. (2001). No right to speak? The relationship between object naming and semantic impairment: Neuropsychological evidence and a computational model. *Journal of Cognitive Neuroscience, 13*(3), 341–356.

Lantos, P. L., & Cairns, N. J. (2001). Neuropathology. In J. R. Hodges (Ed.), *Early-onset dementia: A multidisciplinary approach* (pp. 227–262). Oxford, UK: Oxford University Press.

Le Rhun, E., Richard, F., & Pasquier, F. (2005). Natural history of primary progressive aphasia. *Neurology, 65*, 887–891.

Lubinski, R. (Ed.). (1995). *Dementia and communication*. San Diego, CA: Singular.

Lubinski, R., & Orange, J. B. (2000). A framework for the assessment and treatment of functional communication in dementia. In L. E. Worrall & C. M. Frattali (Eds.), *Neurogenic communication disorders: A functional approach* (pp. 220–246). New York: Thieme.

Mackenzie, I. R. A., & Feldman, H. H. (2005). Ubiquitin immunohistochemistry suggests classic motor neuron disease, motor neuron disease with dementia, and frontotemporal dementia of the motor neuron disease type represent a clinicopathologic spectrum. *Journal of Neuropathology and Experimental Neurology, 64*(8), 730–739.

McKhann, G. M., Albert, M. S., Grossman, M., Miller, B., Dickson, D., & Trojanowski, J. Q. (2001). Clinical and pathological diagnosis of frontotemporal dementia: Report of the Work Group on Frontotemporal Dementia and Pick's Disease. *Archives of Neurology, 58*, 1803–1809.

McLean, C. A., Beyreuther, K., & Masters, C. L. (2001). Molecular pathology of early-onset dementia. In J. R. Hodges (Ed.), *Early-onset dementia: A multidisciplinary approach* (pp. 165–189). Oxford, UK: Oxford University Press.

McNeil, M. R., & Duffy, J. R. (2001). Primary progressive aphasia. In R. Chapey (Ed.), *Language intervention strategies in adult aphasia*. (4th ed., pp. 472–486). Baltimore: Lippincott, Williams & Wilkins.

McNeil, M. R., Small, S. L., Masterson, R. J., & Tepanta, R. D. (1995). Behavioural and pharmacological treatment of lexical-semantic deficits in a single patient with primary progressive aphasia. *American Journal of Speech-Language Pathology, 4*, 76–93.

Mendez, M. F., & Perryman, K. M. (2002). Neuropsychiatric features of frontotemporal dementia: Evaluation of consensus criteria and review. *Journal of Neuropsychiatry and Clinical Neurosciences, 14*(4), 424–429.

Mesulam, M.-M. (1982). Slowly progressive aphasia without generalised dementia. *Annals of Neurology, 11*, 592–598.

Mesulam, M.-M. (1987). Primary progressive aphasia – Differentiation from Alzheimer's disease. *Annals of Neurology, 22*(4), 533–534.

Mesulam, M.-M. (1990). Large-scale neurocognitive networks and distributed processing for attention, language and memory. *Annals of Neurology, 28*, 597–613.

Mesulam, M.-M. (2001). Primary progressive aphasia. *Annals of Neurology, 49*, 425–432.

Mesulam, M.-M. (2003). Primary progressive aphasia – A language-based dementia. *New England Journal of Medicine, 349*(16), 1535–1542.

Mesulam, M.-M., Grossman, M., Hillis, A. E., Kertesz, A., & Weintraub, S. (2003). The core and halo of primary progressive aphasia and semantic dementia. *Annals of Neurology, 54*(Suppl. 5), S11–S14.

Mesulam, M.-M., & Weintraub, S. (1992). Spectrum of primary progressive aphasia. *Bailliere's Clinical Neurology: International Practice and Research, 1*(3), 583–609.

Mummery, C. J., Patterson, K., Wise, R. J. S., Vandenbergh, R., Price, C. J., & Hodges, J. R. (1999). Disrupted temporal lobe connections in semantic dementia. *Brain, 122*, 61–73.

Neary, D. (1999). Overview of frontotemporal dementias and the consensus applied. *Dementia & Geriatric Cognitive Disorders, 10*(Suppl. 1), 6–9.

Neary, D., Snowden, J. S., Gustafson, L., Passant, U., Stuss, D., Black, S., et al. (1998). Frontotemporal lobar degeneration: A consensus on clinical criteria. *Neurology, 51*, 1546–1554.

Oertel, W. H., & Quinn, N. P. (1996). Parkinsonism. In T. Brandt, L. R. Caplan, J. Dichgans, H. C. Diener, & C. Kennard (Eds.), *Neurological disorders: Course and treatment*. San Diego, CA: Academic Press.

Price, C. J., Warburton, E. A., Moore, C. J., Frackowiak, R. S., & Friston, K. J. (2001). Dynamic diaschesis: Anatomically remote and context-sensitive human brain lesions. *Journal of Cognitive Neuroscience, 13*, 419–429.

Rascovsky, K., Salmon, D. P., Ho, G. J., Galasko, D., Peavy, G. M., Hansen, L. A., et al. (2002). Cognitive profiles differ in autopsy-confirmed frontotemporal dementia and AD. *Neurology, 58*, 1801–1808.

Reed, D. A., Johnson, N. A., Thompson, C., Weintraub, S., & Mesulam, M.-M. (2004). A clinical trial of bromocriptine for treatment of primary progressive aphasia. *Annals of Neurology, 56*(5), 750.

Robinson, K. M. (2001). Rehabilitation applications in caring for patients with Pick's disease and frontotemporal dementias. *Neurology, 56*(Suppl. 4), S56–S58.

Ripich, D. N. (1994). Functional communication with AD patients: A caregiver training programme. *Alzheimer Disease and Related Disorders, 8*(Suppl. 3), 95–109.

Ripich, D. N., & Horner, J. (2004). The neurodegenerative dementias: Diagnosis and interventions. *The ASHA Leader*, *9*(8), 4–5, 14.

Roberson, E. D., Hesse, J. H., Rose, K. D., Slama, H., Johnson, J. K., Yaffe, K., et al. (2005). Frontotemporal dementia progresses to death faster than Alzheimer's disease. *Neurology*, *65*, 719–725.

Rogers, M. A., King, J. M., & Alarcon, N. B. (2000). Proactive management of primary progressive aphasia. In D. R. Beukelman, K. M. Yorkston, & J. Reichle (Eds.), *Augmentative and alternative communication for adults with acquired neurologic disorders* (pp. 305–337). Baltimore, MD: Brookes.

Rosen, H. J., Hartikainen, K. M., Jagust, W., Kramer, J. H., Reed, B. R., Cummings, J. L., et al. (2002). Utility of clinical criteria in differentiating frontotemporal lobar degeneration (FTLD) from AD. *Neurology*, *58*, 1608–1615.

Rowland, L. P. (2006). Frontotemporal dementia, Chromosome 17 and progranulin. *Annals of Neurology*, *60*(3), 275–277.

Royal College of Speech and Language Therapists (2005). *Speech and language therapy provision for people with dementia*. Retrieved 25 January 2007 from www.rcslt.org/resources/publications/dementia_paper.pdf).

Schneider, S. L., Thompson, C. K., & Luhring, B. (1996). Effects of verbal plus gestural matrix training on sentence production in a patient with primary progressive aphasia. *Aphasiology*, *10*, 297–317.

Schwartz, M., De Bleser, R., Poeck, K., & Weis, J. (1998). A case of primary progressive aphasia: A 14-year follow-up study with neuropathological findings. *Brain*, *121*, 115–126.

Sinnatamby, R., Antoun, N. A., Freer, C. E., Miles, K. A., & Hodges, J. R. (1996). Neuroradiological findings in primary progressive aphasia: CT, MRI and cerebral perfusion in SPECT. *Neuroradiology*, *38*, 232–238.

Snowden, J. S., Goulding, P. J., & Neary, D. (1989). Semantic dementia: A form of circumscribed cerebral atrophy. *Behavioural Neurology*, *2*, 167–182.

Snowden, J. S., & Griffiths, H. (2000). Semantic dementia: Assessment and management. In W. Best, K. Bryan, & J. Maxim (Eds.), *Semantic processing: Theory and practice* (pp. 180–203). London: Whurr.

Snowden, J. S., Neary, D., & Mann, D. M. A. (1996). *Fronto-temporal lobar degeneration: Fronto-temporal dementia, progressive aphasia, semantic dementia*. New York: Churchill Livingstone.

Sonty, S. P., Mesulam, M. -M., Thompson, C. K., Johnson, N. A., Weintraub, S., Parrish, T. B., et al. (2002). Primary progressive aphasia: PPA and the language network. *Annals of Neurology*, *53*, 35–49.

Taylor, C., Kingma, R., Croot, K., & Nickels, L. (2009). Speech pathology services for progressive aphasia: Exploring an emerging area of practice. *Aphasiology*, *22*, 161–174.

The Lund and Manchester Groups (1994). Clinical and neuropathological criteria for frontotemporal dementia. *Journal of Neurology, Neurosurgery and Psychiatry*, *57*, 416–418.

The National Institute on Aging and Reagan Institute Working Group on Diagnostic Criteria for the Neuropathological Assessment of Alzheimer's disease (1997). Consensus recommendations for the postmortem diagnosis of Alzheimer's disease. *Neurobiology of Aging*, *18*(Suppl. 4), S1–S2.

Thompson, C. K., & Johnson, N. (2006). Language interventions in dementia. In D. K. Attix & K. A. Welsh-Bohmer (Eds.), *Geriatric neuropsychology: Assessment and intervention* (pp. 315–332). New York: Guilford Press.

Varma, A. R., Snowden, J. S., Lloyd, J. J., Talbot, P. R., Mann, D. M. A., & Neary, D. (1999). Evaluation of the NINCDS-ADRA criteria in the differentiation of Alzheimer's disease and frontotemporal dementia. *Journal of Neurology, Neurosurgery and Psychiatry*, *66*, 184–188.

Weintraub, S., Rubin, N. P., & Mesulam, M. M. (1990). Primary progressive aphasia: Longitudinal course, neuropsychological profile, and language features. *Archives of Neurology*, *47*(12), 1329–1335.

Whitwell, J. L., Josephs, K. A., Rossor, M. N., Stevens, J. M., Revesz, T., Holton, J. L., et al. (2005). Magnetic resonance imaging signatures of tissue pathology in frontotemporal dementia. *Archives of Neurology*, *62*(9), 1402–1408.

Subject Index

T - #0284 - 101024 - C0 - 246/174/11 [13] - CB - 9781848727014 - Gloss Lamination